Surgical Critical Care

Editor

BRETT H. WAIBEL

SURGICAL CLINICS
OF NORTH AMERICA

www.surgical.theclinics.com

Consulting Editor
RONALD F. MARTIN

February 2022 • Volume 102 • Number 1

ELSEVIER

1600 John F. Kennedy Boulevard • Suite 1800 • Philadelphia, Pennsylvania, 19103-2899

http://www.surgical.theclinics.com

SURGICAL CLINICS OF NORTH AMERICA Volume 102, Number 1
February 2022 ISSN 0039–6109, ISBN-13: 978-0-323-84856-5

Editor: John Vassallo, j.vassallo@elsevier.com
Developmental Editor: Arlene Campos

Surgical Clinics of North America (ISSN 0039–6109) is published bimonthly by Elsevier Inc., 360 Park Avenue South, New York, NY 10010-1710. Months of publication are February, April, June, August, October, and December. Business and Editorial Offices: 1600 John F. Kennedy Blvd., Suite 1800, Philadelphia, PA 19103-2899. Periodicals postage paid at New York, NY and additional mailing offices. Subscription prices are $456.00 per year for US individuals, $1240.00 per year for US institutions, $100.00 per year for US & Canadian students and residents, $547.00 per year for Canadian individuals, $1283.00 per year for Canadian institutions, $552.00 for international individuals, $1283.00 per year for international institutions and $250.00 per year for foreign students/residents. To receive student/resident rate, orders must be accompanied by name of affiliated institution, date of term, and the *signature* of program/residency coordinator on institution letterhead. Orders will be billed at individual rate until proof of status is received. Foreign air speed delivery is included in all *Clinics* subscription prices. All prices are subject to change without notice. POSTMASTER: Send address changes to *Surgical Clinics*, Elsevier Health Sciences Division, Subscription Customer Service, 3251 Riverport Lane, Maryland Heights, MO 63043. **Customer Service (orders, claims, online, change of address): Telephone: 1-800-654-2452 (U.S. and Canada); 314-447-8871 (outside U.S. and Canada). Fax: 314-447-8029. E-mail: journalscustomerservice-usa@elsevier.com (for print support); journalsonlinesupport-usa@elsevier.com (for online support).**

Reprints. For copies of 100 or more, of articles in this publication, please contact the Commercial Reprints Department, Elsevier Inc., 360 Park Avenue South, New York, New York 10010-1710. Tel. 212-633-3874, Fax: 212-633-3820, E-mail: reprints@elsevier.com

The Surgical Clinics of North America is also published in Spanish by McGraw-Hill Interamericana Editores S.A., P.O. Box 5-237 06500 Mexico D.F. Mexico; and in Portuguese by Interlivros Edicoes Ltda., Rua Comandante Coelho 1085, CEP 21250, Rio de Janeiro, Brazil; and in Greek by Paschalidis Medical Publications, Athens Greece.

The Surgical Clinics of North America is covered in *MEDLINE/PubMed (Index Medicus), EMBASE/Excerpta Medica, Current Contents/Clinical Medicine, Current Contents/Life Sciences, Science Citation Index,* and *ISI/BIOMED.*

Contributors

CONSULTING EDITOR

RONALD F. MARTIN, MD, FACS
Colonel (Retired), United States Army, Department of General Surgery, Pullman Regional Hospital and Clinic Network, Pullman, Washington

EDITOR

BRETT H. WAIBEL, MD
Associate Professor of Surgery, Division of Acute Care Surgery, Department of Surgery, University of Nebraska Medical Center, Omaha, Nebraska

AUTHORS

ZACHARY M. BAUMAN, DO, MHA, FACOS, FACS
Surgery, University of Nebraska Medical Center, Omaha, Nebraska

JANA M. BINKLEY, MD
General Surgery Resident, Department of Surgery, University of Nebraska Medical Center, Omaha, Nebraska

SAMUEL CEMAJ, MD, FACS, FCCM
Surgery, University of Nebraska Medical Center, Omaha, Nebraska

SHAUN CHANDNA, DO, FACP
Assistant Professor of Medicine, Division of Gastroenterology and Hepatology, Department of Medicine, University of Utah School of Medicine, Salt Lake City, Utah

CARL R. CHRISTENSON, MD
Clinical Instructor, Department of Anesthesiology, University of Cincinnati College of Medicine, Cincinnati, Ohio

MATTHEW DALE, MD, PhD
Surgical Resident, Department of Surgery, Creighton University, School of Medicine, Omaha, Nebraska

PETER E. FISCHER, MD
University of Tennessee Health Science Center, Memphis, Tennessee

NATHAN ALAN FOJE, MD
General Surgery Resident, Department of Surgery, University of Nebraska Medical Center, Omaha, Nebraska

JUAN F. GALLEGOS-OROZCO, MD, AGAF
Associate Professor of Medicine, Medical Director of Hepatology and Liver Transplant, Division of Gastroenterology and Hepatology, Department of Medicine, University of Utah School of Medicine, Salt Lake City, Utah

NICOLE M. GARCIA, MD
ACS Fellow, Trauma/Surgical Critical Care/Acute Care Surgery, Department of Surgery, East Carolina University, Brody School of Medicine, Greenville, North Carolina

DIH-DIH HUANG, MD
University of Tennessee Health Science Center, Memphis, Tennessee

DANIEL W. JOHNSON, MD, FCCS
Surgery, University of Nebraska Medical Center, Omaha, Nebraska

ABIGAIL P. JOSEF, MD
Clinical Assistant Professor, Trauma/Surgical Critical Care/Acute Care Surgery, Department of Surgery, East Carolina University, Brody School of Medicine, Greenville, North Carolina

KEVIN M. KEMP, MD
Assistant Professor of Surgery, Division of Acute Care Surgery, Department of Surgery, University of Nebraska Medical Center, Omaha, Nebraska

MEHREEN KISAT, MD, MS
Assistant Professor, Division of Acute Care and Regional General Surgery, Department of Surgery, University of Wisconsin School of Medicine and Public Health, Madison, Wisconsin

KENJI LEONARD, MD
Clinical Assistant Professor, Division of Trauma, Surgical Critical Care, and Acute Care Surgery, Department of Surgery, East Carolina University - Vidant Medical Center, Greenville, North Carolina

IAN MONROE, MD
Surgical Resident, Department of Surgery, Creighton University, School of Medicine, Omaha, Nebraska

THOMAS ARTHUR NICHOLAS IV
Associate Professor, Director of Acute Pain Service, Anesthesiology, University of Nebraska Medical Center, Omaha, Nebraska

PATRYCJA POPOWICZ, MD, MS
Department of General Surgery, East Carolina University - Vidant Medical Center, Greenville, North Carolina

RAIME ROBINSON
Anesthesiology, University of Nebraska Medical Center, Omaha, Nebraska

PAUL J. SCHENARTS, MD, FACS
Department of Surgery, Professor of Surgery, Creighton University, School of Medicine, Omaha, Nebraska

RACHEL SCHENKEL, MD
Surgical Resident, Department of Surgery, Creighton University, School of Medicine, Omaha, Nebraska

MICHAEL SCHWABE, MD
Surgical Resident, Department of Surgery, Creighton University, School of Medicine, Omaha, Nebraska

SALMA SHAIKHOUNI, MD
Division of Nephrology, Department of Medicine, University of Michigan, Ann Arbor, Michigan

OLABISI OLOLADE SHEPPARD, MD
Assistant Professor of Surgery, Division of Acute Care Surgery, Department of Surgery, University of Nebraska Medical Center, Omaha, Nebraska

SHAUN L. THOMPSON, MD
Assistant Professor, Department of Anesthesiology, Division of Critical Care Medicine, University of Nebraska Medical Center, Omaha, Nebraska

MICHAEL R. VISENIO, MD, MPH
Surgery, University of Nebraska Medical Center, Omaha, Nebraska

WILLIAM C. WRISINGER, MD
Department of Anesthesiology, Division of Critical Care Medicine, University of Nebraska Medical Center, Omaha, Nebraska

LENAR YESSAYAN, MD, MS
Division of Nephrology, Department of Medicine, University of Michigan, Ann Arbor, Michigan

MOHSIN A. ZAIDI, MD
Assistant Professor, Anesthesiology and Critical Care Medicine, Department of Anesthesiology, University of Cincinnati College of Medicine, Cincinnati, Ohio

EDUARDO RODRÍGUEZ ZARATE, MD, FACP
Assistant Professor of Medicine, Division of Gastroenterology and Hepatology, Department of Medicine, University of Utah School of Medicine, Salt Lake City, Utah

BEN ZARZAUR, MD, MPH
Professor and Chair, Division of Acute Care and Regional General Surgery, Department of Surgery, University of Wisconsin School of Medicine and Public Health, Madison, Wisconsin

Contents

> COVID-19 continues to rampage around the world. Noncritical care–trained physicians may be deployed into the intensive care unit to manage these complex patients. Although COVID-19 is primarily a respiratory disease, it is also associated with significant pathology in the brain, heart, vasculature, lungs, gastrointestinal tract, and kidneys. This article provides an overview of COVID-19 using an organ-based, systematic approach.

 Video content accompanies this article at http://www.surgical.theclinics.com.

> Overview: The use of extracorporeal membrane oxygenation (ECMO) is becoming commonplace worldwide in ICUs for the care of patients with respiratory and/or cardiac failure. Understanding the use of ECMO and the management of these complex patients will be vital to current and future clinicians as ECMO use continues to grow.

> The ideal device for hemodynamic monitoring of critically ill patients in the intensive care unit (ICU) or the operating room has not yet been developed. This would need to be affordable, consistent, have a very low margin of error (<30%), be minimally or noninvasive, and allow the clinician to make a reasonable therapeutic decision that consistently led to better outcomes. Such a device does not yet exist. This article will describe the distinct options we, as critical care physicians, currently possess for this Herculean endeavor.

Patients with cirrhosis account for 3% of intensive care unit admissions with hospital mortality exceeding 50%; however, improvements in survival among patients with acutely decompensated cirrhosis and organ failure have been described when treated in specialized liver transplant centers. Acute-on-chronic liver failure is a distinct clinical syndrome characterized by decompensated cirrhosis associated with one or more organ failures resulting in a significantly higher short-term mortality. In this review, we will discuss the management of common life-threatening complications in the patient with cirrhosis that require intensive care management including neurologic, cardiovascular, gastrointestinal, pulmonary, and renal complications.

In the intensive care unit, delirium is a major contributor to morbidity and mortality in adult patients. Patients with delirium have been shown to have increased length of stay, decreased functional outcomes, and increased risk for requiring placement at the time of discharge. In addition, decreased cognitive function and dementia have been shown to be long-term complications from delirium. The mainstay of treatment and prevention include therapy- and behavioral-based interventions, including frequent orientation, cognitive stimulation, mobilization, sleep restoration, and providing hearing and visual aids. Refractory delirium may require pharmacologic intervention with antipsychotics or alpha-2 agonists.

Noninvasive ventilation (NIV) provides respiratory support without the use of invasive ventilation with techniques that do not bypass the upper airway. NIV is particularly attractive given its associated reduced risk of complications associated with intubation. Available NIV modes include nasal cannula, simple mask, nonrebreather, high flow nasal cannula, continuous positive airway pressure (CPAP), and bi-level positive airway pressure (BPAP). Acute exacerbation of COPD, cardiogenic pulmonary edema, and COVID-19 are conditions for which NIV has shown to be beneficial, whereas there is no consensus among the use of NIV in trauma patients and ARDS.

Antibiotic resistance is a public health concern. A critical care clinician is faced with a clinical dilemma of using the appropriate treatment without compromising the antibiotic armamentarium. Postoperative and trauma patients in the intensive care unit (ICU) pose a unique challenge of mounting a systemic inflammatory response, which makes it even more difficult to differentiate inflammation from infection. The decision for type of empirical therapy should be individualized to the patient and local ecology data and resistance profiles. After initiation of empirical therapy, deescalation should be done once microbiology data are available. Antibiotic stewardship programs are essential in the ICU.

Mass casualty incidents are increasingly common. They are defined by large numbers of patients arriving nearly simultaneously, overwhelming available resources needed for optimal care. They require rapid mobilization of resources to provide optimal outcomes and limit disability and death. Because the mechanism of injury in a mass casualty incident is often traumatic in nature, surgeons should be aware of the critical role they play in planning and response. The coronavirus disease 2019 pandemic is a notable, resulting in a sustained surge of critically ill patients. Initial response requires local mobilization of resources; large-scale events potentially require a national response.

Common causes of acute kidney injury (AKI) in the ICU setting include acute tubular necrosis (due to shock, hemolysis, rhabdomyolysis, or procedures that compromise renal perfusion), abdominal compartment syndrome, urinary retention, and interstitial nephritis. Treatment is geared toward addressing the underlying cause. Dialysis may be required if renal injury does not resolve. Early initiation of dialysis based on the stage of AKI alone has not been shown to provide a mortality benefit. Dialysis modalities are based on the dialysis indication and the patient's clinical status. Providers should pay close attention to nutritional requirements and medication dosing according to renal function and dialysis modality.

SURGICAL CLINICS OF NORTH AMERICA

SERIES OF RELATED INTEREST

Advances in Surgery
https://www.advancessurgery.com/
Surgical Oncology Clinics
https://www.surgonc.theclinics.com/
Thoracic Surgery Clinics
http://www.thoracic.theclinics.com/

THE CLINICS ARE AVAILABLE ONLINE!
Access your subscription at:
www.theclinics.com

Foreword

Critical Care

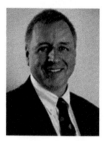

Ronald F. Martin, MD, FACS
Consulting Editor

One of the issues that has been plaguing me of late is, how do we best distribute and apportion limited medical resources. As I type this foreword, we are approaching the 2-year mark into the global SARS-CoV-2 COVID-19 pandemic. I vividly remember when this pandemic began that I felt like it would take us a good long while to sort ourselves out and get back to something resembling normal living—but I did not imagine that 2 years in we would be struggling this hard with no clear path to normalcy in sight.

I rack my brain trying to understand how the United States of America—with all its resources and capabilities—can be one of the most affected nations by this disease. On some levels, it makes sense. The United States is a country with unfettered travel within its borders and historically high volumes of people traversing its borders for myriad reasons. This country has had historical insulation from many world problems given its bicoastal geography, which may have lulled us into a false sense of security. We are used to solving problems and getting the results (more or less) that we want. On the other hand, globalization is real, and oceans aren't as protective as they used to be. Our domestic investment in infrastructure and reserves has dwindled in service to short-term economic indicators favored by many "leaders." While all those shortcomings have played their parts, perhaps the reason that concerns me most is that we have simply crossed over to a society that shuns collectivism in favor of a notion of individualism—which more accurately would be described as tribalism, in my opinion. In fact, if it were only individualists that failed to be part of the solution to our larger problems, this discussion would not be necessary. It takes a group or a tribe to successfully thwart a collective effort.

Tribalism exists across all sectors of the economy, all socioeconomic classes, and among and between all political ideologies—and always has. While most groups are quick to point out that the "other" should change their ways, I don't see a lot of introspection for groups to look inward at how they could change. The unfortunate net

Surg Clin N Am 102 (2022) xiii–xv
https://doi.org/10.1016/j.suc.2021.11.001
0039-6109/21/© 2021 Published by Elsevier Inc.

result of large sections of the population pulling in a diametrically opposed fashion is a compromised ability to plan for and deal with the consequences of our choices.

As of the writing of this foreword, the COVID-19 infection has been listed as the cause of death for over 5 million people worldwide and over 750,000 persons in the United States alone. I repeat, 750,000 persons dead—well over 200 iterations of the 9/11 attacks. And still, we can't come to uniformity of purpose on how to respond. And while the mortality has been horrible, the resource utilization required to treat the sick has not only taxed or exceeded the capacity to treat those ill from COVID but has reduced our capacity to treat and manage other diseases as well. It may be decades before we can accurately assess the excess mortality related to this pandemic.

Of course, not all these deaths were preventable, though some fraction was. Furthermore, thanks to the dedication and brilliance of countless people and organizations, many people survived infection and many more were prevented from becoming ill thanks to a previously inconceivable vaccine development and implementation program. We all owe these people an enormous debt of gratitude.

On the treatment side of the equation, those in the intensive care unit (ICU) setting truly standout. I mean no disrespect to our colleagues in the emergency departments, or general medical care teams, or our first responders—they have all done so much and received so little recognition for their efforts. Yet, the ICU world has had to learn to fix the airplane while still in flight. So much had to be learned so quickly, and much of what was learned was somewhat counterintuitive.

In the past, I have written that in the ICU one must always remember these principles: air goes in and out; blood goes around and around; and oxygen is good. For the most part, all that is still true. What has changed is the complex bits of how we view each of those simple aphorisms have expanded to new levels.

This issue of the *Surgical Clinics* on critical care as put together by Dr Brett Waibel and his colleagues is designed to help us revisit and reimagine what we need to know about critical care and how we can use its principles to benefit not just patients with COVID-19 but also patients with any severe physiologic derangement. We have asked much of them for this issue, and they have delivered. The reader of this issue will benefit from facts and analysis that will help to make a huge difference for someone in perhaps their most perilous moments. We are deeply indebted for their efforts and for their sharing of their wisdom.

This pandemic has taught us (hopefully) many things: we can do what we can to prevent people from becoming ill; we can do what we can to mitigate illness once it occurs; and we can try to improve the survival of those most greatly afflicted with disease. It has also taught us that our resources are limited. We cannot simply absorb an unlimited quantity of ill persons and provide all of them with the care they need at all times. Our system of health care in the United States is not designed to effectively transfer patients all over the country when bed shortages occur. At that level of population health, collective engagement of the communities, the states, the regions, and the nation is required to mitigate the burdens. Decisions made at the collective level have real impacts on individuals. Conversely, individual decisions can have significant impact on the collective society. In order for civilization to function, we must find a mechanism to balance these competing desires and needs.

The current wave of this pandemic is slightly on the downturn at this instant. I would be hesitant to assume another wave is not in the offing at some time. Even if we were to significantly turn the corner on this disease, I would hold off on declaring victory just yet. The fractious state of our health care apparatus, the lack of strategic and operational reserve we hold, and the lack of ability we have shown to unify have all been undeniably demonstrated. At present, we are not as prepared as we need to be for the next challenge, COVID related or otherwise. We must be thinking about the future events as we continue to manage this crisis.

In my opinion, the best way to prepare is to become educated. This issue of the *Surgical Clinics* should greatly help in that regard. Once we have become educated, we must find a way to educate others. Perhaps most importantly, we, as subject matter experts, need to find a way to instill trust in our communities and regain our ability to be helpful as an institution. As difficult as this may be, the alternatives are likely to be far worse.

Ronald F. Martin, MD, FACS
Colonel (retired), United States Army
Department of General Surgery
Pullman Surgical Associates
Pullman Regional Hospital and Clinic Network
825 SE Bishop Blvd, Suite 130
Pullman WA 99163
United States

E-mail address:
rfmcescna@gmail.com

Preface

Surgical Critical Care

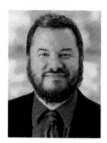

Brett H. Waibel, MD
Editor

I would like to start by thanking Dr Martin and the staff at Elsevier (especially Arlene Campos and John Vassallo, who made this first foray into editing relatively pain free) for the opportunity to edit this issue of *Surgical Clinics*. However, Dr Martin charged me with the daunting task of Surgical Critical Care. While not the first time I have been asked to talk on the subject, I find this request to be equivalent to being requested to quickly cover other broad fields like Surgical Oncology or Trauma. Thus, I tried to create a sampling of different areas in surgical critical care, using different inspirations.

First comes the classical areas in critical care, the management of failing essential organs, such as the kidneys and heart. The aging population in the United States makes keeping up-to-date on the advances in these areas essential. This was the inspiration for many of the articles in this issue.

My second inspiration is more personal in nature, my residents and students. While surgical residents are given the Sisyphean task of learning the breadth of surgery in only a few years, they tend to focus more on the technical aspects of surgery. I find areas such as perioperative management tend to get pushed to the side, creating such beliefs that nonrebreathers or BiPAP (bilevel positive airway pressure) is the go-to for all oxygenation issues, especially at night. This was the motivation for articles such as topical coagulant agents (it kills me when they don't know what they are using on their patients) and noninvasive ventilation and oxygenation strategies.

Finally comes the ever-changing nature of the field. Technical advances, such as ECMO (extracorporeal membrane oxygenation) and advanced hemodynamic monitoring modalities, and changing views of practice, such as pain management with the ongoing opioid epidemic, both have effects upon the field. At the time this issue was prepared, an infectious pandemic, COVID-19, has been ravaging the country. This disease has put critical care in the forefront, along with how we manage limited resources during an emergency.

Surg Clin N Am 102 (2022) xvii–xviii
https://doi.org/10.1016/j.suc.2021.09.009
0039-6109/22/© 2021 Published by Elsevier Inc.

I would like to finish by thanking all the authors for their hard work in creating this issue. The devotion and time they have expended to produce these articles have made the editing process easy. I could not have asked for a better group of experts in preparation of this issue.

Brett H. Waibel, MD
Division of Acute Care Surgery
Department of Surgery
University of Nebraska Medical Center
983280 Nebraska Medical Center
Omaha, NE 68198-3280, USA

E-mail address:
Brett.waibel@unmc.edu

The COVID-19 Patient in the Surgical Intensive Care Unit

Ian Monroe, MD, Matthew Dale, MD, PhD, Michael Schwabe, MD,
Rachel Schenkel, MD, Paul J. Schenarts, MD*

KEYWORDS

- COVID-19 • SARS-CoV-2 • Critical care management
- Multiple organ system failure • Respiratory failure • ARDS

KEY POINTS

- The COVID-19 pandemic continues to surge around the globe. Nonintensive care–trained surgeons may be called on to deploy into the critical care unit to care for these complex patients.
- Acute respiratory failure is the most common manifestation of severe COVID-19 infection.
- COVID 19 may be considered an endothelial disease, causing pathologic changes in the brain, heart, lungs, gastrointestinal tract, and kidneys.
- Our understanding of the pathophysiology and treatment of COVID-19 in the critical care setting continues to evolve at a rapid pace.

Coronaviruses, a name derived from their crownlike morphology observed on electron microscope, have been described in literature for over 70 years.[1] They are enveloped, positive single-stranded RNA viruses. These viruses are known to bind to host cells' membrane via a spike protein that facilitates fusion between the virus and host cell. On entry into the cell, their genome is replicated and packaged for delivery to other cells.[1,2]

Coronaviruses are known to cause a variety of symptoms. Many are nonspecific, including fever, cough, and generalized fatigue. They are often responsible for upper and lower respiratory tract infections that can vary from mild to severe, with acute hypoxic respiratory failure and acute respiratory distress syndrome (ARDS) being known sequalae of these respiratory infections.[1,3,4] Enteric, central nervous system (CNS), renal, cardiac, and hematologic diseases can also develop as a result of coronaviruses.[5]

Department of Surgery, Creighton University, School of Medicine, Medical Education Building, Suite 501, 7710 Mercy Road, Omaha, NE 68124-2368, USA
* Corresponding author.
E-mail address: pjschenartsmd@gmail.com

Surg Clin N Am 102 (2022) 1–21
https://doi.org/10.1016/j.suc.2021.09.015
surgical.theclinics.com

Within the last 2 decades, multiple variants have been responsible for widespread outbreaks of primarily respiratory infections, including SARS-CoV and MERS-CoV in 2003 and 2012, respectively.[2,3]

In 2019, reports of a new variant called SARS-CoV-2 began circulating, and its resulting disease was named COVID-19.[6] By March 2020, the World Health Organization declared this infection a global pandemic.[7] At the time of this submission, COVID-19 infected more than 230 million people, of which approximately 4.7 million have died.[8] Despite other counties having larger populations, the United States accounts for the greatest number of deaths (more than 43 million).[8]

Because the number of patients with COVID-19 has surged, noncritical care–trained and even junior physicians have been redeployed from their normal area of practice into the intensive care unit (ICU) to mange patients with this complex disease.[9–11] Organizations such as the Society for Critical Care Medicine,[12] The American Thoracic Society,[13] and universities[14] have rushed to fill this educational and experience gap with "just-in-time" training.

There is a high likelihood that surgical intensivists and noncritical care–trained surgeons may be called up to provide critical care for patients who would typically be cared for in a medical ICU. The purpose of this article, therefore, is to provide an overview of the pathophysiology, disease manifestations, and treatment options for patients with COVID-19 admitted to a surgical ICU. To accomplish this, an organ-based, systematic approach will be used. Despite the importance of long-term complications of this infection,[15] the primary focus of this article is critical care.

It is important for the reader to understand that the concepts and strategies presented here are based on the best available current information. Given the rapid evolution of our understanding of this complex disease, updated recommendations may occur between manuscript submission and publication.

THE NEUROLOGIC SYSTEM

During the COVID-19 epidemic, one of the first known neurologic changes was anosmia, leading to a worry in otherwise asymptomatic individuals of an upcoming worse symptomatic infection. With ongoing publications, additional neurologic manifestations have been identified and are still being reported. Anosmia, encephalopathy, and stroke were the most common neurologic syndromes associated with SARS-CoV-2 infection.[16] Dizziness, fatigue, headache, nausea, and confusion have also been reported. Postinfectious complications of acute demyelinating encephalomyelitis, generalized myoclonus, acute transverse myelitis, Guillain–Barré syndromes, and variants have been reported.[17] With the vast array of symptoms reported in lethal and nonlethal COVID-19 infections, an infection with the SARS-CoV-2 virus must be included in the differential diagnosis. Imaging studies of patients with anosmia and COVID-19 revealed hyperintensity and swelling of the olfactory bulb, consistent with inflammation.[18] Biopsy samples of anosmic patients showed SARS-CoV-2 infection in the olfactory epithelium with associated local inflammation.[18]

Theories behind the mechanism of SARS-CoV-2 to cause neurologic changes are ongoing. Entry into the CNS may be due to a "trojan horse" theory, where the SARS-CoV-2 virus directly attaches to inflammatory cells such as lymphocytes, granulocytes, and monocytes, which all express angiotensin-converting enzyme 2 (ACE2). The virus is then picked up by the lungs and transported throughout the body.[19] The virus is then either deposited into the CNS or targets vascular endothelial cells in the CNS causing coagulopathy and vascular endothelial cell dysfunction, with resulting small vessel occlusions and microhemorrhages contributing to subtle neurologic and neuropsychiatric changes.[20] Postmortem studies on cerebral pathology show that the virus can directly cross the blood-brain barrier, directly infiltrating astrocytes and microglia.[21] With the ACE2 receptor widely expressed in brain microvascular and endothelial cells, the SARS-CoV-2 spike protein can directly bind to the receptor and either damage the blood brain barrier or induce a cytokine storm causing inflammation and neuronal damage.[22,23] The subsequent neurologic changes may also be secondary due to direct retrograde travel of the SARS-CoV-2 virus up the axons to reach the CNS.[24]

The long-term sequalae of COVID-19 infections are needing continued evaluation. With the exaggerated response of the CNS to infection leading to meningitis, encephalitis, and meningoencephalitis, continued neurologic manifestations are likely to be associated with a COVID-19 infection if otherwise unexplained.[25] A high proportion of patients with COVID-19 in the ICU develop delirium, suggesting microvascular and inflammatory pathologies to cause neurologic changes.[26] The long recovery of anosmic patients points toward long-term neurologic changes. The more severely affected patients with strokes, microvascular changes, and brain damage may have ongoing chronic issues, and further studies will elucidate associations with the COVID-19 pandemic.

THE CARDIAC SYSTEM

There is an emerging body of evidence to show that cardiac involvement is not uncommon among patients with COVID-19.[27–29] The range of cardiac manifestations of the COVID-19 disease is quite broad and requires a high degree of suspicion in order to diagnose and adequately treat the cardiac manifestations of COVID-19. Here, the authors briefly summarize the proposed pathophysiology of COVID-19 cardiac involvement, discuss the range of cardiac manifestations of the SARS-CoV-2 virus, and briefly discuss potential treatment options relevant to the surgeon caring for patients with COVID-19.

Cardiac Pathophysiology

As described in the pulmonary section of this publication, the SARS-CoV-2 virus binds to ACE2 receptors in type 1 and type 2 pneumocytes as well as other ACE2-expressing cell types, then subsequently enter those ACE2-expressing cells.[30] The ACE2 receptor is found in high amounts in pericytes within adult human hearts, indicating that the heart itself is susceptible to infection by the SARS-CoV-2 virus.[31,32] Indeed, there is evidence to suggest that COVID-19 causes viral myocarditis via direct myocardial cell injury.[33] Compared with patients who have no underlying comorbidities, patients with cardiovascular disease, diabetes, chronic obstructive pulmonary disease, hypertension, and cancer have been shown to have a higher incidence of severe/fatal COVID-19 disease. It has been shown that patients with conditions that result in high levels of activation of the renin-angiotensin system, such as heart failure, hypertension, and atherosclerosis, have higher expression of ACE2 receptors on their cardiac pericytes, possibly predisposing them to more severe manifestations of cardiac disease.[31,32]

In addition to direct infection, COVID-19 is known to cause a systemic inflammatory response in severe disease states, which results in high levels of circulating cytokines that cause injury to a host of tissues, including the reticuloendothelial system as well as cardiomyocytes.[27–30] Endothelial dysfunction is a well-established mechanism of myocardial ischemia and dysfunction, and damage to the endothelial system caused by this cytokine storm may result in increased metabolic demand and decreased cellular perfusion to the stressed myocardium, depressing cardiac systolic function and inducing myocardial ischemia. The systemic inflammation/endothelial dysregulation seen in COVID-19 has also been linked to plaque rupture and acute coronary syndromes in patients with underlying coronary artery disease.[28,34]

Patients with COVID-19 are also at risk of secondary cardiac complications. Medications used to treat COVID, such as steroids, antivirals, and other immunologic drugs, can have cardiotoxic effects. All patients with severe illness, including patients with COVID-19, are at risk for electrolyte disturbances that may trigger arrythmias. Given the interaction of the SARS-CoV-2 virus with the renin-angiotensin-aldosterone *system* system, hypokalemia is of particular concern and is well known to increase susceptibility to a variety of arrythmias.[28,35]

Cardiac Manifestations and Treatments

Acute coronary syndrome

There have been some studies that have shown an association between COVID-19 and acute coronary syndrome (ACS).[36,37] In some case series, patients presented with classic ST-segment elevation myocardial infarction (STEMI) symptoms without prior COVID-19 symptoms, suggesting that their ACS was not caused by severe systemic inflammation.[38] The pathophysiology of how COVID-19 may lead to ACS is still uncertain; however, it seems to involve endothelial damage with resultant subendocardial microthrombi (in the case of nonepicardial obstruction) or systemic inflammation leading to plaque rupture or coronary spasm (in the case of epicardial coronary vessel obstruction).[39]

The treatment of ACS in the setting of COVID-19 illness is similar to the algorithm for ACS from any other cause. In the case of STEMI presentation, early cardiac catheter laboratory activation and coronary angiography is essential. A thorough workup including electrocardiogram, cardiac biomarkers, coagulation studies, and possibly echocardiography all may be indicated. In patients with demand-induced cardiac ischemia (type II NSTEMI), treatment should focus on optimizing myocardial oxygen delivery and reducing myocardial oxygen demand by treating the underlying disease process. Referral to centers capable of angiography/percutaneous coronary intervention is essential for patients with any history of coronary artery disease who have severe COVID-19 features.

Heart failure

Multiple studies that have emerged over the last 18 months have described a link between COVID-19 and new-onset heart failure. Studies have shown that among patients with severe COVID-19, 23% to 33% of patients developed new-onset cardiomyopathy, depressed ejection fraction, or cardiogenic shock.[40–42]

In some of the early studies out of Wuhan, China, nearly 50% of the patients who died of COVID-19 developed heart failure.[42] COVID-19 is well known to cause hypoxia and acute lung injury, resulting in significant pulmonary hypertension, and this can lead to development of right heart failure, and the clinician caring for COVID-19 patient must maintain a high degree of suspicion for developing right ventricular failure.

Workup for potential COVID-19–induced heart failure consists of obtaining a congestive heart failure peptide, troponin biomarkers, transthoracic or transesophageal echocardiography, and in some cases cardiac MRI. For patients with suspected right ventricular failure, hemodynamic monitoring via a pulmonary arterial catheter may be indicated.

Treatment of COVID-19–induced heart failure is similar to that of other types of acute heart failure. Limiting preload as well as reducing afterload, particularly in patients with right heart failure, is essential. Inotropic agents such as epinephrine or dobutamine can be used to increase the contractile function of the myocardium. In patients with right ventricular failure, particularly due to pulmonary hypertension, milrinone seems to be an effective medication at reducing the pulmonary vasoconstriction while significantly increasing the contractile force of the right ventricle. Inhaled vasodilators such as epoprostenol may also be used to reduce the afterload experienced by the right heart. In severe cases, venoarterial extracorporeal membranous oxygenation (ECMO) may be used to provide both hemodynamic and ventilatory support; however, the indications for initiation of VA-ECMO in patients with COVID-19 are highly individualized and beyond the scope of this publication.

Arrythmia/sudden cardiac death

As described earlier, COVID-19 can cause injury to the heart via several mechanisms, including hypoxia, exacerbation of underlying coronary artery disease, direct cellular damage, and systemic inflammation.[36] All types of cardiac injury can induce an arrythmia within the cardiac conduction system. Patients with COVID-19 are particularly prone to deviations in serum potassium levels due to the interaction of the SARS-CoV-2 virus with the renin-angiotensin-aldosterone pathway.[36]

Various types of arrhythmias have been seen in patients with COVID-19, including high-grade atrioventricular blocks, supraventricular tachyarrythmias, and ventricular tachyarrhythmias.[43] It is imperative that clinicians be mindful of the proclivity for patients with COVID-19 to develop arrythmias, particularly in light of the various QT-prolonging medications that may be given to these patients. Cardiac monitoring with telemetry is essential, and regular assessment of the QTc is imperative.

Treatment of these cardiac arrythmias is no different than if they were to arise in a non–COVID-19 patient. Correction of underlying electrolyte derangements, hemodynamic stabilization, and possibly correction of the arrythmia are all warranted.

Thromboembolism/hypercoagulability

Studies have shown that COVID-19 tends to cause a hypercoagulable state in affected patients.[44] The hypercoagulability is likely caused by a combination of severe systemic inflammation, extensive cytokine release, and endothelial damage, all of which produce additive effects in patients with baseline hypercoagulable comorbidities.[45,46] This hypercoagulable state can lead to multiple pulmonary emboli and subsequent right heart failure and can even lead to microthrombi within the myocardium itself, presenting as an acute STEMI.[44]

There is some early evidence to suggest that early anticoagulation is of benefit in patients with COVID-19.[47] Retrospective studies have suggested that use of enoxaparin or other low-molecular-weight heparins was associated with increased survival in patients with clinical coagulopathy or elevated D-dimer.[48] Recent studies are still mixed with regard to the optimal anticoagulation strategy. One recent study showed no benefit to intermediate-dose enoxaparin (1 mg/kg daily) compared with standard prophylactic dosing (40 mg daily),[49] whereas other observational studies have suggested a mortality benefit to treatment-dose anticoagulation, particularly in patients with more severe disease.[47] The European Heart Journal has proposed an algorithmic approach to the level of anticoagulation based on severity of disease, serum biomarkers, level of care, and presence of thromboembolism on point-of-care ultrasound.[50] In general, more severe cases of COVID-19 seem to necessitate higher levels of anticoagulation; however, the optimal strategy is still yet to be determined.[51,52]

THE PULMONARY SYSTEM
Pathophysiology of COVID-19–Induced Lung Injury

The role of angiotensin-converting enzyme 2 in the lung

ACE2 has been repeatedly demonstrated to be the host receptor of SARS-CoV-2. ACE2 is an essential component of the renin-angiotensin system (RAS). ACE is the enzyme responsible for catalyzing the conversion of angiotensin I to angiotensin II, which promotes the synthesis of aldosterone, vasoconstriction, and increased sodium reabsorption in the kidney's nephrons.[2,53] Meanwhile, ACE2 inactivates angiotensin II and cleaves it into angiotensin I. Therefore, ACE2 provides a counterbalance to ACE, thus regulating the effect of the RAS system on the body. ACE/ACE2 also play a role in the inflammation process, and a careful balance between proinflammatory and antiinflammatory pathways is maintained in healthy patients.[53] In contrast to its proinflammatory counterpart, the antiinflammatory responsibility of ACE2 provides necessary protection to the lung against injury.

In the lungs, ACE2 is expressed in the alveolar epithelial cells. It has mainly been detected in type II alveolar cells. The role of these cells includes surfactant production, movement of water across the epithelium, and restoration and regeneration of damaged lung alveolar epithelium.[54] The lung's substantial surface area and large concentration of ACE2 contribute to the lung's significant vulnerability to COVID-19 in comparison to other organs.

Sars-CoV-2 and receptor binding

The interaction between ACE2 and SARS-CoV-2 has been thoroughly investigated. Research into its binding kinetics show a 10 to 20x higher receptor preference for SARS-CoV-2 in comparison to SARS-CoV-1, which may provide insight into why the virus is so easily transmissible.[53] Similar to how other coronaviruses bind to host cells, it is thought the spike protein of SARS-CoV-2 interacts with ACE2, which initiates the release of viral RNA into the epithelial cells.[55]

Hyperinflammation, the cytokine storm, and fibrosis

Once SARS-CoV-2 binds to ACE2, the virus is replicated and cell apoptosis occurs. Consequently, proinflammatory cytokines are released, which upregulate the inflammatory reaction.[55,56] ACE2 is also downregulated, reducing its antiinflammatory capabilities in the lung. This local emission of cytokines, including tumor necrosis factor alpha, interleukin-1 (IL-1), IL-6, IL-8, and *monocyte chemoattractant protein 1*, is then released into systemic circulation. Homeostasis is progressively lost between proinflammatory and antiinflammatory pathways, which leads to widespread release of cytokines and damage to tissues, including the lung.[55,56] In addition, this cytokine storm also produces a collapse of T cells, and cellular-mediated adaptive immune response fails to produce meaningful protection for patients with COVID-19.[55] In the lung, ARDS is a common sequela after this widespread cytokine storm. Downregulation of ACE2 also leads to an increase in angiotensin II. Angiotensin II is proinflammatory and profibrotic, thus contributing to the development of pulmonary fibrosis.

Pathophysiologic Modulators of COVID-19 Severity in the Lungs

Age

Age is the strongest predictor of severity of COVID-19 disease in patients.[53] One study found that patients with COVID-19 younger than 60 years had a 1.38% mortality rate compared with 6.4% for those aged 60 years and older[57]; this may occur for a few reasons. First, ACE2 expression may increase with age, thus creating a greater susceptibility to COVID-19 in the elderly population.[58] Moreover, it is widely acknowledged that innate and adaptive immune responses weaken with aging, predisposing older populations to a more severe COVID-19 infection.

OBESITY

Evidence supports an association between obesity and higher mortality from COVID-19, with obese patients having 3.4-fold greater odds of developing severe COVID-19.[59] ACE2 is widely expressed in adipocytes. As a result, when SARS-CoV-2 binds to ACE2, the adipocytes release proinflammatory mediators that are then released systemically andaffect other organs, including the lungs. Furthermore, it is thought that ACE2 also downregulates pulmonary fibrosis, thus pulmonary fibrosis tends to develop more often in obese patients.[59,60]

Diabetes Mellitus

Diabetic patients have a 2.95x higher risk of mortality from COVID-19 in comparison with patients without diabetes, and they are more likely to develop a severe COVID-19 infection, with an odds ratio of 2.58 compared with nondiabetic patients.[61] Diabetes mellitus is known to involve a constant low-grade proinflammatory state that consequently compounds inflammatory damage on the lungs. Furthermore, hyperglycemia associated with diabetes mellitus promotes dysregulation of innate and adaptive immune responses. Studies have demonstrated a higher prevalence of ARDS in patients with hyperglycemia.[62]

Immunosuppression

Intuitively immunosuppression would be predicted to increase the risk of developing COVID-19. A recent metanalysis did not show any significant increased risk of COVID-19 infection for chronically immunosuppressed patients.[63] The pathophysiology of COVID-19 involves upregulation of proinflammatory pathways. However, with immunosuppressed patients, immunosuppressants modulate the proinflammatory pathways, which then limits the damage that COVID-19 can have on the lungs and the rest of the body. Although, the investigators did admit that their study may have been susceptible to selection bias, as immunosuppressed patients are more likely to adhere to precautions to limit transmission of SARS-CoV-2.[63]

MANAGEMENT OF COVID-19–INDUCED RESPIRATORY FAILURE

Management of acute respiratory failure due to COVID-19 may be thought of as a therapeutic pyramid,[64] staring with conventional oxygen therapy, progressing to high-flow nasal canula, noninvasive mechanical ventilation, intubation, conventional and if needed advanced mechanical ventilation, and ultimately extracorporeal membrane oxygenation.

High-Flow Nasal Cannula and Noninvasive Mechanical Ventilation

High-flow nasal cannula has emerged as treatment of hypoxic respiratory failure due to COVID-19. Although data continue to evolve, this technique seems to be an effective alternative to noninvasive mechanical ventilation, delay or reduce the need for intubation, and reduce mortality.[65,66]

Noninvasive ventilation, including continuous positive airway pressure and bilevel positive airway pressure, has been successfully and safely used to treat moderate-to-severe acute hypoxemic respiratory failure and ARDS.[67,68] Preventing the need for invasive ventilation and its potential complications, including ventilator associated pneumonia and lung injury, is undoubtedly beneficial. In patients with acute hypoxemic respiratory failure treated with noninvasive ventilation, only 28% of patients required eventual endotracheal intubation.[67] Meanwhile, noninvasive ventilation was successful in 48.1% of patients with ARDS secondary to COVID-19.[68]

Invasive Mechanical Ventilation

The next step up in the management of respiratory failure in patients with COVID-19 is intubation and conventional mechanical ventilation. Similar to other types of patients with ARDS, it is recommended that patients with CVOID-19 undergo traditional lung protective ventilation, as outlined in the ARDS net study published in 2000.[69] This type of ventilation is characterized by low tidal volume (4–8 mL/kg), high and individualized positive end-expiratoty pressure, and plateau pressures less than 30 cm H_2O.[69–71] It should be noted that although this approach is commonly used, some data suggest that it may also have detrimental effects.[72]

Extracorporeal Membrane Oxygenation

Should invasive mechanical ventilation failure occur, ECMO may be an option. However, evidence on the utilization of ECMO to treat the pulmonary complications of COVID-19 is inconclusive. A recent meta-analysis of 25 peer-reviewed journal articles on the subject showed that further research needs to be performed to determine the effectiveness of ECMO on COVID-19 pulmonary complications because a most of the available research are case reports or case series.[73]

Venovenous (VV) ECMO is the most common form of ECMO used in reported studies. Indications that were used to initiate VV-ECMO included refractory hypoxia and hypercapnia or single organ failure. Meanwhile, venoarterial ECMO was very rarely used in reported studies. Indications that were used included cardiogenic shock due to cardiac injury.[73] Because of the limited amount of data available, the investigators of the meta-analysis recommended caution with using ECMO in the setting of COVID-19 until studies with larger sample sizes are performed to investigate its efficacy.

FLUID MANAGEMENT IN PATIENTS WITH COVID-19 ACUTE RESPIRATORY DISTRESS SYNDROME

In ARDS, regardless of cause, fluid overload can detrimentally affect patients' outcomes, and, consequently, conscientious fluid management is essential. Positive pressure ventilation is known to contribute to pulmonary vasoconstriction, which produces fluid retention and interstitial edema.[70,71] As a result, restrictive fluid management is recommended, as it is associated with greater ventilator-free days.[74] Unfortunately, fluid management in patients with ARDS secondary to COVID-19 has not been thoroughly investigated.

PRONE POSITIONING

Prone positioning has long been used for ARDS and acute hypoxic respiratory failure.[75,76] Over the years, when and how to use this strategy has been refined.[77] Prone positioning has now been implemented as a treatment of COVID-19 respiratory sequelae.

Prone positioning is thought to improve oxygenation through several means. First, lung recruitment and perfusion are optimized. Second, the functional lung size is greatly improved. Third, evidenced on echocardiography, right heart strain is significantly reduced by decreasing overall pulmonary resistance.[70]

For awake, nonintubated patients, it has been demonstrated that simply giving these patients supplemental oxygen in the emergency department and placing them in prone position increases oxygen saturation from a median of 80% to 94%.[78] However, studies have shown that on resupination the increased oxygenation continues in only approximately one-half of patients.[79] Even more, studies have not demonstrated a significant difference in rates of intubation when comparing prone awake patients with supine awake patients, although a delay to intubation has been noted.[80,81] Also, significant changes in 28-day mortality were not evidenced when comparing proned versus supine patients.[81]

Prone positioning has also been used for intubated patients with COVID-19.[82] In ventilated patients, timing of initiating prone positioning is essential. If patients are placed into prone position early in the disease course, then they are less likely to experience in-hospital mortality.[83] Use of early use of the prone position seems to lead to better oxygenation and an earlier pulmonary recovery.

THE ENTERIC SYSTEM
The Gastrointestinal System and Nutrition

Although known primarily as a respiratory ailment, COVID-19 infection has been implicated in the dysfunction of every major organ system, and the gastrointestinal (GI) organs are no exception. An estimated 4% of patients with COVID infection present solely with GI complaints,[84] including diarrhea, abdominal pain, nausea and vomiting, and loss of appetite. Large meta-analyses with thousands of subjects have shown that prevalence of gastrointestinal symptoms among patients with COVID-19 ranged from 10% to 17.6%,[85] and one study found that patients who did present with GI symptoms (nausea, vomiting, or diarrhea) had significantly more severe symptoms of fever, fatigue, and shortness of breath[86] as well as delayed presentation.[87] These gastrointestinal symptoms begin to make sense when examining the pathophysiology of infection; ACE2 is a known cellular attachment receptor for the COVID-19 virion, and transmembrane protease serine 2 (TMPRSS2) has been shown to cleave the spike protein of COVID-19, together facilitating entry into the cell.[88,89] These effects are marked in the lung tissue, whose high expressions of ACE-2 and TMPRSS2 are likely responsible for the characteristic pulmonary symptoms of the disease. High expressions of ACE-2 and TMPRSS2 are also found throughout the gastrointestinal tract, especially in the small intestine and colon,[89] and may be the culprit behind the GI effects of COVID-19.

COVID-19 virions are known to be shed in stool, creating a potential reservoir of infectious virus particle.[90] Seventy percent of those with fecal RNA shedding testing fecal positive after their respiratory specimens cleared the virus,[88] leading to concerns that patients who test negative on a nasopharyngeal swab could still expose others to active disease through fecal-oral transmission. The Centers for Disease Control and Prevention recommends using separate bathrooms for COVID-19–positive patients.[91] COVID has been shown to replicate virus in enterocytes,[85] adding to the concern that endoscopies could be high-risk aerosolizing procedures. All major GI societies have recommended to delay any nonurgent endoscopies during the height of the pandemic.[92] Internationally, upper endoscopy and colonoscopy rates decreased by 85%,[84] concerning for delayed diagnoses or progression of cancer. It has been suggested that alternatives to endoscopy, such as FIT testing for colorectal cancer screening or calprotectin for inflammatory bowel disease (IBD) diagnosis, be used to reduce risk during the pandemic while minimizing harm from delaying endoscopic procedures. Modeling has found that widespread FIT testing would prevent 90% of life years lost due to cancer diagnosis delay.[84] Coronaviruses are known to be transmittable through a fecal-oral routes; one study in mice found exaggerated symptoms and pathology in infected mice that had been treated with a proton pump inhibitors. This group of mice demonstrated increased pulmonary inflammation histologically,[93] raising questions about proton pump inhibitor usage and infectivity in humans but further research is needed. ACE2 and TMPRSS2 both are key receptors involved in cellular entry of COVID-19 virions; ACE2 is overexpressed in states of bowel inflammation,[94] and TMPRSS2 is overexpressed in the ileal inflammation,[84] possibly increasing the likelihood of cellular entry and infection. Direct absorptive enterocyte injury due to COVID-related inflammation can lead to malnutrition and secretory diarrhea.[87] Malnutrition, whether from enterocyte injury or from poor oral intake during acute illness, can lead to atrophied lymphoid tissue and increased bacterial translocation.[95] Loss of appetite is noted to be common ($\sim 26\%$)[94] during COVID infections with a high prevalence of gustatory dysfunction, which may contribute to this[90]; early enteral nutrition is recommended in patients with COVID by the American and European Societies for Parental and Enteral Nutrition, even in proned patients.[95] There are multiple cytokines released in the course of infection that are known to alter gut microbiota[94]; some patients demonstrate decreased intestinal probiotics[92] and increased opportunistic gut bacteria that have been known to cause bacteremia, changes that were shown to persist even after clearance of COVID-19.[85]

GI bleeding does not seem to be increased among patients with COVID but a study among New York patients with GI bleeds found that they tended to have significantly poorer outcomes during the pandemic, possibly related to patient's reluctance to present to hospital during an outbreak along with an increased threshold to perform endoscopy in the setting of widespread COVID-19.[84]

A special population to consider in the COVID era is patients with IBD. ACE2 expression has been shown to be elevated during active IBD.[94] An analysis of patients on the SECURE-IBD registry found that in patients with IBD, steroid and mesalamine use has been shown to be associated with higher rates of mortality from COVID-19, with almost 20% of patients with COVID who require steroid use for their IBD experiencing ICU admission, mechanical ventilation, or death as part of their clinical course of COVID-19.[84] In contrast, only 2% to 3% of patients on biological monotherapy for their IBD experienced these adverse events.

The Liver

In the setting of patients without preexisting liver disease, COVID-19–associated liver injury tends to be mild in most cases. Elevated aspartate transaminase/alanine aminotransferase has been found to be the most common hepatic manifestation of the disease at an estimated rate of 20% to 30%.[92]. However, Hajifathalian and colleagues[96] reported that an association between risk of ICU admission/mortality and the presence of acute liver injury on admission. Potential mechanisms to explain this process include drug-induced liver injury, direct COVID-induced hepatitis/myositis, and ACE2-mediated binding and damage. ACE2 receptors were found to be high in cholangiocytes,[97] and although normally were low in hepatocytes their expression has been shown to be inducible by hypoxia and inflammation or preexisting liver disease,[98] hypoxic injury, indirect injury due to systemic inflammation and cytokines, ventilator-associated hepatic congestion, and aggravation of preexisting viral hepatitis.[99] Remdesivir has been found in a large trial (n = 1073) to increase liver enzymes[88] with 2.5% and 3.6% of patients in the 5- and 10-day courses, respectively, discontinuing treatment due to these elevated liver enzymes.[100]

Other drugs commonly used in the off-label treatment of COVID-19 such as hydroxychloroquine, corticosteroids, and acetaminophen also have known hepatotoxic potential.[98] Systemic inflammatory response syndrome–induced markers of cholestasis, such as bile duct proliferation, bile plugs, and inflammatory infiltrates, have been found in autopsy studies of patients with COVID.[98] Beyond the frequently encountered mild acute liver injury, COVID-19 can have severe implications for patients with preexisting liver problems. Chronic liver disease was associated with a 60% increased risk of mortality from COVID-19, and frequent hepatic decompensation has been reported among this population during acute infection.[84]

Chronic liver disease can also affect COVID treatment options for patients; for example, patients with decompensated cirrhosis are recommended to not receive remdesivir, one of the only antivirals approved to treat COVID-19.[84]

The pandemic has also affected liver transplant programs around the globe; for prospective transplant candidates, it is recommended that transplant be limited to high MELD score patients or those with high risk of decompensation/hepatocellular carcinoma progression, especially given the decreased number of organs procured during the pandemic.[101] It is also unanimously recommended to continue immunosuppressive therapy in postliver transplant patients throughout the COVID pandemic, given the increased risk for rejection.[101]

The Pancreas

Pancreatic acinar cells do express ACE2 receptors, and it was theorized that this could lead to direct viral-mediated pancreatic damage, but despite several early reports of COVID-associated acute pancreatitis, acute pancreatitis seems to be a rare finding in people infected with COVID. One retrospective study of 63,000 patients with COVID in Spain found an incidence of only 0.07% of acute pancreatitis among these patients.[102] However, patients with COVID were much more likely to be diagnosed with idiopathic pancreatitis versus gallstone or alcoholic pancreatitis (69% compared with 21%), although this was thought to be related to pancreatitis due to widespread multiorgan failure. Many early studies did not use uniform definitions of pancreatitis but instead used elevated serum amylase as an indicator even in the absence of abdominal symptoms.[103] Amylase was found to be elevated in 17.9% of severe COVID cases versus only 1.9% of nonsevere COVID-19 cases, although most of these had no other signs of pancreatitis[104]; elevated amylase is not specific for pancreatitis and could be elevated due to cytokine storm or multiorgan failure that can be seen in severe COVID infection. Lung injury and increased intestinal permeability seen in the setting of COVID infection both could also cause increased serum amylase levels. Pancreatic cancer has been associated with increased ACE2 expression, possibly raising the baseline risk for infection among patients with pancreatic adenocarcinoma.[104] Similar to other cancers, the immunosuppressive effects of chemotherapy can worsen the effects of COVID; one study found a 40% rate of severe adverse events, including death, associated with pancreatic cancer among patients with COVID-19 as opposed to just 8% among those without cancer.[105]

THE RENAL SYSTEM

Acute kidney injury in the setting of COVID-19 may be the result of direct viral injury to the kidney[106] and/or dysfunctions in other organ systems that secondarily affect the kidney.[107] Although exact pathophysiologic mechanisms remain controversial,[108] the development of acute kidney injury or worsening of chronic kidney disease is associated with a worse prognosis.[109] Treatment approaches used for acute kidney injury in patients with COVID-19 are similar to those used in non–COVID-19 patients.[110]

THE VASCULAR AND HEMATOLOGICAL SYSTEMS

During normal times of health, the vascular endothelium has many roles: immune competence, inflammatory equilibrium, maintaining tight junctional barriers, and aiding in hemodynamic stability. It is well known that the vascular endothelium also plays a significant role in the thrombotic and fibrinolytic pathways. During the COVID-19 epidemic, studies have been able to elucidate many vascular complications associated with infection with this novel virus apart from the known respiratory problems. Thromboembolic complications have been reported affecting not just the vasculature of the lungs[111] but also the brain,[112] heart,[113] and extremities.[114] The incidence of thrombotic complications in the ICU ranges from 16% to 69%.[114] Current clinical data indicate both deep vein thrombosis and pulmonary embolisms are the most frequent thrombotic events.[115,116] The mechanisms by which this occurs is related to the damage caused by virus on endothelial cells and subsequent inflammatory reaction and activation of the coagulation cascade. The vascular endothelial cells have vast expression of ACE2, including alveolar cells of the lung.[117] Entry of the SARS-CoV-2 virus into the endothelial cell occurs by binding of the spike (S) protein to the ACE2 receptors, where the SARS-CoV-2 virus has a nearly 10-fold greater affinity for ACE2 versus its SARS-CoV-1, also known as severe acute respiratory syndrome.[118] This entry into the endothelial cell then triggers activation of the immune system followed by cytokine release and subsequent activation of macrophages. This hyperinflammatory state leads to expression of IL-1, IL-6, damage-associated molecular patterns, and recruitment of macrophages to the infected cells leading to endothelial injury. Damaged endothelial cells increase vascular permeability and activate the coagulation cascade.[119] In patients with COVID-19, this heightened innate immune system creates a prothrombotic state and endothelial cell injury. Injury then leads to plasminogen activator inhibitor-1 upregulation, which inhibits fibrinolysis. Tissue factor is increased, leading to procoagulation, as well as release of von Willebrand factor creating intraluminal thrombus. Studies have demonstrated an increase in fibrinogen levels as well.[120,121] D-dimer levels have been elevated, as well as fibrin degradation products increased.[122,123]

Autopsy reports in patients with COVID-19 revealed increased pulmonary endothelial inclusions and increased capillary microthrombi.[124,125] Questions on how to best treat this hypercoagulative state remain active. An observational study found a lower mortality and risk of intubation in patients with COVID-19 with either therapeutic or prophylactic anticoagulation compared with no anticoagulation.[126] No benefit was seen comparing prophylactic with therapeutic anticoagulation. A recent recommendation for patients with COVID-19 recommends prophylactic low-molecular-weight heparin given for all patients with COVID-19 in the absence of active bleeding, low platelet counts less than 25,000, and fibrinogen levels less than 0.5 g/L.[127]

Other hematologic issues may also occur in patients with COVID-19. Lymphopenia does develop in more than 50% of patients with COVID-19 infection.[128] The O and Rh blood groups may be associated with a slightly lower risk for SARS-CoV-2 infection and severe COVID-19 illness. However, the reasons why and the significance of this association have yet to be determined.[129]

PHARMACOLOGIC TREATMENTS AND CONVALESCENT PLASMA
Lopinavir-Ritonavir

Lopinavir-ritonavir is a protease inhibitor and nucleoside analogue combination medication primarily used to treat human immunodeficiency virus. It was theorized that its dual antiviral nature would be effective in treating COVID-19. However, a systematic risk-benefit analysis of 7 peer reviewed journal articles did not demonstrate a clear benefit to using this medication for severe COVID-19 infection. Dangerous side effects include prolonged QT interval and inhibitor of cytochrome P450.[130]

Chloroquine and Hydroxychloroquine

Chloroquine and hydroxychloroquine are medications that have multiple antiviral mechanisms, including inhibition of viral entry and release of virus into the cell, along with immunomodularity activities.[130] Despite its increase in popularity in 2020 as a treatment of COVID-19, data are inconclusive in terms of its potential benefit. Dangerous side effects include prolonged QT interval and hypoglycemia.[130–132]

Dexamethasone

Dexamethasone is a corticosteroid that has been used to treat COVID-19. A 10-day course has been demonstrated by multiple studies and trials, including the RECOVERY and CoDEX trials, to have a significant decrease in 28-day mortality, number of ventilator-free days, and incidence of hypoxia.[133,134] As a result, dexamethasone has become standard of care in the treatment of COVID-19.[135] Despite its benefit in the treatment of COVID-19, dexamethasone is also associated with several complications including glaucoma, hyperglycemia, and hypertension.[136]

Remdesivir

Remdesivir is an antiviral nucleoside analogue known to inhibit RNA polymerase that has also been used to treat COVID-19. It has been shown to significantly reduce recovery time and has been associated with higher odds of clinical improvement.[137–140] Side effects are generally mild, but more severe ones include hypotension and cardiac arrythmias.

CONVALESCENT PLASMA

Convalescent plasma treatment of infectious diseases is characterized by immediate immunity through the administration of passive antibodies.[141] A systematic report of 5 studies on convalescent plasma and COVID-19 demonstrated there may be clinical benefit, and it seems to be safe. Almost all patients who were administered convalescent plasma had symptomatic improvement, and zero mortality was reported.[142] However, a recommendation was made for a large multicenter clinical trial to provide stronger evidence. Recommendations for ideal plasma donors include donors who donate 28 days after the onset of symptoms and had fevers for more than 3 days.[143]

SUMMARY

COVID-19 continues to ebb and flow, as waves, across the globe. During times of surge, nonintensive care–trained surgeons may be deployed into a critical care setting, to care for patients who would normally be treated in a medical ICU. Although primarily a pulmonary disease, COVID-19 has many extrapulmonary manifestations. The interaction between different organ systems and COVID-19's effect on each create difficulty in managing these patients. This difficulty is further exacerbated by our incomplete understanding and constantly evolving guidelines. The authors wish health for our patients and safety for those who provide care at this historically challenging time.

CONFLICT OF INTEREST

None of the authors have any conflicts of interest related to this article.

REFERENCES

1. Weiss SR, Navas-Martin S. Coronavirus pathogenesis and the emerging pathogen severe acute respiratory syndrome coronavirus. Microbiol Mol Biol Rev 2005;69(4):635–64.
2. Rezaei M, Ziai SA, Fakhri S, et al. ACE2: Its potential role and regulation in severe acute respiratory syndrome and COVID-19. J Cell Physiol 2021;236(4): 2430–42.
3. Meyerholz DK, Perlman S. Does common cold coronavirus infection protect against severe SARS-CoV-2 disease? J Clin Invest 2021;131(1):e144807.
4. Gengler I, Wang JC, Speth MM, et al. Sinonasal pathophysiology of SARS-CoV-2 and COVID-19: A systematic review of the current evidence. Laryngoscope Investig Otolaryngol 2020;5(3):354–9.
5. Paules CI, Marston HD, Fauci AS. Coronavirus Infections-More Than Just the Common Cold. JAMA 2020;323(8):707–8.
6. Coronavirus disease (COVID-19) outbreak. World Health Organization. Available at: http://www.euro.who.int/en/health-topics/health-emergencies/coronavirus-COVID -19/novel-coronavirus-2019-ncov. Accessed on 15 Sept 2021.
7. 2019-nCoV outbreak is an emergency of international concern. World Health Organization. Available at: http://www.euro.who.int/en/health-topics/health-emergencies/international-health-regulations/news/news/2020/2/2019-ncov-outbreak-is-an-emergency-of-international-concern. Accessed on 17 Sept 2021.
8. COVID-19 live update. Available at: https://www.worldometers.info/coronavirus. Accessed on 21 Sept 2021.
9. Engberg M, Bonde J, Sigurdsson ST, et al. Training non-intensivist doctors to work with COVID-19 patients in intensive care units. Acta Anaesthesiol Scand 2021;65(5):664–73.
10. Dhar SI. An Otolaryngologist Redeployed to a COVID-19 Intensive Care Unit: Lessons Learned. Otolaryngol Head Neck Surg 2020;163(3):471–2.
11. Coughlan C, Nafde C, Khodatars S, et al. COVID-19: lessons for junior doctors redeployed to critical care. Postgrad Med J 2021;97(1145):188–91.
12. Critical Care for the Non-ICU Clinician. Available at: https://www.covid19.sccm.org/nonicu/. Accessed on 21 Sept 2021.
13. An international Virtual COVID-19 critical care training Forum for Healthcare Workers. Available at. https://www.atsjournals.org/doi/full/10.34197/ats-scholar.2020-0154IN. Accessed on 21 Sept 2021.
14. Critical Care Primer: Educational Resources for Non-ICU Clinicians. Available at: https://guides.himmelfarb.gwu.edu/criticalcareprimer. Accessed on 21 Sept 2021.
15. Higgins V, Sohaei D, Diamandis EP, et al. COVID-19: from an acute to chronic disease? Potential long-term health consequences. Crit Rev Clin Lab Sci 2021;58(5):297–310.

16. Ellul MA, Benjamin L, Singh B, et al. Neurological associations of COVID-19. Lancet Neurol 2020;19(9):767–83.
17. Maury A, Lyoubi A, Peiffer-Smadja N, et al. Neurological manifestations associated with SARS-CoV-2 and other coronaviruses: A narrative review for clinicians. Rev Neurol (Paris) 2021;177(1–2):51–64.
18. Solomon T. Neurological Infection with SARS-CoV-2 - the Story so Far. Nat Rev Neurol 2021;17(2):65–6.
19. Wang F, Kream RM, Stefano GB. Long-Term Respiratory and Neurological Sequelae of COVID-19. Med Sci Monit 2020;26:e928996.
20. Beyrouti R, Adams ME, Benjamin L, et al. Characteristics of ischaemic stroke associated with COVID-19. J Neurol Neurosurg Psychiatr 2020;91(8):889–91.
21. Matschke J, Lütgehetmann M, Hagel C, et al. Neuropathology of patients with COVID-19 in Germany: a post-mortem case series. Lancet Neurol 2020; 19(11):919–29.
22. Pezzini A, Padovani A. Lifting the mask on neurological manifestations of COVID-19. Nat Rev Neurol 2020;16(11):636–44.
23. Tsai LK, Hsieh ST, Chang YC. Neurological manifestations in severe acute respiratory syndrome. Acta Neurol Taiwan 2005;14(3):113–9.
24. Li YC, Bai WZ, Hashikawa T. The neuroinvasive potential of SARS-CoV2 may play a role in the respiratory failure of COVID-19 patients. J Med Virol 2020; 92(6):552–5.
25. Yachou Y, El Idrissi A, Belapasov V, et al. Neuroinvasion, neurotropic, and neuro-inflammatory events of SARS-CoV-2: understanding the neurological manifestations in COVID-19 patients. Neurol Sci 2020;41(10):2657–69.
26. Helms J, Kremer S, Merdji H, et al. Delirium and encephalopathy in severe COVID-19: a cohort analysis of ICU patients. Crit Care 2020;24(1):491.
27. Zheng YY, Ma YT, Zhang JY, et al. COVID-19 and the cardiovascular system. Nat Rev Cardiol 2020;17(5):259–60.
28. Xiong TY, Redwood S, Prendergast B, et al. Coronaviruses and the cardiovascular system: acute and long-term implications. Eur Heart J 2020;41(19): 1798–800.
29. Clerkin KJ, Fried JA, Raikhelkar J, et al. COVID-19 and Cardiovascular Disease. Circulation 2020;141(20):1648–55.
30. Xu Z, Shi L, Wang Y, et al. Pathological findings of COVID-19 associated with acute respiratory distress syndrome. Lancet Respir Med 2020;8(4):420–2.
31. Chen L, Li X, Chen M, et al. The ACE2 expression in human heart indicates new potential mechanism of heart injury among patients infected with SARS-CoV-2. Cardiovasc Res 2020;116(6):1097–100.
32. Tikellis C, Thomas MC. Angiotensin-Converting Enzyme 2 (ACE2) Is a Key Modulator of the Renin Angiotensin System in Health and Disease. Int J Pept 2012;2012:256294.
33. Halushka MK, Vander Heide RS. Myocarditis is rare in COVID-19 autopsies: cardiovascular findings across 277 postmortem examinations. Cardiovasc Pathol 2021;50:107300.
34. Schoenhagen P, Tuzcu EM, Ellis SG. Plaque vulnerability, plaque rupture, and acute coronary syndromes: (multi)-focal manifestation of a systemic disease process. Circulation 2002;106(7):760–2.
35. Bansal M. Cardiovascular disease and COVID-19. Diabetes Metab Syndr 2020; 14(3):247–50.
36. Basu-Ray I, Almaddah Nk, Adeboye A, et al. Cardiac manifestations of Coronavirus (COVID-19) [Updated 2021 May 19]. In: StatPearls [Internet]. Treasure

Island (FL): StatPearls Publishing; 2021. Available at: https://www.ncbi.nlm.nih. gov/books/NBK556152/. Accessed on 21 Sept 2021.

37. Bangalore S, Sharma A, Slotwiner A, et al. ST-Segment Elevation in Patients with Covid-19 - A Case Series. N Engl J Med 2020;382(25):2478–80.

38. Stefanini GG, Montorfano M, Trabattoni D, et al. ST-Elevation Myocardial Infarction in Patients With COVID-19: Clinical and Angiographic Outcomes. Circulation 2020;141(25):2113–6.

39. Mahmud E, Dauerman HL, FGP Welt, et al. Management of acute myocardial infarction during the COVID-19 pandemic: A Consensus Statement from the Society for Cardiovascular Angiography and Interventions (SCAI), the American College of Cardiology (ACC), and the American College of Emergency Physicians (ACEP). Catheter Cardiovasc Interv 2020;96(2):336–45.

40. Zhou F, Yu T, Du R, et al. Clinical course and risk factors for mortality of adult inpatients with COVID-19 in Wuhan, China: a retrospective cohort study. Lancet 2020;395:1054–62.

41. Arentz M, Yim E, Klaff L, et al. Characteristics and Outcomes of 21 Critically Ill Patients With COVID-19 in Washington State. JAMA 2020;323(16):1612–4.

42. Chen T, Wu D, Chen H, et al. Clinical characteristics of 113 deceased patients with coronavirus disease 2019: retrospective study. BMJ 2020;368:m1091.

43. Kochav SM, Coromilas E, Nalbandian A, et al. Cardiac Arrhythmias in COVID-19 Infection. Circ Arrhythm Electrophysiol 2020;13(6):e008719.

44. Pellegrini D, Kawakami R, Guagliumi G, et al. Microthrombi as a Major Cause of Cardiac Injury in COVID-19: A Pathologic Study. Circulation 2021;143(10): 1031–42.

45. Panigada M, Bottino N, Tagliabue P, et al. Hypercoagulability of COVID-19 patients in intensive care unit: A report of thromboelastography findings and other parameters of hemostasis. J Thromb Haemost 2020;18(7):1738–42.

46. Tang N, Li D, Wang X, et al. Abnormal coagulation parameters are associated with poor prognosis in patients with novel coronavirus pneumonia. J Thromb Haemost 2020;18(4):844–7.

47. Paranjpe I, Fuster V, Lala A, et al. Association of Treatment Dose Anticoagulation With In-Hospital Survival Among Hospitalized Patients With COVID-19. J Am Coll Cardiol 2020;76(1):122–4.

48. Tang N, Bai H, Chen X, et al. Anticoagulant treatment is associated with decreased mortality in severe coronavirus disease 2019 patients with coagulopathy. J Thromb Haemost 2020;18(5):1094–9.

49. INSPIRATION Investigators, Sadeghipour P, Talasaz AH, et al. Effect of Intermediate-Dose vs Standard-Dose Prophylactic Anticoagulation on Thrombotic Events, Extracorporeal Membrane Oxygenation Treatment, or Mortality Among Patients With COVID-19 Admitted to the Intensive Care Unit: The INSPIRATION Randomized Clinical Trial. JAMA 2021;325(16):1620–30.

50. Atallah B, Mallah SI, AlMahmeed W. Anticoagulation in COVID-19. Eur Heart J Cardiovasc Pharmacother 2020;6(4):260–1.

51. Hadid T, Kafri Z, Al-Katib A. Coagulation and anticoagulation in COVID-19. Blood Rev 2021;47:100761.

52. The Lancet Haematology. COVID-19 coagulopathy: an evolving story. Lancet Haematol 2020;7(6):e425.

53. Bourgonje AR, Abdulle AE, Timens W, et al. Angiotensin-converting enzyme 2 (ACE2), SARS-CoV-2 and the pathophysiology of coronavirus disease 2019 (COVID-19). J Pathol 2020;251(3):228–48.

54. Castranova V, Rabovsky J, Tucker JH, et al. The alveolar type II epithelial cell: a multifunctional pneumocyte. Toxicol Appl Pharmacol 1988;93(3):472–83.
55. Singh SP, Pritam M, Pandey B, et al. Microstructure, pathophysiology, and potential therapeutics of COVID-19: A comprehensive review. J Med Virol 2021; 93(1):275–99.
56. Ryabkova VA, Churilov LP, Shoenfeld Y. Influenza infection, SARS, MERS and COVID-19: Cytokine storm - The common denominator and the lessons to be learned. Clin Immunol 2021;223:108652.
57. Verity R, Okell LC, Dorigatti I, et al. Estimates of the severity of coronavirus disease 2019: a model-based analysis. Lancet Infect Dis 2020;20(6):669–77.
58. Chen Y, Li L. SARS-CoV-2: virus dynamics and host response. Lancet Infect Dis 2020;20(5):515–6.
59. Wang J, Sato T, Sakuraba A. Coronavirus Disease 2019 (COVID-19) Meets Obesity: Strong Association between the Global Overweight Population and COVID-19 Mortality. J Nutr 2021;151(1):9–10.
60. Kruglikov IL, Scherer PE. The Role of Adipocytes and Adipocyte-Like Cells in the Severity of COVID-19 Infections. Obesity (Silver Spring) 2020;28(7): 1187–90.
61. Wu J, Zhang J, Sun X, et al. Influence of diabetes mellitus on the severity and fatality of SARS-CoV-2 (COVID-19) infection. Diabetes Obes Metab 2020; 22(10):1907–14.
62. Fleming N, Sacks LJ, Pham CT, et al. An overview of COVID-19 in people with diabetes: Pathophysiology and considerations in the inpatient setting. Diabet Med 2021;38(3):e14509.
63. Tassone D, Thompson A, Connell W, et al. Immunosuppression as a risk factor for COVID-19: a meta-analysis. Intern Med J 2021;51(2):199–205.
64. Cinesi Gómez C, Peñuelas Rodríguez Ó, Luján Torné M, et al. Clinical consensus recommendations regarding non-invasive respiratory support in the adult patient with acute respiratory failure secondary to SARS-CoV-2 infection. Arch Bronconeumol 2020;56:11–8.
65. Matthay MA, Aldrich JM, Gotts JE. Treatment for severe acute respiratory distress syndrome from COVID-19. Lancet Respir Med 2020;8:433–4.
66. Chavarria AP, Lezama ES, Navarro MG, et al. High-flow nasal cannula therapy for hypoxemic respiratory failure in patients with COVID-19. Ther Adv Infect Dis 2021;8. 20499361211042959.
67. Franco C, Facciolongo N, Tonelli R, et al. Feasibility and clinical impact of out-of-ICU noninvasive respiratory support in patients with COVID-19-related pneumonia. Eur Respir J 2020;56(5):2002130.
68. Menzella F, Barbieri C, Fontana M, et al. Effectiveness of noninvasive ventilation in COVID-19 related-acute respiratory distress syndrome. Clin Respir J 2021; 00:1–9.
69. The Acute Respiratory Distress Syndrome Network: Ventilation with lower tidal volumes as compared with traditional tidal volumes for acute lung injury and the acute respiratory distress syndrome. N Engl J Med 2000;342:1301–8.
70. Welker C, Huang J, Gil IJN, et al. 2021 Acute Respiratory Distress Syndrome Update, With Coronavirus Disease 2019 Focus. J Cardiothorac Vasc Anesth 2021;(21):00188–9. S1053-S0770.
71. Griffiths MJD, McAuley DF, Perkins GD, et al. Guidelines on the management of acute respiratory distress syndrome. BMJ Open Respir Res 2019;6(1):e000420.
72. Tsolaki V, Zakynthinos GE, Makris D. The ARDSnet protocol may be detrimental in COVID-19. Crit Care 2020;24(1):351.

73. Haiduc AA, Alom S, Melamed N, et al. Role of extracorporeal membrane oxygenation in COVID-19: A systematic review. J Cardiovasc Surg 2020; 35(10):2679–87.

74. Vignon P, Evrard B, Asfar P, et al. Fluid administration and monitoring in ARDS: which management? Intensive Care Med 2020;46(12):2252–64.

75. Guérin C, Reignier J, Richard JC, et al, PROSEVA Study Group. Prone positioning in severe acute respiratory distress syndrome. N Engl J Med 2013; 368(23):2159–68.

76. Scholten EL, Beitler JR, Prisk GK, et al. Treatment of ARDS With Prone Positioning. Chest 2017;151(1):215–24.

77. Guérin C, Albert RK, Beitler J, et al. Prone position in ARDS patients: why, when, how and for whom. Intensive Care Med 2020;46(12):2385–96.

78. Caputo ND, Strayer RJ, Levitan R. Early Self-Proning in Awake, Non-intubated Patients in the Emergency Department: A Single ED's Experience During the COVID-19 Pandemic. Acad Emerg Med 2020;27(5):375–8.

79. Coppo A, Bellani G, Winterton D, et al. Feasibility and physiological effects of prone positioning in non-intubated patients with acute respiratory failure due to COVID-19 (PRON-COVID): a prospective cohort study. Lancet Respir Med 2020;8(8):765–74.

80. Padrão EMH, Valente FS, Besen BAMP, et al. Awake Prone Positioning in COVID-19 Hypoxemic Respiratory Failure: Exploratory Findings in a Single-center Retrospective Cohort Study. Acad Emerg Med 2020;27(12):1249–59.

81. Ferrando C, Mellado-Artigas R, Gea A, et al, COVID-19 Spanish ICU Network. Awake prone positioning does not reduce the risk of intubation in COVID-19 treated with high-flow nasal oxygen therapy: a multicenter, adjusted cohort study. Crit Care 2020;24(1):597.

82. Elharrar X, Trigui Y, Dols AM, et al. Use of Prone Positioning in Nonintubated Patients With COVID-19 and Hypoxemic Acute Respiratory Failure. JAMA 2020; 323(22):2336–8.

83. Mathews KS, Soh H, Shaefi S, et al. Prone Positioning and Survival in Mechanically Ventilated Patients With Coronavirus Disease 2019-Related Respiratory Failure. Crit Care Med 2021;49(7):1026–37.

84. Hunt RH, East JE, Lanas A, et al. COVID-19 and Gastrointestinal Disease: Implications for the Gastroenterologist. Dig Dis 2021;39(2):119–39.

85. Trottein F, Sokol H. Potential Causes and Consequences of Gastrointestinal Disorders during a SARS-CoV-2 Infection. Cell Rep 2020;32(3):107915.

86. Jin X, Lian JS, Hu JH, et al. Epidemiological, clinical and virological characteristics of 74 cases of coronavirus-infected disease 2019 (COVID-19) with gastrointestinal symptoms. Gut 2020;69(6):1002–9.

87. Patel KP, Patel PA, Vunnam RR, et al. Gastrointestinal, hepatobiliary, and pancreatic manifestations of COVID-19. J Clin Virol 2020;128:104386.

88. Thuluvath PJ, Alukal JJ, Ravindran N, et al. What GI Physicians Need to Know During COVID-19 Pandemic. Dig Dis Sci 2020;1–11.

89. Dong M, Zhang J, Ma X, et al. ACE2, TMPRSS2 distribution and extrapulmonary organ injury in patients with COVID-19. Biomed Pharmacother 2020;131:110678.

90. Su S, Shen J, Zhu L, et al. Involvement of digestive system in COVID-19: manifestations, pathology, management and challenges. Therap Adv Gastroenterol 2020;13. 1756284820934626.

91. Soetikno R, Teoh AYB, Kaltenbach T, et al. Considerations in performing endoscopy during the COVID-19 pandemic. Gastrointest Endosc 2020;92(1):176–83.

92. Kopel J, Perisetti A, Gajendran M, et al. Clinical Insights into the Gastrointestinal Manifestations of COVID-19. Dig Dis Sci 2020;65(7):1932–9.

93. Zhou J, Li C, Zhao G, et al. Human intestinal tract serves as an alternative infection route for Middle East respiratory syndrome coronavirus. Sci Adv 2017;3(11): eaao4966.

94. Perisetti A, Gajendran M, Mann R, et al. COVID-19 extrapulmonary illness - special gastrointestinal and hepatic considerations. Dis Mon 2020;66(9):101064.

95. Aguila EJT, Cua IHY, Fontanilla JAC, et al. Gastrointestinal Manifestations of COVID-19: Impact on Nutrition Practices. Nutr Clin Pract 2020;35(5):800–5.

96. Hajifathalian K, Krisko T, Mehta A, et al, WCM-GI research group*. Gastrointestinal and Hepatic Manifestations of 2019 Novel Coronavirus Disease in a Large Cohort of Infected Patients From New York: Clinical Implications. Gastroenterology 2020;159(3):1137–40.e2.

97. Galanopoulos M, Gkeros F, Doukatas A, et al. COVID-19 pandemic: Pathophysiology and manifestations from the gastrointestinal tract. World J Gastroenterol 2020;26(31):4579–88.

98. Nardo AD, Schneeweiss-Gleixner M, Bakail M, et al. Pathophysiological mechanisms of liver injury in COVID-19. Liver Int 2021;41(1):20–32.

99. Kunutsor SK, Laukkanen JA. Markers of liver injury and clinical outcomes in COVID-19 patients: A systematic review and meta-analysis. J Infect 2021; 82(1):159–98.

100. Goldman JD, Lye DCB, Hui DS, Marks KM, Bruno R, Montejano R, Spinner CD, Galli M, Ahn MY, Nahass RG, Chen YS, SenGupta D, Hyland RH, Osinusi AO, Cao H, Blair C, Wei X, Gaggar A, Brainard DM, Towner WJ, Muñoz J, Mullane KM, Marty FM, Tashima KT, Diaz G, Subramanian A; GS-US-540-5773.

101. Mohammed A, Paranji N, Chen PH, et al. COVID-19 in Chronic Liver Disease and Liver Transplantation: A Clinical Review. J Clin Gastroenterol 2021;55(3): 187–94.

102. de-Madaria E, Capurso G. COVID-19 and acute pancreatitis: examining the causality. Nat Rev Gastroenterol Hepatol 2021;18(1):3–4.

103. Jabłońska B, Olakowski M, Mrowiec S. Association between acute pancreatitis and COVID-19 infection: What do we know? World J Gastrointest Surg 2021; 13(6):548–62.

104. Samanta J, Gupta R, Singh MP, et al. Coronavirus disease 2019 and the pancreas. Pancreatology 2020;20(8):1567–75.

105. Patel R, Saif MW. Management of Pancreatic Cancer During COVID-19 Pandemic: To Treat or Not to Treat? JOP 2020;21(2):27–8.

106. Batlle D, Soler MJ, Sparks MA, et al. Acute kidney injury in COVID-19: emerging evidence of a distinct pathophysiology. J Am Soc Nephrol 2020;31(7): 1380-1383.

107. Ahmadian E, Hosseiniyan Khatibi SM, Razi Soofiyani S, et al. Covid-19 and kidney injury: Pathophysiology and molecular mechanisms. Rev Med Virol 2021; 31(3):e2176.

108. Lau WL, Zuckerman JE, Gupta A, et al. The COVID-Kidney Controversy: Can SARS-CoV-2 Cause Direct Renal Infection? Nephron 2021;145(3):275–9.

109. Titus T, Rahman A. SARS-CoV-2 and the kidney. Aust J Gen Pract 2021;50(7): 441–4.

110. Ronco C, Reis T, Husain-Syed F. Management of acute kidney injury in patients with COVID-19. Lancet Respir Med 2020;8(7):738–42.

111. Wichmann D, Sperhake JP, Lütgehetmann M, et al. Autopsy Findings and Venous Thromboembolism in Patients With COVID-19: A Prospective Cohort Study. Ann Intern Med 2020;173(4):268–77.

112. Oxley TJ, Mocco J, Majidi S, et al. Large-Vessel Stroke as a Presenting Feature of Covid-19 in the Young. N Engl J Med 2020;382(20):e60.

113. Juthani P, Bhojwani R, Gupta N. Coronavirus Disease 2019 (COVID-19) Manifestation as Acute Myocardial Infarction in a Young, Healthy Male. Case Rep Infect Dis 2020;2020:8864985.

114. Klok FA, Kruip MJHA, van der Meer NJM, et al. Confirmation of the high cumulative incidence of thrombotic complications in critically ill ICU patients with COVID-19: An updated analysis. Thromb Res 2020;191:148–50.

115. Gómez-Mesa JE, Galindo-Coral S, Montes MC, et al. Thrombosis and Coagulopathy in COVID-19. Curr Probl Cardiol 2021;46(3):100742.

116. Hanff TC, Mohareb AM, Giri J, et al. Thrombosis in COVID-19. Am J Hematol 2020;95(12):1578–89.

117. Letko M, Marzi A, Munster V. Functional assessment of cell entry and receptor usage for SARS-CoV-2 and other lineage B betacoronaviruses. Nat Microbiol 2020;5(4):562–9.

118. Wrapp D, Wang N, Corbett KS, et al. Cryo-EM structure of the 2019-nCoV spike in the prefusion conformation. Science 2020;367(6483):1260–3.

119. Siddiqi HK, Libby P, Ridker PM. COVID-19 - A vascular disease. Trends Cardiovasc Med 2021;31(1):1–5.

120. Han H, Yang L, Liu R, et al. Prominent changes in blood coagulation of patients with SARS-CoV-2 infection. Clin Chem Lab Med 2020;58(7):1116–20.

121. Goshua G, Pine AB, Meizlish ML, et al. Endotheliopathy in COVID-19-associated coagulopathy: evidence from a single-centre, cross-sectional study. Lancet Haematol 2020;7(8):e575–82.

122. Levi M, Thachil J, Iba T, et al. Coagulation abnormalities and thrombosis in patients with COVID-19. Lancet Haematol 2020;7(6):e438–40.

123. Helms J, Tacquard C, Severac F, et al. CRICS TRIGGERSEP Group (Clinical Research in Intensive Care and Sepsis Trial Group for Global Evaluation and Research in Sepsis). High risk of thrombosis in patients with severe SARS-CoV-2 infection: a multicenter prospective cohort study. Intensive Care Med 2020 Jun;46(6):1089–98.

124. Ackermann M, Verleden SE, Kuehnel M, et al. Pulmonary Vascular Endothelialitis, Thrombosis, and Angiogenesis in Covid-19. N Engl J Med 2020;383(2):120–8.

125. Varga Z, Flammer AJ, Steiger P, et al. Endothelial cell infection and endotheliitis in COVID-19. Lancet 2020;395(10234):1417–8.

126. Nadkarni GN, Lala A, Bagiella E, et al. Anticoagulation, Bleeding, Mortality, and Pathology in Hospitalized Patients With COVID-19. J Am Coll Cardiol 2020;76(16):1815–26.

127. Rosovsky RP, Sanfilippo KM, Wang TF, et al. Anticoagulation Practice Patterns in COVID-19: A Global Survey. Res Pract Thromb Haemost 2020;4(6):969–78.

128. Carpenter CR, Mudd PA, West CP, et al. Diagnosing COVID-19 in the Emergency Department: A Scoping Review of Clinical Examinations, Laboratory Tests, Imaging Accuracy, and Biases. Acad Emerg Med 2020;27(8):653–70.

129. Ray JG, Schull MJ, Vermeulen MJ, et al. Association Between ABO and Rh Blood Groups and SARS-CoV-2 Infection or Severe COVID-19 Illness : A Population-Based Cohort Study. Ann Intern Med 2021;174(3):308–15.

130. Osborne V, Davies M, Lane S, et al. Lopinavir-Ritonavir in the Treatment of COVID-19: A Dynamic Systematic Benefit-Risk Assessment. Drug Saf 2020; 43(8):809–21.
131. Meyerowitz EA, Vannier AGL, Friesen MGN, et al. Rethinking the role of hydroxychloroquine in the treatment of COVID-19. FASEB J 2020;34(5):6027–37.
132. Fteiha B, Karameh H, Kurd R, et al. QTc prolongation among hydroxychloroquine sulphate-treated COVID-19 patients: An observational study. Int J Clin Pract 2020;e13767.
133. Welker C, Huang J, Gil IJN, et al. 2021 Acute Respiratory Distress Syndrome Update, With Coronavirus Disease 2019 Focus. J Cardiothorac Vasc Anesth 2021;(21):00188. S1053-S0770.
134. Hosseinzadeh MH, Shamshirian A, Ebrahimzadeh MA. Dexamethasone vs COVID-19: An experimental study in line with the preliminary findings of a large trial. Int J Clin Pract 2020;e13943.
135. Tomazini BM, Maia IS, Cavalcanti AB, et al. COALITION COVID-19 Brazil III Investigators. Effect of Dexamethasone on Days Alive and Ventilator-Free in Patients With Moderate or Severe Acute Respiratory Distress Syndrome and COVID-19: The CoDEX Randomized Clinical Trial. JAMA 2020;324(13):1307–16.
136. Mattos-Silva P, Felix NS, Silva PL, et al. Pros and cons of corticosteroid therapy for COVID-19 patients. Respir Physiol Neurobiol 2020;280:103492.
137. Davies M, Osborne V, Lane S, et al. Remdesivir in Treatment of COVID-19: A Systematic Benefit-Risk Assessment. *Drug Saf* 2020;43(7):645–56.
138. Jiang Y, Chen D, Cai D, et al. Effectiveness of remdesivir for the treatment of hospitalized COVID-19 persons: A network meta-analysis. J Med Virol 2021; 93(2):1171–4.
139. Beigel JH, Tomashek KM, Dodd LE, et al. ACTT-1 Study Group Members. Remdesivir for the Treatment of Covid-19 - Final Report. N Engl J Med 2020; 383(19):1813–26.
140. Jorgensen SCJ, Kebriaei R, Dresser LD. Remdesivir: Review of Pharmacology, Pre-clinical Data, and Emerging Clinical Experience for COVID-19. Pharmacotherapy 2020;40(7):659–71.
141. Tiberghien P, de Lamballerie X, Morel P, et al. Collecting and evaluating convalescent plasma for COVID-19 treatment: why and how? Vox Sang 2020;115(6): 488–94.
142. Rajendran K, Krishnasamy N, Rangarajan J, et al. Convalescent plasma transfusion for the treatment of COVID-19: Systematic review. J Med Virol 2020;92(9): 1475–83.
143. Li L, Tong X, Chen H, et al. Characteristics and serological patterns of COVID-19 convalescent plasma donors: optimal donors and timing of donation. Transfusion 2020;60(8):1765–72.

Basics of Extracorporeal Membrane Oxygenation

William C. Wrisinger, MD, Shaun L. Thompson, MD*

KEYWORDS

- ECMO • Respiratory failure • Cardiac failure • ARDS • Cardiogenic shock
- Lung-protective ventilation

KEY POINTS

- Understand the use of extracorporeal membrane oxygenation (ECMO) and patients that may benefit from this treatment.
- Discuss the components of ECMO and how it provides respiratory and cardiac support.
- Review management strategies for patients requiring ECMO support.
- Discuss weaning and discontinuation from ECMO support.

 Video content accompanies this article at http://www.surgical.theclinics.com.

HISTORY OF EXTRACORPOREAL MEMBRANE OXYGENATION

Extracorporeal life support is the ability to supplement native pulmonary and/or cardiac function in the setting of native system failure. Development of modern extracorporeal life support devices began with the invention of the cardiopulmonary bypass (CPB) circuit by John Gibbon, successfully used in cardiac surgery for the first time in 1953 when extracorporeal support was used to repair an atrial septal defect in an 18-year-old patient.[1] Soon after, bubble oxygenators were invented by C. Walton Lillehei, MD and Richard DeWall. However, these early bubble oxygenators caused significant hemolysis thus limiting the use of a bubble oxygenator for prolonged gas exchange.[2] The development of silicone in 1957, a rubber material that allows for efficient gas exchange, led to the development of the "membrane oxygenator" and the coined phrase 'extracorporeal membrane oxygenation' (ECMO). This, along with the recognition that ECMO required continuous anticoagulation allowed for prolonged extracorporeal support to become a reality.[3]

The first successful use of ECMO in the ICU was reported in a 24-year-old trauma patient who was cannulated due to posttraumatic ARDS.[4] Modern ECMOs roots,

Department of Anesthesiology, Division of Critical Care Medicine, University of Nebraska Medical Center, 984455 Nebraska Medical Center, Omaha, NE 68198-4455, USA
* Corresponding author.
E-mail address: slthomps@unmc.edu

Surg Clin N Am 102 (2022) 23–35
https://doi.org/10.1016/j.suc.2021.09.001
0039-6109/22/© 2021 Elsevier Inc. All rights reserved.
surgical.theclinics.com

however, are in neonatal critical care whereby Dr Robert Bartlett pioneered its use in pediatric cardiopulmonary failure and published the first randomized controlled trial comparing ECMO to standard care in 1985.[5] ECMO became more ubiquitous in the late 2000s during the H1NI influenza epidemic as ECMO was used successfully in many patients for treatment of ARDS. Since that time, ECMO utilization has expanded globally and thus clinicians in the critical care realm must possess a basic understanding of indications, contraindications, and complications of ECMO support.

COMPONENTS OF THE EXTRACORPOREAL MEMBRANE OXYGENATION CIRCUIT

Veno-venous (VV) or veno-arterial (VA) ECMO requires the drainage of deoxygenated blood from the venous system, moving it across a membrane oxygenator that removes carbon dioxide (CO_2), replenishes oxygen, and returns oxygenated blood back to the patient's venous or arterial system depending on the use of VV or VA, respectively. This process is facilitated by a simple system of cannulas, a blood pump, a nonmicroporous polymethylpentene oxygenator, and a heat exchanger.[6]

Multiple brands of pumps are commercially available. All are centrifugal pumps and provide an efficient flow for ECMO support. To provide oxygenation and ventilation for the patient, all ECMO circuits have an oxygen supply (Fio_2) and "sweep gas" flowmeters in line with the circuit. (**Fig. 1**) This oxygen flow will be the source of oxygen used for gas exchange in the membrane lung. The sweep gas allows for the removal of CO_2 in an efficient manner and allows low tidal volume ventilation and lung rest to allow for patient recovery. Lung-protective ventilation strategies are paramount to lung recovery and full utilization of ECMO can help facilitate recovery. (**Fig. 2**)

VENO-VENOUS EXTRACORPOREAL MEMBRANE OXYGENATION
Indications and Overview

Veno-venous extracorporeal membrane oxygenation (VV-ECMO) is indicated in primary respiratory failure that is refractory to conventional medical therapy and mechanical ventilation.[7](**Box 1**) Many candidates will have failed use of deep sedation, paralytics, prone position, inhaled pulmonary vasodilators, and diuretics.[7]

The primary goal of supporting a patient with VV-ECMO is to promote lung rest via lung-protective ventilation.[8,9] Lung-protective ventilation aims to decrease the incidence and severity of ventilator-induced lung injury (VILI) associated triggers such as volutrauma, barotrauma, atelectrauma, and biotrauma.[8] The advent of currently accepted lung-protective ventilation strategies arose from the recognition in animal

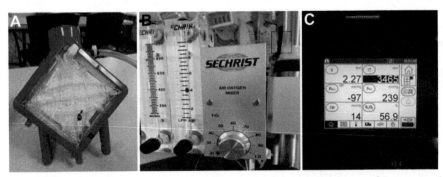

Fig. 1. Examples of (A) membrane lung, (B) flowmeters for oxygen deliver and "sweep gas" regulation, and (C) ECMO pump device.

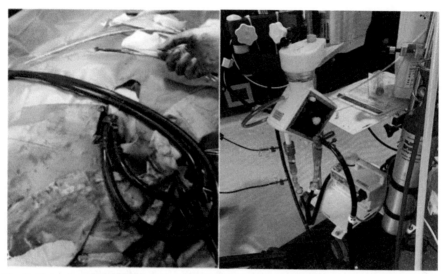

Fig. 2. Picture on the left showing completed dual lumen cannula in the RIJ with deoxygenated and oxygenated blood shown. Picture on the right showing a complete ECMO circuit with oxygen and medical-grade air connected to the flowmeters to control Fio_2 and sweep gas flows. Tubing can be seen connected to the membrane oxygenator.

models of acute lung injury, large tidal volumes (V_t) lead to lung endothelial, and epithelial disruption resulting in inflammation, atelectasis, hypoxemia, and inflammatory mediator release.[10] Brower and colleagues[10] first recommended the use of lower V_t in patients with acute lung injury/ARDS after finding significantly reduced mortality and increased ventilator-free days in patients treated with lower V_t than traditionally accepted volumes of 10 to 15 mL/kg. The decrease in stretch-induced lung injury thought to be occurring with lower V_t was supported by finding significantly decreased levels of the inflammatory mediatory interleukin-6 (IL-6) in these patients, suggesting that lower V_t led to decreased lung inflammation, contributing to their improved clinical outcomes. Later meta-analysis and Cochrane Reviews have provided further support using lung-protective ventilation with lower V_t ($\sim$7 mL/kg ideal body weight) and plateau pressures less than 30 cm H_2O, resulting in lower 28-day mortality and morbidity by avoiding VILI.[11,12]

Box 1
Indications for VV ECMO[8,9]
Acute respiratory distress syndrome (ARDS)
Bronchopleural fistula
Status asthmaticus
Bridge to lung transplant
Refractory viral/bacterial pneumonia
Acute lung injury
Refractory hypoxia/hypercarbia

Lung-protective ventilation strategies have been shown to improve outcomes and perhaps prevent progression to ARDS in patients without preexisting ARDS.[12] By using lung-protective ventilation strategies during VV-ECMO runs, VILI can be minimized, facilitating earlier ventilator weaning, liberation, and mobilization of patients with VV-ECMO, decreasing the likelihood of multiorgan dysfunction and decreasing mortality.[8,13]

Patient Selection

Patients being considered for cannulation onto VV-ECMO, or any form of ECLS, should be thoroughly investigated to rule out irreversible disease processes that would contraindicate the use of ECMO(**Box 2**). Echocardiography should be obtained before cannulation to rule-out cardiac etiologies of respiratory failure and to ensure near-normal cardiac function as VV-ECMO is dependent on the patient's cardiovascular system to maintain pulmonary and systemic perfusion.[7,8] If evidence of severe cardiac dysfunction is present, veno-arterial extracorporeal oxygenation (VA-ECMO) should be considered. Approximately 10% of patients with primary respiratory failure will develop right ventricular (RV) dysfunction secondary to hypoxemia, hypercarbia, and acidosis in ARDS.[14] Patients with RV dysfunction can oftentimes be managed with inotropes, pulmonary vasodilators, diuretics, and optimization of their acid/base status to reduce RV afterload and promote gas exchange without the need for VA-ECMO. In some patients requiring multiple inotropic/vasoactive medications before cannulation, VV-ECMO may not lead to worse outcomes or increased complication rates with some authors suggesting that VA-ECMO being reserved for patients with refractory hypotension after VV-ECMO cannulation.[15]

Clinicians evaluating a patient for possible VV-ECMO cannulation, or treating an already cannulated patient, can use the respiratory ECMO survival prediction (RESP) score to assist with predicting survival (respscore.com) Given that VV-ECMO is a scarce medical resource, labor-intensive, and expensive tool for health care systems, the use of a validated predictive mortality model may assist clinicians better allocate these resources and create risk/benefit benchmarks.[16] (**Table 1**) Although the RESP score can aid in predicting survival in patients with adult respiratory failure requiring ECMO, it should not replace bedside clinical decision making or be the sole determinant of whether or not to use ECMO.[1]

Cannulation and Cannula Selection

Two cannulas are required to perform ECMO: an inflow and outflow cannula. The cannulae are named based on relation to the blood pump. That is, blood flowing from the patient to the blood pump is via the inflow cannula and blood returning

---

Box 2
Contraindications to VV ECMO

Overwhelming sepsis/septic shock

Multi-system organ failure

End-stage chronic disease (ie, end-stage COPD)

Nonsurvivable neurologic injury

Advanced malignancy diagnosis

Eldery over the age of 70

Family refusal

Table 1
RESP score criteria and their associated points

RESP Score Criteria[a]			
Age	18–49 (0)	50–59 (−2)	>60 (−3)
Immunocompromised status	No (0)	Yes (−2)	
Mechanically ventilated before ECMO initiated	>7 d (0)	48 h - 7 d (+1)	<48 h (+3)
Diagnosis	Viral pneumonia (+3)		
	Bacterial pneumonia (+3)		
	Asthma (+11)		
	Trauma or burn (+3)		
	Aspiration pneumonitis (+5)		
	Other acute respiratory diagnoses (+1)		
	Nonrespiratory or chronic respiratory diagnosis (0)		
History of CNS dysfunction	No (0)	Yes (−7)	
Acute associated nonpulmonary infection	No (0)	Yes (−3)	
Neuromuscular blockade before ECMO	No (0)	Yes (+1)	
Nitric oxide before ECMO	No (0)	Yes (−1)	
Bicarbonate infusion before ECMO	No (0)	Yes (−2)	
Cardiac arrest before ECMO	No (0)	Yes (−2)	
$Paco_2$ >75 mm Hg	No (0)	Yes (−1)	
Peak inspiratory pressure >42 cm H2O	No (0)	Yes (−1)	

[a] Adopted from www.respscore.com.

from the blood pump to the patient is via the outflow cannula. It should be noted that cannula nomenclature can be institutionally dependent.

VV-ECMO cannulation can be performed in multiple settings including emergency rooms, ICUs, ORs, and cardiac cath laboratories. Most VV-ECMO cannulations are performed percutaneously via Seldinger or modified Seldinger techniques.[8] Before cannulation, the patient's airway should be secured, arterial access should be obtained for hemodynamic management, and central venous access should be obtained, preferentially sparing the right internal jugular vein (RIJ) as this may be used for outflow cannula placement.[7] Cannula placement is typically confirmed under echocardiographic or radiographic image guidance. (**Fig. 3**)

Anatomic site of cannulation for VV-ECMO is primarily dictated by the patient's clinical stability, mode of ECMO to be used, and the experience of the treating team. A common cannulation strategy for VV-ECMO is a femoral-RIJ approach whereby the inflow cannula is placed in the femoral vein with its tip inferior to the RA-IVC junction and the outflow cannula is placed in the RIJ with its tip at the SVC-RA junction.[17] Another cannulation configuration is femoral-femoral whereby an inflow cannula is placed distal to the RA-IVC junction and the outflow cannula is placed in the opposite femoral vein with the cannula positioned at the SVC-RA junction. A femoral-femoral strategy can be more prone to recirculation whereby oxygenated blood being returned to the patient does not enter the pulmonary circulation but is immediately drained back into the ECMO circuit through the inflow cannula.[17,18] If this configuration is selected,

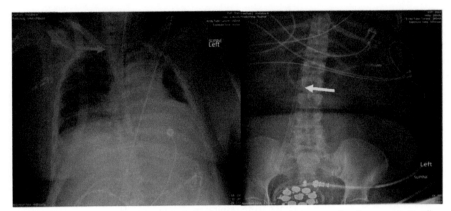

Fig. 3. Chest and abdominal radiographs showing appropriate cannula placement. Outflow cannula in the image on left noted by blue arrow and inflow cannula in image on right noted by yellow arrow.

the inflow cannula should be secured at approximately the level of the diaphragm or lower to prevent recirculation.

Alternatively, a single dual-lumen cannula approach with cannulation of the right IJ vein may accommodate faster ventilator weaning, liberation, decreased risk of groin site infections, and ultimately mobilization of a patient requiring VV-ECMO. A commonly used dual lumen device is the Avalon Elite (Maquet, Germany), sized 16 to 31 Fr. Additionally, this approach reduces the likelihood of recirculation, particularly at higher ECMO flow rates.[19]

Selecting appropriately sized cannulas for both inflow and outflow is vital to maintain adequate flows and provide sufficient support to the patient. To facilitate adequate oxygen saturation on VV-ECMO, flow rates of approximately 60 to 80 mL/kg should be targeted.[17] Determinants of achieving blood flow targets include cannula size, hemoglobin level, Fio_2 of the circuit, ECMO flow (L/min) relative to native cardiac output, metabolic demands, and the degree of recirculation occurring.[20] CO_2 removal alone requires approximately 20% of the flow required for oxygenation.

Maintenance and Complications

Caring for a patient on VV-ECMO requires a team composed of physicians, surgeons, respiratory therapists, nurses, perfusionists, pharmacists, nutritionists, and other personnel. All play a key role in maintaining safety and optimal function of the ECMO circuit.[20] Patients with VV-ECMO support should be monitored by many variables including ventilatory settings and pressures, arterial blood pressure monitoring, central venous pressures, and frequent laboratories including arterial blood gases to make adjustments to sweep gas flows and/or ECMO flows. Based on arterial blood gas findings, changes can be made to correct issues with oxygenation and ventilation and not require changes to the ventilator that may result in further mechanical damage to the lungs from mechanical ventilation. If hypercarbia and resultant respiratory acidosis are encountered, the sweep gas flow can be increased to eliminate more CO_2 through the membrane oxygenator. If hypoxemia is the issue, then increasing the flow on ECMO, administration of blood, or increasing Fio_2 on the ventilator can be tried to correct the hypoxemia. Issues resulting in refractory hypoxemia on VV ECMO such as recirculation will be discussed later in this article.

Complications during treatment with mechanical support are often either medical or mechanical in nature. In a systematic review of studies examining VV-ECMO used in ARDS by Vaquer and colleagues[21] (2017), medical complications were found to occur in 40.2% of patients with bleeding being the most common (29.3%). Complications involving mechanical support circuits including inflow/outflow cannula and the oxygenator occurred in 10.9% of patients with 12.8% of them requiring oxygenator replacement during their treatment period.

Recognizing evolving complications through constant communication with clinical staff and physical examination of the patient and ECMO circuit is essential. As mentioned, recirculation is a common problem encountered during VV-ECMO. Its classic presentation includes refractory hypoxemia and high pre-oxygenator oxygen saturation (SpreO2). Although multiple factors can affect recirculation percentage, greater separation of inflow, and outflow cannulae tips should be performed if a two-site cannulation strategy is used to reduce recirculation. If the cannula's tips cannot be further separated, either switching to a single dual lumen catheter or addition of an additional venous drainage catheter can be performed.[20,22]

When native cardiac output exceeds the flow rate of the ECMO circuit, mixing of deoxygenated blood with oxygenated blood returning from the ECMO circuit occurs, potentially leading to poor systemic oxygenation and low SaO2. To maintain SpO2 greater than 88%, it is recommended for ECMO flows to be at least 60% of total systemic flow.[23] The most common etiology of increased cardiac output during treatment with ECMO is sepsis, with approximately 13.5% of patients with adult VV-ECMO developing antimicrobial-resistant bloodstream infections.[24] In addition to organic pathologies, iatrogenic supra-normal cardiac output due to inadequate sedation or analgesia should be avoided.

ECMO circuit components are prone to failure including the cannulas, blood pump, membrane oxygenator, and other tubing. They must be continually assessed by both clinicians and other ancillary bedside providers.

The inflow cannula can commonly vibrate or "chatter". This is due to high negative pressures in the inflow cannula due to collapse of the vein around the cannula and vibrations within the tubing to occur. (Video 1) A common etiology of this is hypovolemia that can be corrected with the administration of either colloid or crystalloid solution.

Membrane oxygenator failure is due to either oxygen supply failure or thrombus formation.[20] After ensuring that oxygen supply is intact, findings suggestive of thrombus formation include direct visualization of thrombus, particularly on the preoxygenator side of the membrane along with a large pressure gradient across the membrane (normal gradient is < 50 mm Hg).[25]

Complications from bleeding account for a large majority of morbidity and mortality during ECMO. Maintaining circuit patency while preventing thromboembolic complications with systemic anticoagulation can be challenging. Absolute anticoagulation strategies for VV-ECMO do not yet exist.[26] Anticoagulation with systemic heparin is typically initiated at the time of cannulation and monitored with serial activated clotting time (ACT), activated partial thromboplastin time (aPTT), anti-factor Xa (aXa) assays, and thromboelastography (TEG). Monitoring approaches are oftentimes institutionally dependent, with aPTT being the predominately monitored laboratory value. However, concordance between monitoring techniques should be seen regardless. If contraindication to anticoagulation develops or is present from the time of cannulation, VV-ECMO may be performed without anticoagulation, though flows should be at least 3.5 L/min[20,27,28]

Weaning Veno-Venous-Extracorporeal Membrane Oxygenation

ECMO support should be discontinued as soon as safe to do so. Determining the optimal time to decannulate is not well described or protocolized and is oftentimes institutional and provider dependent. In general, once native lung function has improved to the point that ECMO sweep gas flow can be reduced to minimal allowed settings and the patient's V_t, respiratory rate, peak pressures, and plateau pressures are acceptable, the patient can be decannulated and supported with mechanical ventilation until extubation is deemed appropriate.

VENO-ARTERIAL EXTRACORPOREAL MEMBRANE OXYGENATION
Indications and Overview

VA-ECMO provides not only the gas exchange capabilities of VV-ECMO but also provides mechanical circulatory support, in parallel to native cardiac function, in the setting of either isolated cardiac failure or combined cardiopulmonary failure.[29] The components of the VA-ECMO circuit are similar to VV-ECMO. The difference is that the outflow cannula is placed into an artery to provide circulatory support to the patient. Cannulation for VA-ECMO can either be central or peripheral. Central cannulation, whereby a venous inflow cannula is placed in the right atrium and the outflow cannula is placed in the ascending aorta, primarily occurs postcardiotomy in patients who are failing to wean from CPB despite high dose inotropic and vasopressor support.[17] These patients often have preexisting heart failure, incomplete revascularization, poor intraoperative myocardial protection, or underwent a technically difficult surgery.[30] Peripheral cannulation for cardiogenic shock and cardiac arrest is commonly accomplished by placing a venous inflow cannula in either a femoral vein or the right IJ vein and placing an arterial outflow cannula in either the femoral artery or grafting it onto the right subclavian or axillary artery.[7]

Patient Selection

Rao and colleagues outline 5 considerations that should be made before offering VA-ECMO to a patient: (I) the indication, (II) the cannulation strategy, (III) LV distension/venting strategy, (IV) distal limb ischemia/perfusion strategy, and (V) exit strategy.[29] Indications for initiation of VA-ECMO are listed in **Box 3**. However, there are currently no society-endorsed evidence-based guidelines for which patients are most likely to benefit from VA-ECMO.[29,31]

Mortality among patients with VA-ECMO is 50% to 60% and 6-month survivorship as low as 30%.[32] Vetting candidates for VA-ECMO cannulation is thus of the utmost importance. Similar to VV-ECMO, irreversible disease processes should be ruled out before cannulation and echocardiography should be obtained to characterize the cardiac pathology. Echocardiographic studies should ensure that no greater than mild aortic insufficiency is present due to increased risk of severe left ventricular (LV) distension. Large bore central venous access along with an arterial line should be placed before cannulation for hemodynamic monitoring and fluid or blood product administration. Similar to the RESP score, the survival after veno-arterial ECMO (SAVE) score may be used before cannulation in attempting to predict survival in refractory cardiogenic shock requiring VA-ECMO therapy.[33]

Cannulation

Central cannulation is primarily performed when a patient fails to wean from CPB. The preexisting venous and arterial cannulas placed for CPB are often used for VA-ECMO initiation, eliminating the need for additional cannula placement. Disadvantages of

Box 3
Indications for VA ECMO
Acute chronic heart failure
Acute heart failure secondary to myocarditis
Massive pulmonary embolism
Mediastinal mass
Refractory cardiogenic shock
Refractory ventricular tachycardia
Postcardiotomy shock
Hypothermia
Cardiac arrest with ongoing CPR (ECPR)

central cannulation include the need to reenter the chest for decannulation, increasing patients' risk of bleeding and infection, and inability to extubate while cannulated, limiting the potential for early mobilization.[2,34] Upper-body peripheral cannulation via arterial cannulation of the subclavian, innominate, or axillary arteries with an end-to-side Dacron graft, may offer the physiologic advantages of central cannulation including decreased potential for LV distension and decreased risk of cerebral hypoxemia but still allow for early extubation and mobilization.[17,35] Although peripheral cannulation via a femoral artery and vein is the most common cannulation strategy, it is not without significant risk including femoral artery occlusion, distal limb ischemia, compartment syndrome, and upper body hypoperfusion.[36]

Appropriate cannula sizing should accommodate the equivalent cardiac index of 2.2 to 2.5 L/m^2/min, considered full flow VA-ECMO.[17] Venous cannulas are typically 19 to 25 Fr although arterial cannulas are 15 to 24 Fr.

Maintenance and Complications

Special considerations for VA-ECMO include the risk of LV distension and pulmonary edema, ensuring adequate distal perfusion of the arterial cannulated leg, Harlequin syndrome, and anticoagulation requirements. Identification of LV distension is essential to promoting myocardial recovery, preventing blood stasis within the LV, and optimizing the patient for weaning.[29,31] Bedside recognition of LV distension may be accomplished in several ways. First, ensuring that the aortic valve is opening can be accomplished with an arterial line tracing, bearing in mind that as ECMO flows increase, the MAP will also increase and lead to lower pulse pressure and stroke volume.[29] Ideally, a right radial arterial line will have been placed to allow for both hemodynamic monitoring and to ensure adequate oxygenation of the right cerebral hemisphere and right arm; however, pulmonary edema due to new or worsening LV distention may be detected by progressively lower Po$_2$ values on the right radial arterial line.[29,37] Third, the presence of spontaneous echo contrast within the LV cavity likely suggests an increased risk of thrombus formation.[38] Lastly, serial chest x-rays may reveal pulmonary edema suggestive of LV distension; however, if chest radiographs alone are used for detection, one must rule out other etiologies of opacities and edema such as ARDS or infection. LV venting strategies include intra-aortic balloon pump (IABP), atrial septostomy, left atria to aortic cannula, and surgical or percutaneous venting with an Impella. Although the advantages and disadvantages of each venting method are beyond the scope of this review, it should be acknowledged that there is not currently a standard-of-care LV venting practice.

Ensuring adequate perfusion to the arterial cannulated leg is paramount as lower extremity ischemia occurs in 12% to 22% of peripherally cannulated patients, potentially resulting in compartment syndrome requiring fasciotomy or amputation.[29,39] At the time of peripheral VA-ECMO cannulation, many centers place a 6 to 8 Fr distal perfusion cannula in either the common femoral or superficial femoral artery to provide antegrade flow distal to the arterial cannulation site. Limb ischemia may not only lead to patients needing additional surgery, it may also contribute to unsuccessful weaning of VA-ECMO and is an independent risk factor for in-hospital death.[40,41]

Given that peripherally cannulated VA-ECMO flow is retrograde, a watershed region, sometimes referred to as a "mixing cloud", of blood may form between the aortic root and the level of the diaphragm depending on the cardiac output relative to VA-ECMO flow.[42] The watershed region is the direct result of impaired pulmonary gas exchange leading to hypoxic blood being ejected by the LV mixing with the well-oxygenated ECMO blood flowing retrograde in the aorta. Higher LV output will push the watershed region more distal, closer to the diaphragm, whereas lower LV output will cause the watershed region to remain closer to the aortic root.[43] The threat posed by the watershed region is that of differential hypoxemia, otherwise known as Harlequin syndrome or North-South syndrome, whereby the upper body is at risk for hypoxic blood flow to the brain, heart, and upper extremities whereas the lower body will be well perfused from the ECMO circuit. Recognition of the phenomenon depends on serial right upper extremity arterial blood gas measurements and continuous cerebral oximetry trends. Treating underlying lung pathology, maximizing ventilator oxygenation support, venting the LV if indicated, and placing a Y-connector onto the arterial outflow cannula to deliver well-oxygenated blood to the venous system through an additional vein cannula (venous-arterial-venous ECMO) should all be considered in treating Harlequin syndrome.[29,44]

VA-ECMO is inherently proinflammatory leading to increased risk of pump thrombosis, oxygenator failure, or thromboembolic events.[45] The risk of thrombosis must be weighed against the risk of major bleeding as up to 27% of patients with VA-ECMO will suffer a major bleeding event, with or without systemic anticoagulation present.[45] Most institutions align with current ELSO recommendations to use unfractionated heparin with a targeted ACT goal of 180 to 220; however, anti-Xa assays are becoming standard of care and a mixed approach to evaluating anticoagulation goals may be best.[1]

Weaning Veno-Arterial-Extracorporeal Membrane Oxygenation

Attempts to wean VA-ECMO should occur as soon as signs of myocardial recovery are noted. However, all organ systems should be optimized, particularly the pulmonary system which will become responsible for gas exchange once ECMO support is discontinued.[31] Inotropic and vasopressor medications should be titrated to low doses, with room to increase, before weaning attempts. Hemodynamic monitors including right upper extremity arterial line and PA catheter should remain in place for perfusion indices to be trended, ensuring that adequate myocardial recovery has occurred to support the end-organs.[31,46] Though there is not a standard-of-care approach to weaning, an algorithmic, step-wise approach is advocated.[31,47] Many centers adopt a 3 step approach consisting of daily weaning studies followed by bedside assessment for decannulation and ultimately a formal turn-down study under TEE guidance for decannulation in the operating room. Fried and colleagues detail daily weaning attempts as incremental decreases in flow by 0.5 LPM to a minimum of 2 LPM. If the patient's MAP does not fall more than 10 to 15 mm Hg and filling pressures do not significantly increase, the patient is allowed to flow at the lowest tolerated rate and hemodynamics are trended for 8 hours.[46] Daily weaning trials are often performed sequentially with serial TTE examinations as successful weaning is associated with an aortic VTI greater than 10 cm, LVEF greater than 20 to 25%, and lateral mitral annulus peak systolic velocity greater than 6 cm/s[48] Once a daily weaning trial is tolerated, a bedside assessment for decannulation is often performed by decreasing ECMO flow to 1 LPM and hemodynamics are assessed. If well tolerated, the patient may be scheduled for a formal ECMO turn down the study in the operating room whereby ECMO flows will be decreased and the cannulae clamped for 30 minutes, up to 4 hours.[1] If this is successful, the patient can be decannulated and this typically involves surgical repair of the arteriotomy site.

SUMMARY

The use of ECMO continues to increase in ICUs across the world and the indications for its use continue to expand. Further investigation into its use in otherwise contraindicated states such as sepsis is ongoing and may lead to improved outcomes in this high-risk category of patients. Other areas whereby ECMO is beginning to show potential for the treatment of patients is in the realm of traumatic injury and burn patients. With this ever-evolving and increasing footprint, knowledge of ECMO and its day-to-day maintenance is going to be important for any clinician who works in the field of critical care medicine.

SUPPLEMENTARY DATA

Supplementary data related to this article can be found online at https://doi.org/10.1016/j.suc.2021.09.001.

REFERENCES

1. Brogan TV, Roberto L, MacLaren G, et al. Extracorporeal life support: the ELSO red Book. In: T.V.B., editor. Extracorporeal life support: the ELSO red book. 5th edition. Ann Arbor (MI): Extracorporeal Life Support Organization; 2017. p. 868.
2. Sangalli F, P.N, Pesenti A. In: S. F., editor. ECMO-extracorporeal life support in adults. Milan (MI): Springer-Verlag Mailand; 2014.
3. Custer JR. The evolution of patient selection criteria and indicatiSons for extracorporeal life support in pediatric cardiopulmonary failure: next time, let's not eat the bones. Organogenesis 2011;7(1):13–22.
4. Hill JD, et al. Prolonged Extracorporeal Oxygenation for Acute Post-Traumatic Respiratory Failure (Shock-Lung Syndrome). New Engl J Med 1972;286(12):629–34.
5. Bartlett RH, et al. Extracorporeal circulation in neonatal respiratory failure: a prospective randomized study. Pediatrics 1985;76(4):479–87.
6. Squiers JJ, Lima B, DiMaio JM. Contemporary extracorporeal membrane oxygenation therapy in adults: Fundamental principles and systematic review of the evidence. J Thorac Cardiovasc Surg 2016;152(1):20–32.
7. Shaheen A, et al. Veno-Venous Extracorporeal Membr Oxygenation (VVECMO):Indications ,Preprocedural Considerations ,and Tech. J Card Surg 2016;31(4):248–52.
8. Brodie D, Slutsky AS, Combes A. Extracorporeal Life Support for Adults With Respiratory Failure and Related Indications: A Review. JAMA 2019;322(6):557–68.

9. Ramanathan K, et al. Extracorporeal Membrane Oxygenation for Adult Community-Acquired Pneumonia: Outcomes and Predictors of Mortality*. Crit Care Med 2017;45(5):814–21.
10. Brower RG, et al. Ventilation with lower tidal volumes as compared with traditional tidal volumes for acute lung injury and the acute respiratory distress syndrome. N Engl J Med 2000;342(18):1301–8.
11. Petrucci N, De Feo C. Lung protective ventilation strategy for the acute respiratory distress syndrome. Cochrane Database Syst Rev 2013;2013(2):Cd003844.
12. Serpa Neto A, et al. Association between use of lung-protective ventilation with lower tidal volumes and clinical outcomes among patients without acute respiratory distress syndrome: a meta-analysis. Jama 2012;308(16):1651–9.
13. Lehr CJ, et al. Ambulatory extracorporeal membrane oxygenation as a bridge to lung transplantation: walking while waiting. Chest 2015;147(5):1213–8.
14. Osman D, et al. Incidence and prognostic value of right ventricular failure in acute respiratory distress syndrome. Intensive Care Med 2009;35(1):69–76.
15. Kon ZN, et al. Venovenous versus venoarterial extracorporeal membrane oxygenation for adult patients with acute respiratory distress syndrome requiring precannulation hemodynamic support: a review of the ELSO registry. Ann Thorac Surg 2017;104(2):645–9.
16. Schmidt M, et al. Predicting survival after extracorporeal membrane oxygenation for severe acute respiratory failure. The respiratory extracorporeal membrane oxygenation survival prediction (RESP) score. Am J Respir Crit Care Med 2014;189(11):1374–82.
17. Jayaraman AL, Shah Pranav, Ramakrishna Harish. Cannulation strategies in adult veno-arterial and veno-venous extracorporeal membrane oxygenation: techniques, limitations, and special considerations. Ann Card Anesth 2017;20(1):S11–8.
18. Lindholm JA. Cannulation for veno-venous extracorporeal membrane oxygenation. J Thorac Dis 2018;10(Suppl 5):S606–12.
19. Ngai C-W, Ng PY, Sin W-C. Bicaval dual lumen cannula in adult veno-venous extracorporeal membrane oxygenation-clinical pearls for safe cannulation. J Thorac Dis 2018;10(Suppl 5):S624–8.
20. Patel B, Arcaro M, Chatterjee S. Bedside troubleshooting during venovenous extracorporeal membrane oxygenation (ECMO). J Thorac Dis 2019;11(Suppl 14):S1698–707.
21. Vaquer S, et al. Systematic review and meta-analysis of complications and mortality of veno-venous extracorporeal membrane oxygenation for refractory acute respiratory distress syndrome. Ann Intensive Care 2017;7(1):51.
22. Allen S, et al. A review of the fundamental principles and evidence base in the use of extracorporeal membrane oxygenation (ECMO) in critically ill adult patients. J Intensive Care Med 2011;26(1):13–26.
23. Schmidt M, et al. Blood oxygenation and decarboxylation determinants during venovenous ECMO for respiratory failure in adults. Intensive Care Med 2013;39(5):838–46.
24. Sun H-Y, et al. Infections occurring during extracorporeal membrane oxygenation use in adult patients. J Thorac Cardiovasc Surg 2010;140(5):1125–32.e2.
25. Sidebotham D. Troubleshooting adult ECMO. J Extra Corpor Technol 2011;43(1):P27–32.
26. Sklar MC, et al. Anticoagulation Practices during Venovenous Extracorporeal Membrane Oxygenation for Respiratory Failure. A Systematic Review. Ann Am Thorac Soc 2016;13(12):2242–50.

27. Fina D, et al. Extracorporeal membrane oxygenation without systemic anticoagulation: a case-series in challenging conditions. J Thorac Dis 2020;12(5):2113–9.
28. Lee YY, et al. Heparin-free veno-venous extracorporeal membrane oxygenation in a multiple trauma patient: A case report. Medicine (Baltimore) 2020;99(5):e19070.
29. Rao P, et al. Venoarterial extracorporeal membrane oxygenation for cardiogenic shock and cardiac arrest. Circ Heart Fail 2018;11(9):e004905.
30. Biancari F, et al. Meta-Analysis of the Outcome After Postcardiotomy Venoarterial Extracorporeal Membrane Oxygenation in Adult Patients. J Cardiothorac Vasc Anesth 2018;32(3):1175–82.
31. Keebler ME, et al. Venoarterial Extracorporeal Membrane Oxygenation in Cardiogenic Shock. JACC Heart Fail 2018;6(6):503–16.
32. Takayama H, et al. Clinical outcome of mechanical circulatory support for refractory cardiogenic shock in the current era. J Heart Lung Transpl 2013;32(1):106–11.
33. Schmidt M, et al. Predicting survival after ECMO for refractory cardiogenic shock: the survival after veno-arterial-ECMO (SAVE)-score. Eur Heart J 2015;36(33):2246–56.
34. Abrams D, et al. Early mobilization of patients receiving extracorporeal membrane oxygenation: a retrospective cohort study. Crit Care 2014;18(1):R38.
35. Javidfar J, et al. Subclavian artery cannulation for venoarterial extracorporeal membrane oxygenation. Asaio j 2012;58(5):494–8.
36. Stulak JM, et al. ECMO cannulation controversies and complications. Semin Cardiothorac Vasc Anesth 2009;13(3):176–82.
37. Su Y, et al. Hemodynamic monitoring in patients with venoarterial extracorporeal membrane oxygenation. Ann Transl Med 2020;8(12):792.
38. Douflé G, et al. Echocardiography for adult patients supported with extracorporeal membrane oxygenation. Crit Care 2015;19:326.
39. Cheng R, et al. Complications of extracorporeal membrane oxygenation for treatment of cardiogenic shock and cardiac arrest: a meta-analysis of 1,866 adult patients. Ann Thorac Surg 2014;97(2):610–6.
40. Aubron C, et al. Factors associated with outcomes of patients on extracorporeal membrane oxygenation support: a 5-year cohort study. Crit Care 2013;17(2):R73.
41. Hei F, et al. Five-year results of 121 consecutive patients treated with extracorporeal membrane oxygenation at Fu Wai Hospital. Artif Organs 2011;35(6):572–8.
42. Hoeper Marius M, et al. Extracorporeal Membrane Oxygenation Watershed. Circulation 2014;130(10):864–5.
43. Napp LC, et al. Heart against veno-arterial ECMO: Competition visualized. Int J Cardiol 2015;187:164–5.
44. Cakici M, et al. Controlled flow diversion in hybrid venoarterial-venous extracorporeal membrane oxygenation. Interact Cardiovasc Thorac Surg 2018;26(1):112–8.
45. Sy E, et al. Anticoagulation practices and the prevalence of major bleeding, thromboembolic events, and mortality in venoarterial extracorporeal membrane oxygenation: A systematic review and meta-analysis. J Crit Care 2017;39:87–96.
46. Fried JA, et al. How I approach weaning from venoarterial ECMO. Crit Care 2020;24(1):307.
47. Cavarocchi NC, et al. Weaning of extracorporeal membrane oxygenation using continuous hemodynamic transesophageal echocardiography. J Thorac Cardiovasc Surg 2013;146(6):1474–9.
48. Aissaoui N, et al. Predictors of successful extracorporeal membrane oxygenation (ECMO) weaning after assistance for refractory cardiogenic shock. Intensive Care Med 2011;37(11):1738–45.

Ultrasound and Other Advanced Hemodynamic Monitoring Techniques in the Intensive Care Unit

Samuel Cemaj, MD, FCCM*, Michael R. Visenio, MD, MPH,
Olabisi Ololade Sheppard, MD, Daniel W. Johnson, MD, FCCS,
Zachary M. Bauman, DO, MHA

KEYWORDS

- Intensive care unit • Echocardiography • Hemodynamic

KEY POINTS

- Physical examination continues to be the primary strategy for the hemodynamic assessment of critically ill patients.
- When hemodynamic monitoring for shock is needed, echocardiography is an important skill set with a steep learning curve. It is a critical skill that any intensive care unit (ICU) care provider should familiarize themselves with.3.- In complex patients, other advanced modalities of hemodynamic monitoring should be chosen.
- These techniques are not exclusive, but rather inclusive and should be used concurrently as we do not yet have the holy grail of hemodynamic monitoring.

INTRODUCTION

The ideal device for hemodynamic monitoring of critically ill patients in the intensive care unit (ICU) or the operating room has not yet been developed.

This would need to be affordable, consistent, have a very low margin of error (<30%), be minimally or noninvasive, and allow the clinician to make a reasonable therapeutic decision that consistently led to better outcomes. Such a device does not yet exist. This article will describe the distinct options we, as critical care physicians, currently possess for this Herculean endeavor.

This article is divided into 2 sections. The first section will address different tools, whether invasive or noninvasive, to assess the hemodynamic status of the patient. The second section will consist of an overview of point of care ultrasonography (POCUS) in the ICU.

Surgery, University of Nebraska Medical Center, Omaha, NE 68198, USA
* Corresponding author.
E-mail address: Samuel.cemaj@unmc.edu

Surg Clin N Am 102 (2022) 37–52
https://doi.org/10.1016/j.suc.2021.09.010
0039-6109/22/© 2021 Elsevier Inc. All rights reserved.

ADVANCED HEMODYNAMIC MONITORING TECHNIQUES

Shock is an entity known throughout history, in particular, hypovolemic shock during multiple wars. Shock causes symptoms like clammy and mottled skin, hypothermia, weak pulse, decreased capillary filling, skin changes, mental status changes, and oliguria. These are often considered the hallmark signs of shock and remain valid despite significant advances in technology.

Over the last 2 decades, hemodynamic monitoring has moved from pressure-focused and noninvasive techniques such as the measurement of vital signs to invasive monitoring with the use of various catheters. The pendulum has swung from noninvasive to invasive techniques, and now is swinging back to more noninvasive techniques as technology continues to advance.[1] The key is to make sure the information provided via noninvasive techniques is as adequate and reliable as invasive techniques.[1]

The goal of patient-centered hemodynamic monitoring is to make accurate and timely therapeutic decisions and optimize the cardiovascular system in patients undergoing surgery or in the ICU. The goal of this optimization is to avoid secondary injury to other organs, as well as to provide timely administration of intravenous (IV) fluids or the use of other strategic therapies like vasopressors or inotropes.[2] The ideal monitoring device should be continuous, with real-time measurements, and if possible, be minimally or noninvasive.[3] Over the past few decades and with the advancement of technology, these technologic strategies have transitioned from pressure-based to flow-based parameters.[2,4]

A recent study polling intensivist from Brazil showed that the most trusted hemodynamic monitoring device used by them was a pulmonary artery catheter (PAC) (56.9%) followed by echocardiogram (22.3%). However, the most ubiquitous resource was echocardiogram, as half of the physicians used routine treatment protocols using echocardiogram. Furthermore, it was noted in this study that private institutions had more access to hemodynamic devices than public ones.[5]

The PAC is the most invasive monitoring technique and one of the oldest modalities available. Often considered the gold standard than newer techniques, PAC is also associated with multiple complications and fewer practitioners today are familiar with PAC interpretation outside of cardiac surgery.[2] Furthermore, with its infrequent use and training, the risk of complications from its placement goes up substantially. Thus, we will not discuss this modality further.

Physical Examination Noninvasive Vital Sign Measurements and Laboratory Values

This is the cornerstone and least invasive method for hemodynamic monitoring and should be first applied to critically ill patients. The first device using an inflatable non-expanding occluding upper arm cuff attached to a mercury manometer was described in 1896. This has evolved into the automated sphygmomanometer using oscillometer which is widely used today. It can be conducted in an intermittent way with a cuff or continuously with automated electronically placed sensors.[2]

Another noninvasive but uncommonly used technique is arterial applanation tonometry.[2,6] Aside from systolic and diastolic blood pressure (SBP and DBP), mean arterial pressure (MAP) can be calculated by using the formula $MAP = SBP+2(DBP)/3$. Most monitors calculate this value automatically. Blood pressure should be individualized with higher blood pressures being acceptable for patients with a history of hypertension and lower blood pressures being a permissive strategy for patients with penetrating injuries.

Arterial pulse pressure is commonly used and calculated by subtracting SBP by DBP, which is directly proportional to stroke volume.[5,7]

Stroke volume is the amount of milliliters that the heart ejects with every beat in milliliters and multiplied by the heart rate is the cardiac output (CO).

The clinical examination is useful but does have a limited value. A low blood pressure not necessarily means poor perfusion. It must be taken in the general context of the clinical situation.

The laboratory work done on the initial evaluation of an unstable patient is lactic production which depends mostly on the balance between its production and clearance and occasionally can be misleading.[8] Lactic acidosis seen in shock is due to circulatory failure associated with inadequate tissue oxygenation. It usually includes but is not limited to the presence of hypotension (MAP <65 mm Hg). The prognostic value of lactate exceeds that of blood pressure.[9] Other laboratory values are CBC, BMP, arterial, and venous or central venous blood gases.

Arterial and Central Lines

Arterial line is an invasive way to measure blood pressure. It has been a useful tool in hemodynamic monitoring since the eighteenth century. This requires arterial cannulation to obtain a blood pressure waveform through a pressure transducer and allows for blood sampling as well (ie, blood gases analysis). Several arteries can be used for cannulation including the radial (usually the preferred site), radial, brachial, axillary, femoral, or dorsalis pedis arteries. Despite arterial cannulation being a safe procedure, potential complications do include infection, distal ischemia, bleeding, or pseudoaneurysm formation.[2,9]

Central lines are commonly placed in the internal jugular, subclavian, or femoral veins. This is usually conducted via a Seldinger technique, and it is highly encouraged the use of ultrasound guidance to help avoid the various complications that can arise from this procedure. Ideally, the tip should be in the atrio-cava junction. Complications from central lines do include bleeding, pneumothorax (when placing a subclavian or internal jugular vein catheter), infection, line malposition, and in rare cases, fistula with the adjacent artery.

This allows for the measurement of central venous pressure (CVP) and oxygenation. CVP is a helpful indicator of cardiac preload but is not great at measuring preload responsiveness nor does it correlate well with intravascular volume.[4] Despite the short falls of CVP, the authors do feel that there is still utility using CVP, especially when trending it with the rest of the patient's clinical picture. Furthermore, a high CVP could mean volume overload or a depressed heart function. On the contrary, a low CVP could be seen in normal or hypovolemic states. Lastly, the waveform tracing on the continuous monitor in the ICU is also important as it can reflect cardiac and respiratory function.[2]

Transpulmonary Thermodilution Devices

Transpulmonary thermodilution devices (TPTD) is a tool for advanced hemodynamic monitoring in patients with shock. It is used to monitor CO through similar technology as used with the PAC (thermodilution). There are several devices available in the market. All of them with different technology and algorithms like PiCCO, LiDCCO (uses lithium to measure CO), and noninvasive cardiac output (NICO).

A cold fluid bolus is given in a central vein ipsilateral to the arterial line access and above the diaphragm and the change in temperature is picked up by a thermistor at the tip of an arterial line preferably in the femoral artery. This, in turn, allows intermittent CO measurements and if combined with a pulse wave analysis device can measure CO continuously as well as stroke volume variation (SVV) among other parameters.[7]

Given the versatility of TPTD devices (**Fig. 1**), it can be used in cases of severe shock, mixed shock, or acute respiratory distress syndrome. (ARDS). Along with continuous CO monitoring, it can determine, with great accuracy, global end-diastolic volume (GEDV) (normal: 600–800 cc/m2) (volume of blood on all 4 chambers at the end of diastole) which can be used as a marker of cardiac preload. Other parameters measured by TPTD include cardiac function index (CFI) (normal is 4.5–6.5 L/min), which is calculated by the ratio of cardiac index (CI) divided by the GEDV, and the global ejection fraction (GEF) (normal 25%–35%), which serves as a marker. for systolic function. This device, as opposed to an echocardiogram, does not provide structural detail of the heart, and needs frequent calibration.[7]

Extravascular lung water (EVLW) and pulmonary vascular permeability index (PVPI) are also hemodynamic markers provided by TPTD. They calculate the amount of water outside the pulmonary blood system giving an idea of the water in the interstitial tissue of the lung. They are calculated by subtracting the intrathoracic blood volume (GEVDX1.25) by the intrathoracic thermal volume (normal (<10 mL/kg).

The PVPI is the ratio of EVLW to pulmonary blood volume. Pulmonary blood volume is defined as the fluid that has escaped to the extravascular space over the fluid that remains inside the vessels (normal <3). This, in turn, provides a quantitative measure of pulmonary edema and lung capillary leak.[3,7] CO value is similarly obtained with PAC or TPTD devices.[3,7]

Another technology to measure CO is the NICO system. With this system, carbon dioxide (CO_2) is used to calculate CO in sedated and mechanically ventilated patients. This is conducted through a proprietary disposable rebreathing loop attached to the ventilatory circuit. It can calculate CO_2 production (VCO2) and arterial CO_2 content. CO is calculated by the difference between normal and rebreathing ratios of CO_2.[10]

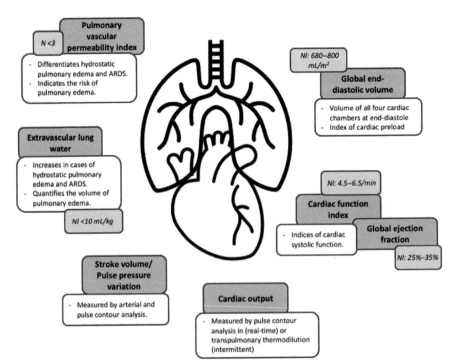

Fig. 1. Algorithm for TPTD (*Adapted from.*[7,11])

Pressure Waveform Analysis Devices (Pulse Contour Analysis)

Pulse contour analysis (PCA) is a dynamic measure based on the relationship between the shape of the aortic pressure curve and the stroke volume. (The amount in milliliters that the heart ejects in every beat). PCA works analyzing the geometry of the pressure waveform of an arterial line through proprietary algorithms[7] and by transferring a pressure signal (arterial waveform) into a flow signal.[2] It is a beat-to-beat continuous analysis and therefore user independent.[2] It requires that the patient is on mechanical ventilation and in sinus rhythm. These measurements have no predictive value in patients that breathe spontaneously or have ongoing arrhythmias.

However, it is suggested that more accurate results are obtained from PCA when the tidal volume on the ventilator is set to 8 cc/kg (10). During a positive pressure breath, right ventricle (RV) filling can decrease between 20% and 70% leading to a decrease in stroke volume, signaling worsening hypovolemia. A value for pulse pressure variation (PPV), or SVV (which we will discuss in a few paragraphs), more than 13% is highly predictive of fluid responsiveness; therefore, additional fluid bolus challenges should be provided to the patient in this situation. The major drawback to PCA is that it requires several calibrations, especially if the results have not been monitored in a one-hour period.

A study of goal-directed therapy using this technology was compared with a control group. The resuscitation intraoperatively was guided by measurements of PPV and CI for the use of fluids, vasopressors, or inotropes. The study group showed less complications like infections, the other measured parameters, however, were similar among groups.[12]

Another hemodynamic monitoring tool is SVV. This parameter is measured during inspiration and expiration and the variability is calculated by the following formula:
SVmax - SVmin x 100/SV mean.[4]

The combination of this technology with echocardiography allows for a better calculation of preload status and in combination with dynamic measures like leg elevation allows to better define the need for IV fluids.[7,11]

Bioimpedance and Bioreactance Devices

These devices were first described in the 1950s using variations in the transthoracic electrical impedance to an alternating current that occurs synchronously to the cardiac cycle. Because of this, it can calculate and relay CO in a continuous manner to the end-user. A modification of the bioimpedance principle is bioreactance, which involves the sum of the electrical resistance, capacitive and inductive properties of blood and tissues used to calculate SV, as well as other parameters. They can likewise measure intracellular, extracellular, and total body water.[2] Although there remain several limitations to this technology, it can provide the health care provider with useful information and trends which allow for the management of the patient's intravascular volume status.[9,10]

Esophageal Doppler Device

This technique is not often used because is partially invasive and the constant movement of the probe necessitates frequent adjustments Conceptually, given its proximity to the heart and accurate data output, it is a reliable monitoring device that can be used to measure CO in a frequent manner as a monitor of global cardiac performance and fluid response. Researchers have found a good correlation between esophageal Doppler monitoring and thermodilution techniques.[13,14] End expiratory occlusion test can be used along esophageal Doppler to calculate CO and to calculate fluid responsiveness.[15]

Other Techniques

With the decrease demand of PAC, the (oxygen saturation in a central venous blood sample) ScvO2 can be a substitute to the SVO2. It can reflect the adequacy of tissue oxygenation. It helps the clinician estimate the CO, the shunt fraction, (amount of blood that goes through the lung without oxygenation). oxygen delivery, consumption, and extraction ratio of oxygen (normal about 25%).[16]

The ScvO2 normally is about 75%, if this measurement is less than 70% to 75% could indicate a hypovolemic state; therefore, the patient might need additional IV fluids or blood products. On the other side, central venous oxygenation values greater than 70% to 75% can signify end organs are starting to shut down and therefore do not extract oxygen from the hemoglobin molecules within the erythrocytes. This is usually not a good sign and can signal impending patient demise.[16]

The SvO2 or ScvO2 can be misleading, especially in septic shock because the oxygen saturation on those samples can look normal with an abnormal extraction of oxygen from the tissues. If low, it indicates poor tissue perfusion, but if high, it is not necessarily reassuring as it can mean that there is shunting (blood going through the lungs without proper oxygenation) or poor use of oxygen by the tissues.[2]

CO2-derived indices: Pco_2 gap is the difference between arterial and mixed venous CO2 content. Basically, arterial Pco_2 measuring CO2 production in the body, and mixed venous Pco_2 is a measurement of lung elimination of CO2. The difference between these 2 values is known as the Pco_2 gap. In practice, when the CO2 gap is > 6 mm Hg, this suggests poor blood flow to the tissues despite a ScvO2 greater than 70%. When this occurs, interventions like assessing fluid responsiveness and/or assessing cardiac contractility need to be considered as illustrated in **Fig. 2.**[8,9]

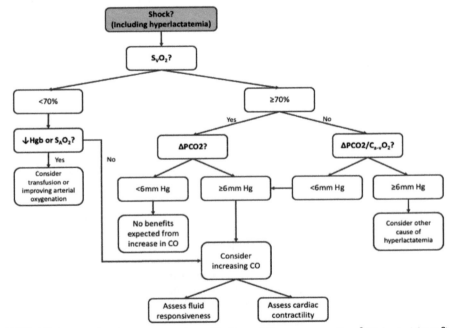

Fig. 2. Algorithm for the interpretation of indices of tissue oxygenation.[8] (*Adapted from.*[8])

Microcirculatory Analysis Devices. (The Future of Hemodynamic Monitoring)

The concept of hemodynamic coherence is a consistency between the macro and the microcirculation. Most of the technology available today for hemodynamic monitoring addresses the macro-circulation with the hope that optimizing the former, will lead to the same effect on the microcirculation. That is, however, not necessarily true. The authors of this concept[17] describe 4 forms of microcirculatory abnormalities that include: (1) heterogeneous microcirculatory flow (due to partial capillary obstruction), (2) reduced capillary density (hemodilution and anemia); (3) microcirculatory flow reduction (vasoconstriction and tamponade), and (4) tissue edema. Its done with the use of hand-held vital microscope to assess the sublingual circulation in real life to guide the clinician choice of therapy (fluid, vasopressors, etc.) that will optimize the microcirculation.[17,18] Another future technology that will have a significant impact on the use of artificial intelligence to predict in advance hemodynamic changes before they occur. This, in turn, will allow the implementation of various therapeutic maneuvers to be performed before cardiovascular collapse. To accomplish this would theoretically require machine learning of big data to obtain predictive analysis. In the anesthesiology field, it has already been used to predict hypotension in the operating room with high sensitivity and specificity, allowing for the prediction of these events about 15 minutes before they happen. The potential use for this technology is endless.[2]

Table 1 indicates the strength and weaknesses of different monitoring devices.

ULTRASOUND TECHNIQUES
Echocardiography

The use of ultrasonography (US) in medicine dates to 1942 on the preliminary works from a neurologist and a psychiatrist who did work on the brain.[19] This technology was popularized for diagnosis in the 1980s.

In the last 10 years, critical care echocardiography has become an essential part of critical care US and has gained widespread acceptance among the ICU Community. One of the most crucial factors is the increased availability of ultrasound (US) machines in many ICUs, emergency departments, and operating rooms. It has emerged, after the physical examination, as the initial modality to establish the presence and type of shock by allowing the bedside clinician to assess the structure and function

Table 1
Strengths and weaknesses of different monitoring devices

	Invasive	Reliability	Ease set up	Record CO
PAC	+++	+++	-	+++
TPTD	+++	+++	+	+++
Arterial PCA	++	+/−	++	+++
Noninvasive PCA	0	+/−	+++	+++
Esophageal Doppler	+	++	+	+++
Bioreactance	0	+/−	+/−	+++

The more pluses indicate that the test is better. +/− means more or less.
Abbreviations: CO, cardiac output; PCA, pulmonary artery catheter; PCA, pulse contour analysis; TPTD, Transpulmonary thermodilution.[3]

of the heart.[3] Its use has increased worldwide thanks to the availability of handheld US devices that can be carried in a physician's pocket.

Several organizations like the American Society of Echocardiography (ASE), The Society of Critical Care Medicine, and the American College of Chest Physicians have outlined the required education and procedures that need to be completed to achieve competency with this technology. The ASE this year will apply the fourth examination for certification in critical care ultrasonography. The purpose of certification on echocardiography is like other certifications, which is to maintain certification and ensure diagnostic accuracy and safety.[3,20]

The core competencies that have been assessed for critical care ultrasound skills are left ventricle (LV) and RV systolic function, assessment of pericardial fluid/tamponade physiology, inferior vena cava (IVC) size, and respiratory variation, basic color, and spectral Doppler to measure red blood cell velocities, basic lung, abdominal, and vascular examination. There is a wide variation between programs with regards to the content and how training is delivered.[21]

POCUS is different from a comprehensive US in the sense that is, used by a critical care specialist, and it is used to address an acute change in the ICU and to guide resuscitation efforts. Can be used as well for therapeutic procedures like drainage of a fluid collection or vascular access. The indications for its use are ever-expanding. Another advantage is its potential to repeat the evaluation as often as necessary.[19]

It has been suggested that a minimum of 30 studies are needed to achieve competency with POCUS.

Most of the POCUS examinations conducted in the ICU are TTE, but TEE is conducted in less than 7% of ICUs.[20] A smaller TEE probe has now been developed that can be left in place for up to 72 hours and allow almost continuous view of 3 principal areas: Two midesophageal views that can assess the superior vena cava (SVC), a 4-chamber view of the heart, and a transgastric view of the heart, allowing users a short-axis view of the heart. Several parameters like cardiac contractility, SVC collapsibility, and preload can be viewed and analyzed with this technology.[14]

Although TEE has an extremely low index of complications, these have been reported. Examples are oropharyngeal or esophageal injuries, or accidental extubation.[22]

In the critical care settings, there are other limitations when performing ultrasound like patient positioning when there are multiple devices, challenging body habitus, fresh wounds or dressings, and subcutaneous air that decreases the quality of the images.[23]

To get an acceptable study, the physician must be familiarized with the basic function of the machine adjusting settings like choosing the right probe, patient identification, gain, depth, focus, use of color, spectral, and tissue Doppler (continuous and pulse wave) and M mode features.[21,24]

Also, the operator should attempt to place and connect EKG leads to the US machine, so it is possible to identify different measurements during systole or diastole.[25]

A detailed description of the performance of echocardiography is beyond the scope of this article.

The Basic Views to Master on echocardiography are

1. Parasternal long-axis view (PLAX): patient should be position ideally on left lateral decubitus. The probe is placed on the left of the sternum around 3 or fourth intercostal space (varies with patient body habitus). The probe is oriented toward the right shoulder.

The structures seen are: RV , aortic valve (AV), left atrium (LA), right ventricular outflow tract (RVOT), and left ventricular outflow tract (LVOT) as well as ascending aorta.

2. Parasternal short-axis view (PSAX): The probe is turned to the left shoulder (90°) and with the probe straight, the first image seen is at the level of the papillary muscles. The structures obtained are RVOT, AV, LV, TV, and pulmonary valve (PV). Depending on how the probe is tilted, one can see the base of the LV and mitral and AV to the apex of the heart.

3. Apical 4 chamber view (A4C): The probe is placed about the left nipple or in the inframammary fold (females) and adjusted to see all 4 chambers by orienting the probe with the index mark at 3 o'clock. The structures seen are LV, RV, LA, RA, TV, MV, and pericardial space.

4. The subcostal view (S4C) is obtained by placing the probe at the subxiphoid area and aligning the marker at 3 o'clock) ideally for this view is best to have the patient in a decubitus position and the structures seen are all the chambers and the pericardial space. This view is facilitated by a liver window.

The probe is turned counterclockwise 90° (12 o'clock) and the entrance of the IVC into the RA.[19]

With the performance of these basic views and practice, the physician can calculate several measurements that allow for a comprehensive hemodynamic evaluation. The basic image interpretation has 4 core elements:

1. Assessment of LV size and systolic function
2. Assessment of RV size and function
3. Assessment of pericardial space for fluid
4. Assessment of IVC size and respiratory variation

Other parameters that help to assess hemodynamic status are[20]:

A. Pulmonary artery systolic pressure, on an A4C view the velocity of TV regurgitation can be calculated and using the simplified Bernoulli equation plus adding the calculated CVP, the PA pressure can be calculated unless there is no TV regurgitation.

Another signs that aids to make this dx is the McConnell's sign (hyperdynamic RV apex and akinetic RV base) as well as paradoxical septal movement (D shaped) on PSAX view.

B. Calculation of the stroke volume: On a PLAX view at the end of systole, the LVOT diameter can be measured and with the formula, Pi square the LVOT volume can be calculated. To this, we add on an A5C view the CW (continuous wave) of the LVOT is used to measure the velocity of the red cells going through the LVOT, and by measuring the VTI (velocity time integral) of that flow and multiplying it by the LVOT volume, the stroke volume can be calculated. If this is multiplied by the HR, the CO can be measured. A normal value of VTI is > 20[24].

It is possible to calculate other parameters of Systolic function like the fractional shortening of the LV on a PLAX or PSAX.[24]

C. Basic measurement of diastolic function can be calculated by measuring the flow at the tip of the mitral valve and therefore measuring E and A velocity as well as with tissue Doppler at the mitral annulus the e' and a' can be measured as well.

The division of the E/e' does give the LA pressure.

D. IVC collapsibility index: On a spontaneously breathing patient, and on an S4C with the probe turned to 12 o'clock, the IVC can be assessed and if it is less than 2 cm and collapses, a diagnosis of hypovolemia can be made whereas if I is > 2 cm and does not collapse, one can assume that the CVP is between 10 and 15 cm of H2O.

The collapsibility index of the IVC is calculated on expiration by subtracting the maximum diameter by the minimum diameter of the IVC and dividing it by its maximum diameter X 100. This measurement can be conducted with M mode as well.

E. Diagnosis of pericardial fluid or tamponade by looking for RA wall systolic collapse for longer than one-third of the cardiac cycle or RV wall diastolic collapse plus dilated IVC.

Doing those maneuvers and settings the above-mentioned values could allow the practitioner to get by echocardiography, most of the values that can be obtained with the PAC whose use has decreased to 7% in the last 20 years.[20,24]

An advanced competency of TTE (transthoracic echocardiography) requires much more detail on the imaging of the structures plus more advanced Doppler spectrum velocity measurements as well as a more in-depth study of the cardiac valves.

TTE can be used to evaluate patients following cardiac arrest as patients on PEA (pulseless electrical activity) who have cardiac activity on ultrasound, have higher chances of achieving ROSC (return of spontaneous circulation).[20]

POCUS can be used in the ICU for a variety of situations (**Table 2**).

Recent studies have shown in a prospective way that an Echocardiogram in the ICU has modified treatment strategies in more than 50% of the times.[22]

TEE with a disposable can be more suitable for hemodynamic monitoring in the ICU on ventilated patients by using abbreviated views like SVC respiratory variation, RV size, LV systolic function, and movement of the septum. By using a disposable probe for up to 72 hours, it is in the author's opinion not a very cost-effective option.[2]

The Rush protocol (rapid ultrasound for shock and hypotension was first introduced in 2006 and published in 2009.

The original RUSH protocol describes 3 physiologic variables called pump (heart and lungs), tank (lungs, IVC, and abdominal compartment) and pipes (aorta and femoral veins) to identify the source of shock and hypotension (**Table 3**).[26,27]

The first part of the RUSH examination is a limited echo focusing on looking for pericardial fluid, contractility of the LV, size of both ventricles, and their relationship.

The second part of the RUSH examination is the determination of volume status by looking in an S4C the collapsibility of the IVC, the status of the IJ, and looking at the lung looking for hemothorax or pneumothorax or pulmonary edema and a FAST examination to look for fluid in the abdomen.

Lastly, the femoral or popliteal veins should be looked for compressibility looking for deep venous thrombosis (DVT).[28]

Another element that could have an impact is the assessment of the stroke volume response that was not identified or measured on the original description of the RUSH protocol. This parameter can measure response to fluid (increase in SV by 15%) or the use of inotropes (increase in SV by 20%). The author's proposal is to measure VTI as a unique surrogate for SV without necessarily measuring the LVOT area.

Limitations to this technique are LVOT obstruction or aortic insufficiency.

In a study of resource-limited areas whereby the RUSH protocol was tested in 97 with SBP less than 90. This study diagnosed 100% correctly the patients with obstructive shock and about 96% cardiogenic shock, 94.4% hypovolemic shock, and 75% distributive shock.[28]

A meta-analysis was conducted to evaluate the ability of the RUSH examination to diagnose the etiology of shock in patients presenting to the emergency room (ER).

This study showed that RUSH examination is more accurate to rule out obstructive shock and least accurate for mixed etiology of shock.[29]

Table 2
Uses of POCUS in critical care[20]

Hemodynamic Monitoring Tool	Cardiac Output SVOT Volume and VTI of the SVOT	Stroke Volume Variation (SVV) IVC Collapsibility Index	Response to Fluid Challenge (Passive leg raising)	Movement and Size of LV and RV
Prognosis of Shock	LV and RV dysfunction	Guidance in the use of IVF	Guidance in the use of vasopressors	Guidance in the use of inotropes
Respiratory Failure	Assessment of RV function	Pulmonary Vascular Resistance	Changes in TV	Changes s in PEEP
Perioperative Setting	During complex abdominal procedures	During Vascular Surgery	During Cardiac Surgery	During Transplant Surgery
Mechanical Circulatory Support ECMO	Insertion of Cannulas	Ongoing Assessment of RV and LV	Weaning of ECMO	Postweaning of ECMO

Table 3
Typical findings on RUSH protocol.[27]

RUSH	Hypovolemic	Cardiogenic	Obstructive	Distributive
Pump	Small chambers and kissing walls.	Decrease contraction and dilated heart.	Increased contractility Pericardial effusion/ tamponade RV strain or thrombus	Increased contractility (early) or deceased contractility (late)
Tank	Flat IVC or IJ Peritoneal or pleural fluid	Distended IVC or IJ B lines Pleural or peritoneal fluid	Distended IVC OR internal jugular vein (IJ) No lung sliding (pneumothorax)	Normal IVC Peritoneal or Pelvic fluid
Pipes	Abdominal Aneurysm or dissection	Normal	DVT	Normal

Lung Ultrasound

Lung ultrasound has popularized a lot in the last decade with the improved way to identify and describe various artifacts as a concrete image of the lung is not entirely possible due to the mingling of air and water in the lung there is increased acoustic impedance and US cannot penetrate the lung and the pleura generates artifacts as well.[29] Most lung US are conducted with the probe in the longitudinal axis and the ideal

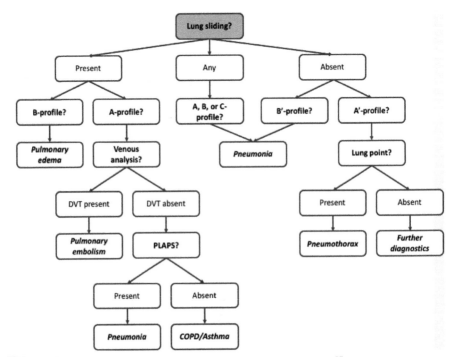

Fig. 3. Modified BLUE protocol. (*Adapted from* Lichtenstein, *et al.*)[25]

view to scan should show the Bat sign whereby the ribs simulate the bat wings but on occasion, to get a better view of the lung the probe is rotated 90° and on a short view this structure can be visualized better.

A score of lung aeration has been created by scanning several areas on each hemithorax (6 per hemithorax) and assessing A or B lines and depending on these findings a score is given from 1 to 3 per area. Its sum allows the clinician to assess the aeration of the lungs and consider maneuvers like recruitment and/or prone positioning of the patient.[30]

Lung US is useful to assess the adequacy of intubation, make ventilatory changes, assess weaning strategies, and aids in procedures like drainage of a pleural effusion.

Patterns of artifacts have been described to explain different situations through the FALLS and the BLUE protocols[27,31,32]

It is used to do a rapid diagnosis of respiratory failure, the lung is examined with an ultrasound probe in 3 different areas of each hemothorax. It is based on the normal artifacts seen on lung ultrasound.

A lines are the normal reverberation artifacts caused by the parietal pleura and consists of horizontal lines. B lines are several vertical lines described as comet tails. Based on the above, several profiles have been described.

A profile defines a normal lung surface, if, in addition, a venous scan is positive for thrombus, gives a diagnosis of pulmonary embolism (PE) (99% sensitivity).

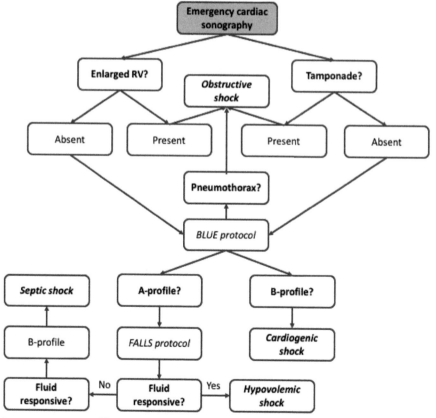

Fig. 4. Falls protocol.[25] (*Adapted from* Lichtenstein, et al.).

The A profile with positive PLAPS (postero-lateral alveolar or pleural syndrome) suggests a diagnosis of pneumonia (96% specificity).

A' (A-prime) profile with no pleural sliding suggests pneumothorax and can be confirmed by finding a lung point sign.

B profile showing lung sliding with rockets (B lines) suggests hemodynamic pulmonary edema (specificity 95%). B lines also suggest a pulmonary artery occlusion pressure of 18 mm Hg.

B' (B-prime) profile absent lung sliding with B lines suggest pneumonia (specificity 100%).

A/B profile combination of A profile on one side and B lines on the other side suggests pneumonia (100% specificity).

C profile: Large anterior lung consolidation and irregularly thickened pleural line suggests pneumonia as well (specificity 99%).[25,31–33] See **Fig. 3**.

The FALLS protocol (fluid administration limited by lung sonography) adds another dimension to the evaluation of the lungs by adding a limited echocardiogram and assessing enlargement of the RV or the presence of tamponade and combines features of the BLUE protocol to differentiate what kind of shock there is.[25] This algorithm sequentially rules out obstructive, cardiogenic hypovolemic and distributive shock[32] See **Fig. 4**.

SUMMARY

The hemodynamic monitoring of a critically ill patient involves many aspects of care like clinical acumen, experience, gut feeling, and use of advanced techniques such as the physical examination, use of monitors of catheters, and ultrasound techniques. It is not just the skill to use these tools but the ability to interpret their findings what leads the clinician to better decisions that in turn leads to better outcomes on critically ill patients.

"One size does not fit all."

REFERENCES

1. Scheeren TWL, Ramsay MAE. New developments in hemodynamic monitoring. J Cardiothorac Vasc Anesth 2019;33(Suppl 1):S67–72.
2. Pinsky M, Teboul JL, Vincent JL. Hemodynamic monitoring. Springer; 2019.
3. Jozwiak M, Monnet X, Teboul JL. Less or more hemodynamic monitoring in critically ill patients. Curr Opin Crit Care 2018;24(4):309–15.
4. Johnson A, Mohajer-Esfahani M. Exploring hemodynamics: a review of current and emerging noninvasive monitoring techniques. Crit Care Nurs Clin North Am 2014;26(3):357–75.
5. Dias FS, Rezende EA, Mendes CL, et al. Hemodynamic monitoring in the intensive care unit: a Brazilian perspective. Rev Bras Ter Intensiva 2014;26(4):360–6.
6. Saugel B, Flick M, Bendjelid K, et al. Journal of clinical monitoring and computing end of year summary 2018: hemodynamic monitoring and management. J Clin Monit Comput 2019;33(2):211–22.
7. Monnet X, Teboul JL. Transpulmonary thermodilution: advantages and limits. Crit Care 2017;21(1):147.
8. Gavelli F, Teboul JL, Monnet X. How can CO2-derived indices guide resuscitation in critically ill patients? J Thorac Dis 2019;11(Suppl 11):S1528–37.
9. Cecconi M, De Backer D, Antonelli M, et al. Consensus on circulatory shock and hemodynamic monitoring. Task force of the European Society of Intensive Care Medicine. Intensive Care Med 2014;40(12):1795–815.

10. Kobe J, Mishra N, Arya VK, et al. Cardiac output monitoring: technology and choice. Ann Card Anaesth 2019;22(1):6–17.

11. Beurton A, Teboul JL, Monnet X. Transpulmonary thermodilution techniques in the haemodynamically unstable patient. Curr Opin Crit Care 2019;25(3):273–9.

12. Salzwedel C, Puig J, Carstens A, et al. Perioperative goal-directed hemodynamic therapy based on radial arterial pulse pressure variation and continuous cardiac index trending reduces postoperative complications after major abdominal surgery: a multi-center, prospective, randomized study. Crit Care 2013;17(5):R191.

13. Cholley BP, Singer M. Esophageal Doppler: noninvasive cardiac output monitor. Echocardiography 2003;20(8):763–9.

14. Nowack T, Christie DB 3rd. Ultrasound in trauma resuscitation and critical care with hemodynamic transesophageal echocardiography guidance. J Trauma Acute Care Surg 2019;87(1):234–9.

15. Depret F, Jozwiak M, Teboul JL, et al. Esophageal doppler can predict fluid responsiveness through end-expiratory and end-inspiratory occlusion tests. Crit Care Med 2019;47(2):e96–102.

16. Walley KR. Use of central venous oxygen saturation to guide therapy. Am J Respir Crit Care Med 2011;184(5):514–20.

17. Hernandez G, Ospina-Tascon GA, Damiani LP, et al. Effect of a resuscitation strategy targeting peripheral perfusion status vs serum lactate levels on 28-day mortality among patients with septic shock: The ANDROMEDA-SHOCK Randomized Clinical Trial. JAMA 2019;321(7):654–64.

18. Ince C. Hemodynamic coherence and the rationale for monitoring the microcirculation. Crit Care 2015;19(Suppl 3):S8.

19. Ali S, Brown CD, Inaba K. Chapter 68 ultrasound imaging for the Surgical intensivist. Springer; 2018.

20. Vieillard-Baron A, Millington SJ, Sanfilippo F, et al. A decade of progress in critical care echocardiography: a narrative review. Intensive Care Med 2019;45(6):770–88.

21. Kanji HD, McCallum JL, Bhagirath KM, et al. Curriculum development and evaluation of a hemodynamic critical care ultrasound: a systematic review of the literature. Crit Care Med 2016;44(8):e742–50.

22. Romero-Bermejo FJ, Ruiz-Bailen M, Guerrero-De-Mier M, et al. Echocardiographic hemodynamic monitoring in the critically ill patient. Curr Cardiol Rev 2011;7(3):146–56.

23. Wong A, Galarza L, Duska F. Critical care ultrasound: a systematic review of international training competencies and program. Crit Care Med 2019;47(3):e256–62.

24. McLean AS. Echocardiography in shock management. Crit Care 2016;20:275.

25. Lichtenstein D, van Hooland S, Elbers P, et al. Ten good reasons to practice ultrasound in critical care. Anaesthesiol Intensive Ther 2014;46(5):323–35.

26. Blanco P, Aguiar FM, Blaivas M. Rapid ultrasound in shock (RUSH) velocity-time integral: a proposal to expand the RUSH protocol. J Ultrasound Med 2015;34(9):1691–700.

27. Perera P, Mailhot T, Riley D, et al. The RUSH exam: rapid ultrasound in SHock in the evaluation of the critically Ill. Emerg Med Clin North Am 2010;28(1):29–56, vii.

28. Rahulkumar HH, Bhavin PR, Shreyas KP, et al. Utility of point-of-care ultrasound in differentiating causes of shock in resource-limited setup. J Emerg Trauma Shock 2019;12(1):10–7.

29. Stickles SP, Carpenter CR, Gekle R, et al. The diagnostic accuracy of a point-of-care ultrasound protocol for shock etiology: A systematic review and meta-analysis. CJEM 2019;21(3):406–17.
30. Mojoli F, Bouhemad B, Mongodi S, et al. Lung ultrasound for critically Ill patients. Am J Respir Crit Care Med 2019;199(6):701–14.
31. Bekgoz B, Kilicaslan I, Bildik F, et al. BLUE protocol ultrasonography in emergency department patients presenting with acute dyspnea. Am J Emerg Med 2019;37(11):2020–7.
32. Lichtenstein DA. BLUE-protocol and FALLS-protocol: two applications of lung ultrasound in the critically ill. Chest 2015;147(6):1659–70.
33. Lichtenstein DA. Current misconceptions in lung ultrasound: a short guide for experts. Chest 2019;156(1):21–5.

Systemic Anticoagulation and Reversal

Abigail P. Josef, MD, Nicole M. Garcia, MD*

KEYWORDS

- Anticoagulant reversal • Warfarin • Heparin • Direct-acting oral anticoagulants
- Prothrombin complex concentrate

KEY POINTS

- Prothrombin complex concentrates (PCC) with vitamin K are recommended for the rapid reversal of Warfarin. If volume expansion is desired and time is not critical, FFP is an appropriate alternative.
- Protamine is recommended as a reversal agent for unfractionated heparin; it is less effective in reversing low-molecular-weight heparin.
- Andexanet alfa is recommended as a specific reversal agent for the reversal of factor Xa inhibitors. When not available, PCC has been used off-label with good effect.
- Idarucizumab is a specific reversal agent recommended for patients on dabigatran with major bleeding or those in need of emergent surgery.

INTRODUCTION

Increasing numbers of patients require anticoagulation for a variety of conditions (**Fig. 1; Table 1**).[5] Indications for chronic anticoagulation currently include[6,7]:

1. Venous thromboembolism (VTE) treatment and prevention
2. Prevention of thromboembolic complications in patients with nonvalvular atrial fibrillation
3. Secondary prevention of arterial ischemic events in high-risk patients with acute coronary syndrome
4. Inherited hypercoagulable states, that is, Factor V Leiden
5. Mechanical heart valves

These conditions are most common diseases of the elderly, and the elderly population is increasing, leading to growing numbers of patients on various forms of anticoagulation. Physicians from many disciplines not only need to understand the

Trauma/Surgical Critical Care/Acute Care Surgery, Department of Surgery, East Carolina University, Brody School of Medicine, 600 Moye Boulevard, Greenville, NC 27858, USA
* Corresponding author.
E-mail address: Garcian16@ecu.edu

Surg Clin N Am 102 (2022) 53–63
https://doi.org/10.1016/j.suc.2021.09.011
0039-6109/22/© 2021 Elsevier Inc. All rights reserved.

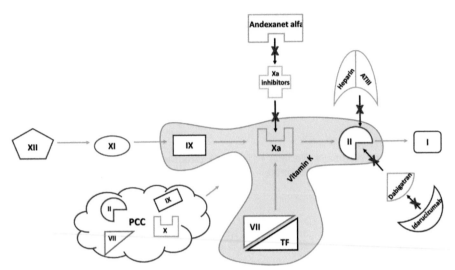

Fig. 1. The clotting cascade, including targets of action of the anticoagulants heparin, the Xa inhibitors, and dabigatran and their reversal agents. ATIII (Antithrombin III).

varying reasons why patients may require anticoagulation but also vitally important is knowledge of how and when reversal is warranted. Patients who present with traumatic injuries or critical illness requiring emergent surgery often have need of immediate reversal of their anticoagulation.

INDICATIONS FOR REVERSAL

The main indications for immediate reversal of anticoagulation include the need for emergent procedures and the presence of life-threatening bleeding.[5] Life-threatening hemorrhage can include the exacerbation of hemorrhage secondary to traumatic injury, or spontaneous hemorrhage such as gastrointestinal bleeding or non-traumatic intracranial hemorrhage.

Reversal of anticoagulation before the procedure is also indicated if the risk of bleeding secondary to the procedure itself is high and cannot be performed without interruption of the anticoagulation. Preprocedural reversal of anticoagulation may differ in that there is often more time to correct coagulopathy before the procedure. With a longer time frame, bridging with intravenous (IV) heparin may be indicated.[6]

Importantly, trauma itself is not an indication for reversal. Studies indicate that without major bleeding, trauma patients on anticoagulation do not suffer worse outcomes when not reversed after a fall (in the absence of intracranial hemorrhage).[8] However, the decision not to reverse therapeutic anticoagulation with direct-acting oral anticoagulants (DOACs) may prolong time to surgery which can lead to higher risks of postoperative complications and readmissions in patients who sustain hip fractures.[9] The need for in-hospital reversal of anticoagulation before time-sensitive procedures is evolving and at this point must be considered on a case-by-case basis.

All patients with life-threatening hemorrhage require supportive care, monitoring, and volume administration including potentially blood product administration for hemorrhagic shock. Local measures should be undertaken for hemostasis (apply pressure dressings, temporary tourniquets, embolization, endoscopy, or surgery[10]).

Table 1
Reversal agents and their targets

Reversal Agent	Anticoagulant	Mechanism of Action	Dose
Vitamin K	Warfarin	Cofactor for production of factors II, VII, IX, and X	10 mg IV
Protamine	Heparin Enoxaparin	Binds bound and unbound heparin	Heparin (based on time from last heparin dose) 0 min: 1–1.5 mg/100 units of heparin 30–60 min: 0.5–0.75mg/100 units of heparin Up to max of 50 mg Enoxaparin 1 mg/mg of enoxaparin up to max of 50 mg
4-factor PCC	Warfarin	Replenishes inactivated factors II, VII, IX, and X	Warfarin Major bleeding: 25 units/kg Minor bleeding: 12.5 units/kg DOACs 2000 units
Activated PCC	Warfarin	Replenishes activated factor VII, and factors II, IX, and X	25–50 units/kg
Idarucizumab	Dabigatran	Binds free and thrombin-bound dabigatran	5 g IV (two 2.5/50 mL vials given 15 minutes apart)
Andexanet alfa	Apixaban Rivaroxaban	Binds to the active site of the Xa inhibitors	High dose: 800 mg IV followed by 8 mg/min for 120 min Low dose: 400 mg IV followed by 4 mg/min for 120 min
Ciraparantag	Heparin Enoxaparin Rivaroxaban Apixaban Dabigatran	Binds anticoagulants	Not available yet, still in clinical trials

Data from:[1–4]

Anticoagulant agents should be stopped, and consideration for reversal should be the next step, depending on the clinical scenario, and severity of the bleeding.

PHARMACOLOGIC AGENTS

Over a century ago, heparin was identified and subsequently isolated and purified for pharmacologic use, bringing the first anticoagulant to the bedside.[11] It was not until 1954 that the first oral anticoagulant, warfarin, was available as a pharmacologic agent after it initial use as a rat poison. Warfarin was long the only available oral anticoagulant agent.[1] Heparin and subsequently, low-molecular-weight heparin (LMWH) were introduced to provide more consistent, nontitrated anticoagulation administered subcutaneously.

Warfarin works by the inhibition of hepatic vitamin K epoxide reductase, leading to the inhibition of vitamin K-dependent clotting factors (II, VII, IX, X, and proteins C and S).[12] Its use requires monitoring of blood international normalized ratios (INR) to maintain an appropriate therapeutic range, and it has many drug and dietary interactions that can prolong or hasten its effect.[13] Normalization of the INR is sufficient to ensure the correction of warfarin-induced coagulopathy.

Heparin binds antithrombin III, which then binds to factor II, irreversibly inhibiting its coagulant properties.[2] The half-life of heparin is 2 hours. LMWH consists of depolymerized heparin, which is itself a penta-saccharide.[14] LMWH activates antithrombin III which inactivates factor Xa, with additional variable effects on factor II. The half-life is 3 to 6 hours after subcutaneous injection.[14] Fondaparinux is another penta-saccharide that binds antithrombin III and leads to the inhibition of factor Xa, without additional effects on factor II.[2]

Argatroban is a direct thrombin inhibitor that binds to the catalytic site of the thrombin molecule.[15] Argatroban is usually used as a continuous infusion for those with heparin-induced thrombocytopenia (HIT) and need for titratable anticoagulation. The half-life is 39 to 51 minutes, and thus stopping the infusion is usually sufficient for the cessation of effect.[16]

The DOACs, also called nonvitamin K antagonist oral anticoagulants or novel oral anticoagulants (NOACs) although this title has fallen out of favor, currently include the direct factor Xa inhibitors rivaroxaban, apixaban, edoxaban, betrixaban, and the direct thrombin inhibitor dabigatran. These medications were introduced with the goal of increased patient compliance as there is more consistent anticoagulant effect without the need for frequent monitoring compared with what is required with warfarin. Rivaroxaban and apixaban are currently the most frequently used in the United States. Betrixaban is an oral agent that is approved for VTE prophylaxis but is not currently available.[1]

Dabigatran is the only oral direct thrombin inhibitor available, which acts by the inhibition of the production of fibrin.[6] It was the first of the DOACs to be invented, and the only currently available oral direct thrombin inhibitor. It binds thrombin competitively, in both the free and clot-bound forms.[17] Laboratory assays to assess the degree of dabigatran-induced anticoagulation are lacking. Ecarin clotting time and thrombin time both demonstrate a linear dose response to serum dabigatran concentrations, but neither of these are widely used clinically.[18]

DOAC use is increasing due to the ease of use and similar safety profiles to warfarin. Some studies indicate less nontraumatic intracranial hemorrhage events on DOACs when compared with warfarin.[19,20] DOAC indications and uses have expanded and now include atrial fibrillation, prevention of ischemic stroke, treatment and prevention of VTE, and in patients with high-risk ischemic heart disease.[7,21] Specific application of DOAC use may be as a primary agent or used after transition from heparin or LMWH.[7] Warfarin remains the drug of choice for anticoagulation in patients with mechanical heart valves, as those patients were excluded from DOAC trials, but future recommendations may change with emerging data.[22] Recently, COVID-19 has been determined to be associated with significant coagulopathy and thrombotic events.[23] Prophylactic enoxaparin in-hospital and DOAC use for high-risk patients for 35 to 45 days is currently recommended to reduce VTE events.[24]

LMWH is still in use most notably by pregnant patients, and until recently remained the drug of choice for oncologic populations for VTE treatment. However, recent studies have suggested that oncologic patients may experience similar efficacy between DOACs and LMWH.[25] Obese patients with a BMI greater than 40 may also still achieve superior anticoagulation with LMWH versus DOACs due to the concern for unpredictable dosing due to the volume of distribution.[1] Kidney failure and various degrees of renal impairment require dose-adjustment of DOACs to varying degrees.[26]

NONSPECIFIC REVERSAL

Although the ability to provide anticoagulant medications has drastically improved the morbidity and mortality of a variety of conditions, it has given rise to an increase in hospitalizations for bleeding either associated with traumatic hemorrhage or secondary to the induced coagulopathy itself.[27] As such, the need to reverse the effects of anticoagulants rapidly has arisen as a significant area of clinical focus. Several earlier solutions have included nonspecific mechanisms of factor replacement and restoration of coagulation in general, or removal of the drug from circulation.

Fresh frozen plasma (FFP) replenishes clotting factors, leading to the reversal of warfarin. FFP often requires the administration of multiple units, which can be useful in a patient who requires volume-expansion, but can be a drawback in the patient who cannot tolerate significant volume (ie, patients with congestive heart failure). In addition, the infusion of FFP should be no faster than 1 hour per unit volume, requiring a significant amount of time for reversal. Volumes of up to 10 to 15 mL/kg (potentially 4–5 units of FFP) can be required for life-threatening bleeding.[2,12] Additionally, the INR of FFP is 1.5, and this is the lowest INR that can be achieved with FFP administration.[28] FFP requires ABO compatibility testing before administration, but not Rh factor.

Prothrombin complex concentrates (PCC) are concentrated volumes of 3 or 4 clotting factors that essentially act in the same way FFP does without the need for excess volume. Kcentra is a four-factor PCC, containing factors II, VII, IX, and X, and also proteins C and S along with antithrombin III and heparin to maintain factors in their inactive state.[12,29] Onset of action is 10 to 30 minutes, with effects lasting 12 to 24 hours.[2] FEIBA is an activated four-factor PCC, containing activated factor VII, with factors II, IX, and X. It does not contain heparin and is therefore indicated for use in patients with HIT.[30] Three-factor PCC (Profilnine-SD) contains factor II, IX, and X was primarily designed for the treatment of life-threatening hemorrhage in patients with hemophilia B to replenish factor IX deficiency. Profilnine was studied off-label for warfarin reversal with unsatisfactory results due to the lack of factor VII in the mix.[3,13] Its use is not currently recommended.

Reversal of DOACs has proved to be more difficult. Simple replenishment of factors via FFP is slow and largely ineffective. Initially, activated charcoal was the only option for the attempted removal of the drug itself. Administration of activated charcoal has been suggested to be effective if administered within 4 hours of DOAC use at a dose of 50g,[31] but it may not be effective beyond 2 hours.[32] Its use is currently suggested for acute overingestion of DOACs in a patient who is awake and alert, as one risk of activated charcoal is aspiration.

Hemodialysis was investigated as a method of direct removal of DOAC agents from circulation. It has been found to be ineffective for apixaban and rivaroxaban as they are highly protein bound.[2] Edoxaban has low protein-binding but is also not cleared well by dialysis. Dabigatran exhibits low protein-binding and high renal excretion and thus may be cleared by dialysis.[31,33] The main drawback to relying on dialysis, in addition to its limited efficacy, is the time it takes to perform.

Tranexamic acid (TXA) is an antifibrinolytic agent that is given as a 1 g bolus followed by an infusion of 1 g over 8 hours. The CRASH-2 trial demonstrated that the administration of TXA significantly reduced death, vascular occlusive events, and the need for blood transfusion in trauma patients with significant hemorrhage.[34] Additionally, the CRASH-3 trial demonstrated that TXA is safe in TBI patients with decreased head-injury related death, and a similar risk of vascular occlusive events in both patient groups who placebo or TXA.[35,36] The use of TXA for OAC-related bleeding is not well-studied directly, however. At this time, TXA is best incorporated into resuscitation protocols for massive transfusion, rather than being considered a reversal agent itself.

SPECIFIC REVERSAL AGENTS

Nonspecific agents still have utility in actively bleeding patients, but pharmacologic agents designed to directly target individual anticoagulants have been introduced with growing interest. Reversal agents with a specific anticoagulant target are likely to be more efficacious and rapid than current nonspecific agents.[12] By basing each of the reversal agents' mechanism of action on its intended target, a predictable reversal pattern can be expected.

Protamine reverses heparin via its inhibition of factor II, but it incompletely reverses the effects on factor Xa, leading to the incomplete reversal of LMWH (only about 60%).[2] Protamine is a positively charged peptide that electrostatically binds to both unbound heparin and after dissociating bound heparin from antithrombin III.[4] Doses of 1 mg of protamine per mg of LMWH administered within the last 8 hours will provide effective anticoagulant reversal, however, doses greater than 50 mg can lead to additional unwanted anticoagulation by inhibition of factor V.[2] Despite its similar mechanism of action to heparin and LMWH, fondaparinux is not reversed by protamine,[37] although activated PCC (aPCC) has some efficacy.[31] There are no effective reversal agents for argatroban currently.[16]

Vitamin K is effective as an adjunct in addition to FFP and/or PCC for warfarin, but using it alone is not sufficient to attain rapid INR reversal. Vitamin K is necessary for the synthesis of factors II, VII, IX, and X, and is necessary for rebuilding stores of these factors once warfarin is stopped. For life-threatening hemorrhage, the IV form achieves faster INR reversal than oral administration.[4] Vitamin K is associated with a very low but severe (0.03%) risk of anaphylaxis and must be infused slowly, 10 mg intravenously over 20 minutes.[2]

Idarucizumab and andexanet alfa are the 2 currently approved specific reversal agents for DOACs. Idarucizumabis a monoclonal antibody fragment that binds both free and bound dabigatran with higher affinity than dabigatran's affinity for factor II.[2] Andexanet alfa is a factor Xa decoy protein that binds Xa inhibitors.[10] Andexanet alfa may theoretically also reverse the factor Xa inhibition of heparin, LMWH, and fondaparinux, but studies are lacking.[2]

Ciraparantag, also known as aripazine or its experimental name PER977, is currently undergoing clinical trials. Ciraparantag is a synthetic molecule that binds and reverses the effects of unfractionated heparin, LMWH, and DOACs including both dabigatran and the Xa inhibitors.[38] It also binds EDTA, citrate, and other in vitro anticoagulants, causing interference with any blood tests that may be desired to measure the degree of anticoagulation after reversal.[1] Further studies are still needed to assess clinical efficacy and safety.

Variants of Factor Xa including Zymogen-like FXa and engineered FXa are currently undergoing in vitro evaluation as potential reversal agents for the Xa inhibitors. They would theoretically provide alternative binding sites for the drugs, removing them from action. Their efficacy in vivo and in situations of severe bleeding is unknown.[1]

TIMING OF REVERSAL

When deciding whether to administer specific reversal agents, knowing when the patient's last dose of their anticoagulant medication can help inform decision-making. In general, if it has been 8 hours or less as the patient has received their last dose, they should be considered fully anticoagulated, whereas after that time drug effect can be more variable.[3] The half-lives of individual medications are important to consider (apixaban 12 hours, rivaroxaban 5–9 hours, and dabigatran 7–9 hours). Reversal agents are currently expensive and their efficacy is greatest when appropriately timed after DOAC dosage. Unfortunately, this information is not always available and best judgment must be used based on the clinical situation. Although it is possible to obtain plasma levels of specific DOACs, it is not recommended to delay treatment of a bleeding patient to await these results.[10] Neither rotational thromboelastometry (ROTEM) nor thromboelastography (TEG) are very reliable indicators of anticoagulation with DOACs, although they can give some indication about the presence of coagulopathy.[39,40] Rapid-assays are under development and likely to soon become available, which would potentially provide near-immediate results.[41] These assays could support the decision for reversal in patients for whom reversal of anticoagulation would be high risk.

COMPLICATIONS

Complications of reversing anticoagulation are highly dependent on the reversal agent used. As with other blood products, there is a risk of viral transmission and transfusion reactions including transfusion-related acute lung injury (TRALI) and allergic reactions with the administration of FFP.[2] Additionally, the risk of volume-overload in patients who cannot tolerate the volume required for reversal of INR should be considered before the use of FFP. Thromboembolic complications including DVT/PE, stroke, and myocardial infarction can also occur, most frequently with larger or frequent doses.[42] PCC that contains heparin can also induce HIT.[2] Protamine has been associated with anaphylactic reactions and cardiac circulatory collapse of unclear mechanism.[43] Vitamin K administration, in addition to a small (0.03%) risk of anaphylaxis, can cause inability to achieve therapeutic INR with the resumption of warfarin for up to 2 weeks.[2] Adverse events experienced after the administration of idarucizumab in study populations included DVT/PE, myocardial infarction, and stroke in 6% to 7% of patients.[44] The observed thrombotic side effects observed with administration of andexanet alfa include myocardial infarction, stroke, TIA, and DVT/PE in 10% of patients, although most events occurred over 10 days from the administration of andexanet.[10,45]

CURRENT CONTROVERSIES

The commonly held belief that the use of OAC places a patient at the higher risk for expansion of intracranial hemorrhage (BIG trial) has been recently challenged by the ongoing accumulation of data retrospectively. Failure to reverse the INR to a normal range within 2 hours of presentation to the hospital with intracranial hemorrhage has previously been found to be an independent predictor of mortality.[46] When compared with warfarin, DOAC use in the presence of mild TBI did not appear to increase in-hospital mortality or increase rates of surgery or intracranial hemorrhage expansion.[20] In a recent multi-institutional review, anticoagulants were found to have minimal impact on rates of TBI, surgery, and overall mortality in elderly patients who suffered a ground level fall.[47] It remains to be seen if it will ultimately prove necessary to reverse every patient who presents with intracranial hemorrhage due to a fall.

Availability of reversal agents in rural and community emergency departments is highly variable. Many small-volume centers do not stock the less commonly used or more expensive DOAC reversal agents, and some do not have clinical volume to support stocking PCC.[48] Nonspecific reversal agents may well continue to have utility, despite their inefficiencies, as long as access to more specific agents is lacking. Current guidelines must continue to include FFP, despite its inefficiency, as long as this continues to be the case.[13]

SUMMARY

The availability of anticoagulants and reversal agents has increased significantly in the last century, especially in the last 20 years with the arrival of DOACs. Much of the available data today comes from retrospective reviews, and prospective, randomized trials would greatly improve our ability to discern those patients who would benefit most from anticoagulation reversal or continuation. The complexity of dosing regimens and reversal strategies will continue to evolve in the years to come.

CLINICS CARE POINTS

- Identification of which anticoagulation medication a patient is on is crucial to identify how to reverse anticoagulation
- Not all patients on anticoagulation require reversal in the presence of bleeding
- The list of anticoagulation medication is expanding and medical providers must be aware of both the mechanism of the medication and the appropriate reversal agent
- Availability of reversal agents is variable and providers must be aware of what their facility has available

DISCLOSURE

The authors have nothing to disclose.

REFERENCES

1. Mujer MTP, Rai MP, Atti V, et al. An update on the reversal of non-vitamin K antagonist oral anticoagulants. Adv Hematol 2020;2020:7636104. https://doi.org/10.1155/2020/7636104.

2. Yee J, Kaide CG. Emergency reversal of anticoagulation. West J Emerg Med 2019;20(5):770–83.

3. Strein M, May S, Brophy GM. Anticoagulation reversal for intracranial hemorrhage in the era of the direct oral anticoagulants. Curr Opin Crit Care 2020;26(2):122–8.

4. Bower MM, Sweiden AJ, Shafie M, et al. Contemporary reversal of oral anticoagulation in intracerebral hemorrhage. Stroke 2019;50(2):529–36.

5. Milling TJ Jr, Ziebell CM. A review of oral anticoagulants, old and new, in major bleeding and the need for urgent surgery. Trends Cardiovasc Med 2020;30(2): 86–90.

6. Cuker A, Burnett A, Triller D, et al. Reversal of direct oral anticoagulants: guidance from the anticoagulation forum. Am J Hematol 2019;94(6):697–709.

7. Burnett AE, Mahan CE, Vazquez SR, et al. Guidance for the practical management of the direct oral anticoagulants (DOACs) in VTE treatment. J Thromb Thrombolysis 2016;41(1):206–32.

8. Chenoweth JA, Johnson MA, Shook L, et al. Prevalence of intracranial hemorrhage after blunt head trauma in patients on pre-injury Dabigatran. West J Emerg Med 2017;18:794–9.

9. Cheung ZB, Xiao R, Forsh DA. Time to surgery and complications in hip fracture patients on novel oral anticoagulants: a systematic review. Arch Orthop Trauma Surg 2021. https://doi.org/10.1007/s00402-020-03701-2.

10. Moia M, Squizzato A. Reversal agents for oral anticoagulation-associated major or life-threatening bleeding. Intern Emerg Med 2019;14(8):1233–9.

11. Wardrop D, Keeling D. The story of the discovery of heparin and warfarin. Br J Haematol 2008;141(6):757–63.

12. Simon EM, Streitz MJ, Sessions DJ, et al. Anticoagulation reversal. Emerg Med Clin Morth Am 2018;36(3):585–601.

13. Milling TJ, Pollack CV. A review of guidelines on anticoagulation reversal across different clinical scenarios- is there a general consensus? Am J Emerg Med 2020; 8(9):1890–903.

14. Hirsh J, Raschke R. Heparin and low-molecular-weight heparin; the seventh ACCP conference on antithombotics and thrombolytic therapy. Chest 2004;126: 188S–203S.

15. McKeage K, Plosker GL. Argatroban. Drugs 2012;61:515–22.

16. Greinacher A, Thiele T, Selleng K. Reversal of anticoagulants: an overview of current developments. Thromb Haemost 2015;113(5):931–42.

17. Wienen W, Stassen JM, Priepke H, et al. In-vitro profile and ex-vivo anticoagulant activity of the direct thrombin inhibitor dabigatran and its orally active prodrug, dabigatran etexilate. Thromb Haemost 2007;98(1):155–62.

18. Ganetsky M, Babu KM, Salhanick SD, et al. Dabigatran: review of pharmacology and management of bleeding complications of this novel oral anticoagulant. J Med Toxicol 2011;7(4):281–7.

19. Caldeira D, Barra M, Pinto FJ, et al. Intracranial hemorrhage risk with the new oral anticoagulants: a systematic review and meta-analysis. J Neurol 2015;262(3): 516–22.

20. Nederpelt CJ, van der Aalst SJM, Rosenthal MG, et al. Consequences of pre-injury utilization of direct oral anticoagulants in patients with traumatic brain injury: a systematic review and meta-analysis. J Trauma Acute Care Surg 2020;88(1): 186–94.

21. Rawal A, Ardeshma D, Minhas S, et al. Current status of oral anticoagulant reversal strategies: a review. Ann Transl Med 2019;7(17):411.

22. Owens RE, Kanra R, Oliphant CS. Direct oral anticoagulant use in nonvalvular atrial fibrillation with valvular heard disease: a systematic review. Clin Cardiol 2017;40(6):407–12.

23. Hasan SS, Radford S, Kow CS, et al. Venous thromboembolism in critically ill COVID-19 patients receiving prophylactic or therapeutic anticoagulation: a systematic review and meta-analysis. J Thromb Thrombolysis 2020;50(4):814–21.

24. McBane RD 2nd, Torres Roldan VD, Niven AS, et al. Anticoagulation in COVID-19: a systematic review, meta-analysis, and rapid guidance from Mayo Clinic. Mayo Clin Proc 2020;95(11):2467–86.

25. Young AM, Marshall A, Thrilwall J, et al. Comparison of an oral factor Xa inhibitor with low molecular weight heparin in patients with cancer with venous thromboembolism: results of a randomized trial (SELECT-D). J Clin Oncol 2018;36(20):2017–23.

26. Harhiharan S, Madabushi R. Clinical pharmacology basis of deriving dosing recommendations for dabigatran in patients with severe renal impairment. J Clin Pharmacol 2012;52(1):119S–25S.

27. Galanaud JP, Laroche JP, Righini M. The history and historical treatments of deep vein thrombosis. J Thromb Haemost 2013;11(3):402–11.

28. Hickey M, Gatien M, Taljaard M, et al. Outcomes of urgent warfarin reversal with frozen plasma versus prothrombin complex concentrate in the emergency department. Circulation 2013;128(4):360–4.

29. US Food and Drug Administration (FDA). Highlights of prescribing information: KCENTRA. Available at: https://www.fda.gov. Accessed April 21, 2021.

30. Franchini M, Lippi G. Prothrombin complex concentrates: an update. Blood Transfus 2010;8:149–54.

31. Dhakal P, Rayamajhi S, Verma V, et al. Reversal of anticoagulation and management of bleeding in patients on anticoagulants. Clin Appl Trhom Hemost 2017;23(5):410–5.

32. van Ryn J, Sieger P, Kink-Eiband M, et al. Adsorption of dabigatran etexilate in water or dabigatran in pooled human plasma by activated charcoal in vitro. Blood 2009;114(22):1065.

33. Chang DN, Dager WE, Chin AI. Removal of dabigatran by hemodialysis. Am J Kidney Dis 2013;61(3):487–9.

34. Perel P, Al-Shahi Salman R, Kawahara T, et al. CRASH-2 intracranial bleeding study: the effect of tranexamic acid in traumatic brain injury—a nested randomized, placebo-controlled trial. Health Technol Assess 2012;16(13):1–54.

35. CRASH-3 trial collaborators. Effects of tranexamic acid on death, disability, vascular occlusive events and other morbidities in patients with acute traumatic brain injury (CRASH-3): a randomized, placebo-controlled trial. Lancet 2019;394(10210):1713–23.

36. Boer C, Meesters MI, Vonk ABA. Anticoagulant and side-effects of protamine in cardiac surgery: a narrative review. Br J Anaesth 2018;120(5):914–27.

37. Glangarande P. Fondaparinux (Arixtra): a new anticoagulant. Int J Clin Pract 2002;56(8):615–7.

38. Kuramatsu JB, Sembill JA, Huttner HB. Reversal of oral anticoagulation in patients with acute intracerebral hemorrhage. Crit Care 2019;23(1):206.

39. Seyve L, Richarme C, Polack B, et al. Impact of four direct oral anticoagulants on rotational thromboelastometry (ROTEM).

40. Kopytek M, Zabczyk M, Natorska J, et al. Effects of direct anticoagulants on thromboelastographic parameters and fibrin clot properties in patients with

venous thromboembolism. J Physiol Pharmacol 2020;71(1). https://doi.org/10.26402/jpp.2020.1.03.

41. Gosselin RC, Adcock DM, Douxfils J. An update on laboratory assessment for direct oral anticoagulants (DOACs). Int J Lab Hematol 2019;41(1):33–9.
42. Baskaran J, Lopez RA, Cassagnol M. Prothrombin complex concentrate. StatPearls Publishing; 2021.
43. US National Library of Medicine. Protamine sulfate-injection, solution. Available at: dailymed.nlm.nih.gov. Accessed April 29, 2021.
44. Pollack C, Reilly P, van Ryn J, et al. Idracizumab for dabigatran reversal-full cohort analysis. N Engl J Med 2017;377:431–41.
45. Connolly SJ, Crowther M, Eikelboom JW, et al. ANNEXA-4 investigators. Full study report of adnexanet alfa for bleeding associated with factor Xa inhibitors. N Engl J Med 2019;380(14):1326–35.
46. Huttner HB, Schellinger PD, Hartmann M, et al. Hematoma growth and outcome in treated neurocritical care patients with intracerebral hemorrhage related to oral anticoagulant therapy: comparison of acute treatment strategies using vitamin K, fresh frozen plasma, and prothrombin complex concentrates. Stroke 2006;37:1465–70.
47. Fakhry SM, Morse JL, Garland JM, et al. Antiplatelet and anticoagulant agents have minimal impact on traumatic brain injury incidence, surgery, and mortality in geriatric ground level falls: a multi-institutional analysis of 33,710 patients. J Trauma Acute Care Surg 2021;90(2):215–23.
48. Faine BA, Amendola J, Homan J, et al. Factors associated with availability of anticoagulation reversal agents in rural and community emergency departments. Am J Health Syst Pharm 2018;75(2):72–7.

Topical Coagulant Agents

Olabisi Ololade Sheppard, MD[a],*, Nathan Alan Foje, MD[b]

KEYWORDS

- Topical coagulant agents • Hemostatic agents • Surgical hemostasis • Thrombin
- Fibrinogen • Chitin • Chitosan • Combat gauze

KEY POINTS

- Bleeding is inevitable in surgical intervention, and the capacity to address bleeding because of different pathways in surgical procedures is important; hence, the need for topical anticoagulant agents.
- Topical anticoagulant agents exist in different forms and are effective based on how they interact with the body's innate coagulation cascade.
- Knowing these different topical anticoagulant agents (how they function, ideal conditions for use, and drawbacks) improves the overall effectiveness of the agents.

BACKGROUND

It is no surprise that most surgical intervention has some degree of bleeding that occurs. Typically, the bleeding is minor and considered acceptable; however, there are times when the situation changes because of pathophysiology, patient disease, or surgical technique (**Fig. 1**). In these situations, it is essential that bleeding is controlled in a timely and safe manner. Ongoing bleeding limits optimal exposure and visualization of the surgical field, and increases the morbidity and mortality of the surgery.[1,2] The body has its own innate mechanism at resolving bleeding; however, surgical procedures can often overwhelm or impair this system. There are various methods to control bleeding in a surgical site including direct compression, electrocautery, and suture ligation. However, surface area, proximity to surrounding structures, patient pathophysiology, and source of bleeding often limit the surgeon's ability to gain control of bleeding using these traditional methods. In these scenarios, topical hemostatic agents can quickly and safely help achieve hemostasis. The earliest topical adjuncts for hemostasis were developed in 1886, and since that time there has been significant advancement in this area as the understanding of coagulation and pathophysiology has increased.[3] Today, there are dozens of topical hemostats that aid in intraoperative

[a] Division of Acute Care Surgery, Department of Surgery, University of Nebraska Medical Center, 983280 Nebraska Medical Center, Omaha, NE 68198, USA; [b] Department of Surgery, University of Nebraska Medical Center, 983280 Nebraska Medical Center, Omaha, NE 68198, USA
* Corresponding author.
E-mail address: Olabisi.Sheppard@unmc.edu

Surg Clin N Am 102 (2022) 65–83
https://doi.org/10.1016/j.suc.2021.09.004
0039-6109/22/© 2021 Elsevier Inc. All rights reserved.

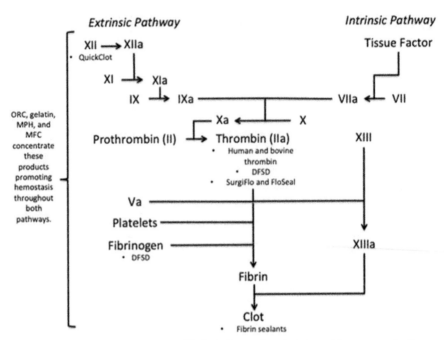

Fig. 1. Coagulation cascade diagram.[52] Clinical use of topical thrombin as a surgical hemostat. DFSD, dry fibrin sealant dressing; MFC, microfibrillar collagen; MPH, microporous polysaccharide hemospheres; ORC, oxidized regenerated cellulose. (*From:* Kustos SA, Fasinu PS. Direct-Acting Oral Anticoagulants and Their Reversal Agents—An Update. Medicines. 2019; 6(4):103. https://doi.org/10.3390/medicines6040103.)

hemostasis. In this article we review the relevant agents (**Box 1**), their roles in surgical hemostasis, and their relevant benefits and drawbacks.

TYPES OF TOPICAL COAGULANT AGENTS
Caustic

Caustic agents are topical hemostats that are applied to the area of bleeding and coagulate tissue by promoting protein precipitation and vessel occlusion.[3] They are predominately used during dermatologic procedures or other procedures confined to the superficial soft tissue. These agents are all stable at room temperature and many have antibacterial properties. As such, these agents are popular for use during in-office procedures.

One of the first caustic agents introduced was Monsel solution, which was developed in the late nineteenth century by a French medic during the Crimean War.[4] Its active ingredient is ferrous sulfate; the ferric ion is a precipitant that promotes local coagulation and provides antibacterial properties.[3] It is still used in dermatologic and gynecologic procedures even today.[3,5] The principal drawbacks of Monsel solution are the tattooing effect that it can have on the skin, the potential injury to surrounding tissues, and possible interference with appropriate histologic interpretation.[5–7]

Mohs paste, first used in 1941 for cutaneous malignancy treatment, has zinc chloride as its active ingredient, which exists in a paste form or impregnated dressings.[3] Another coagulant, silver nitrate, is often used to control local bleeding because the silver ions promote protein precipitation, eschar formation, and coagulation.[3,8] Like

Box 1
Classes of hemostats

Thermal/energy-based methods

Chemical methods
  Systemic pharmacologic agents
  Topical coagulant agents
    Caustic agents
    Mohs paste: zinc chloride
    Monsel solution: 20% ferrous sulfate
    Aluminum chloride
    Silver nitrate
    Noncaustic agents
      Mechanical
      Absorbable
      Cellulose
      Surgicel (Surgicel, Nu-Knit, Surgicel Fibrillar, Surgicel SNOW, and Surgicel Powder)
      Oxycel
      Collagen (bovine)
      Avitene (flour, Ultrafoam, UltraWrap, EndoAvitene)
      Instat
      Helitene
      Helistat
      Gelatin (porcine)
      Gelfoam
      Gelfilm
      Surgifoam
      Ostene
      Polysaccharide sphere: Arista
      Nonabsorbable
      Bone wax
      Hemostatic dressings
      Chitin (medical rapid deployment hemostat)
      Chitosan (HemCon)
      Mineral Zeolite (QuikClot/combat gauze)
      Stasilon
      Dry fibrin sealant dressing
      Pro or Urgent QR Powder

    Active
      Thrombin-JMI (bovine)
      Evithrom (human)
      Recothrom (recombinant)

    Combination agents
      Flowables
        FloSeal (bovine gelatin + thrombin)
        SurgiFlo (porcine gelatin + thrombin)
      Fibrin sealants
        Tisseel
        Evicel (previously Crosseal)
        Vitagel surgical hemostat/Costasis
        Vistaseal

    Synthetic agents
      Cyanoacrylates (Dermabond)
      Polyethylene glycol polymers (Coseal)
      Glutaraldehyde cross-linked albumin (Bioglue)

ferrous sulfate, silver nitrate has local antibacterial benefits. Aluminum chloride is another common topical hemostat. When exposed to water, it causes hydrolysis of hydrogen chloride leading to vasoconstriction and activation of the extrinsic coagulation cascade.[9]

Mechanical and Absorbable

Mechanical hemostatic agents provide a latticework for promotion of platelet aggregation and subsequent fibrin plug formation to stop bleeding expediently. Their function, unlike some other agents, depends on an intact coagulation cascade because they are simply structures to expedite intrinsic coagulation mechanisms. Mechanical agents are further subdivided into absorbable and nonabsorbable mechanical hemostats. Absorbable hemostats have the principal benefit of being able to be left in situ with the product being resorbed over time. Nonabsorbable hemostats, however, are not resorbed by the body and can often be a nidus for infection and/or promote inappropriate inflammation hindering appropriate wound healing.

Hemostatic cellulose products have been used since the 1940s.[3] WoundClot (Core Scientific Creations, Westlake Village, CA) is a commercially available nonoxidized regenerated cellulose product that resorbs water and concentrates coagulation factors to promote clot formation. Unlike its oxidized regenerated counterparts, WoundClot does not rely on acidity to aid in clot formation.[10]

Most commercially available cellulose-based products rely on oxidized cellulose. This includes Surgicel, Nu-Knit, Oxycel, Surgicel Fibrillar, Surgicel SNOW, and Surgicel Powder (Ethicon, Somerville, NJ). The mechanism of action of these products is multifactorial. First, the oxidized cellulose promotes platelet aggregation and adherence to the wound bed. Second, because of its low pH, the product has caustic properties, resulting in coagulative necrosis and clot formation.[3] In addition to promoting hemostasis, the acidity of oxidized cellulose is bacteriostatic against organisms that commonly cause wound infections including methicillin-resistant*Staphylococcus aureus*, vancomycin-resistant *Enterococcus*, and *Staphylococcus epidermidis*.[11] It is worth noting that acidity of oxidized cellulose products can inactivate biologically active hemostatic agents that have been concurrently applied to the area, negatively affecting their efficacy.[12] These products are used ubiquitously in a variety of surgical fields including neurologic, cardiac, and general surgery.[13]

Oxidized regenerated cellulose-based products are some of the most widely used topical hemostats in today's operating rooms. They are readily available, easy to store, and intuitive to apply. Multiple studies have demonstrated that these products reduce blood loss and time to hemostasis compared with other products and placebo.[14,15] The chief adverse effects of these products include local acidity leading to granuloma formation and expansion with blood absorption with subsequent compression of surrounding structures, most importantly, nerves. These adverse effects are mitigated by removing excess product after use; however, this can frequently lead to rebleeding because the adherent clot is also removed. Irrigation with sterile saline can help remove excess product while leaving the newly formed clot in situ. Care should be taken when interpreting postoperative imaging because oxidized regenerated cellulose can be mistaken for abscess formation or malignancy on computed tomography scans.[16,17]

Microfibrillar collagen (MFC) is like cellulose, which is an effective topical hemostat that has been formatted into different forms including powder, sheet, and sponge. Commercially available forms of MFC include Avitene (BD, Franklin Lakes, NJ), Helitene (Integra Life Sciences Corporation, Plainsboro, NJ), Helistat (Integra Life Sciences Corporation), and INSTAT (Ethicon).[1,3,18] MFC is used in similar applications as cellulose products, and it functions by promoting platelet aggregation and degranulation resulting in clot formation via the intrinsic pathway.[3] Importantly, because of its reliance on platelet aggregation to promote coagulation, MFC is of limited utility in patients with thrombocytopenia or platelet dysfunction. Additionally, MFC negatively affects bond strength of methylmethacrylate and should not be used on bone if a prosthesis will be inserted.[3,18] In contrast to some other hemostatic agents, MFC does not have bacteriostatic or bactericidal properties. MFC is most used for application over a broad surface area to decrease bleeding.

Gelatin-based products are also widely used for hemostasis and are often combined with other topical hemostats to enhance overall hemostasis. Gelfoam (Pfizer, New York, NY), the first gelatin-based product, was developed in 1945 and remains in use to this day.[3] Surgifoam (Ethicon) and Gelfilm (Pfizer) were later developed and all products use gelatin from porcine skin.[3] They promote coagulation by contact activation and platelet aggregation.[3] On contact with blood, the gelatin sheet is quickly absorbed leaving behind a highly concentrated area of coagulants. Additionally, the meshwork serves as a framework for promoting further clot formation and granulation tissue formation.[9] For this reason, porcine gelatin products have the benefit of promoting wound healing and granulation tissue formation. Because of its neutral pH, porcine gelatin products are easily combined with other hemostatic agents for a synergistic effect. Common combinations include porcine gelatin with thrombin and porcine gelatin wrapped in oxidized regenerated cellulose.[3] Gelatin-based products are used in a wide variety of applications from vascular surgery to trauma.

Ostene (Baxter Healthcare, Deerfield, IL) is a new and specialized topical hemostatic agent. It was developed as an alternative to bone wax to aid in hemostasis from bony surfaces. In contrast to bone wax, Ostene is readily absorbed and does not interfere with bone healing or promote an inflammatory response. Ostene is available as a semisolid stick, which becomes more pliable as it is warmed. Like bone wax, it is applied directly to the bony surface and functions as a mechanical obstruction to ongoing bleeding. Ostene is often used in cardiothoracic and orthopedic surgery to aid in hemostasis from bony surfaces without promoting inflammation or interfering with bone healing.[19]

Microporous polysaccharide hemospheres (MPH) are a new development in topical hemostasis. These particles consist of cross-linked polysaccharides, which are highly hydrophilic. When these particles touch a bleeding surface their hydrophilic nature promotes concentration of erythrocytes, platelets, and various proteins to form a gelatinous matrix and plug formation via the intrinsic pathway.[3] Additionally, this matrix serves as the framework for early fibrin clot formation. These products are distributed as a powder, which is applied to the surgical site to help control venous, capillary, and arteriolar bleeding in general, cardiac, and orthopedic procedures.[20,21] MPH have not been evaluated for safety in neurologic or ophthalmic procedures.[20,21] These products are favored in certain situations, because they provide good hemostasis even in the setting of underlying coagulopathy. Additionally, MPH are absorbed within 48 to 72 hours of application, and do not carry the risk of immunogenicity or allergic reaction that some other hemostatic agents do.[3,20,21] MPH are commercially available in the United States as Arista (BD) and Perclot (Cryolife Inc, Kennesaw, GA), both of which are distributed in a powder form with various applicators for open and endoscopic use.

Mechanical and Nonabsorbable

Bone wax
Bone wax, a combination of beeswax, salicylic acid, and almond oil was first developed in 1886, and it remains in use today, albeit with a slightly different formula.[3]

Bone wax as used today contains beeswax, palmitate, paraffin, and a softening agent. Bone wax, as its name suggests, is used to achieve hemostasis from bony surfaces. When applied, the compound obstructs and tamponades the flow of blood to achieve hemostasis. Bone wax is instantaneous in its effect because it does not rely on the complex physiology of fibrin clot formation or coagulation. The principal drawback of bone wax is that it is nonabsorbable and identified as a foreign body by the innate immune system.[3,22,23] Consequently, bone wax can possibly serve as a nidus for infection and impairs appropriate bone healing.[22,23] Bone wax is broken down by phagocytes over an extended period of time.[3,23]

Hemostatic dressings

This term has been adopted to describe dressings, usually gauze, which have been combined with some other agent with hemostatic properties. These are often used in first aid applications and must be removed before final wound closure.[3]

Chitin is a polysaccharide naturally found in the exoskeletons of arthropods. When applied to the wound, chitin promotes vasoconstriction and the release of PDGF-AB and transforming growth factor-β1.[3,24] Additionally, the positively charged chitin concentrates negatively charged erythrocytes, platelets, and coagulation factors.[24] Importantly, this process remains intact even in situations where the patient is heparinized or defibrinated. Chitin-based products are not readily available; however, Chitin's cousin, chitosan is commonly used in hemostatic dressings.

Chitosan is the deacylated form of chitin and shares the same mechanism for hemostasis.[3,25] Its dressings are commonly used on today's battlefields because of their durability, analgesic, and antimicrobial properties.[24,25] In vivo animal models have demonstrated significantly shorter time to hemostasis when using chitosan dressings.[26] Likewise, chitosan products continue to function as effective hemostatic agents even in heparinized or otherwise coagulopathic patients.[3,27]

QuikClot (Z-Medica LLC, Wallingford, CT), currently known as combat gauze, is a nonwoven mineral zeolite-coated dressing (specifically, kaolin).[28,29] The initial variant of QuikClot was in powder form; this was replaced by the combat gauze version.[30,31] Kaolin, an aluminum silicate, is a potent coagulation initiator that acts through factor XII surface activation to trigger the intrinsic clotting cascade.[28,29] The substance is inert and does not interact with otherwise intact skin surfaces, thereby eradicating the probability of skin reactions or allergies when used. Given the multiple-ply rayon/polyester construction, it is absorbent. In an in vitro study, QuikClot was found to be effective at decreasing the time to clot formation and increasing clot strength not only in nonanticoagulated individuals but also in patients taking antiplatelet therapy, traditional vitamin K antagonist (warfarin), factor Xa inhibitors, direct thrombin inhibitors, and heparin (including low-molecular-weight heparin).[28] QuikClot has been shown to be the most effective hemostatic agent with success rates of 80% to 90% on first application, and 100% after second application in swine models with exsanguinating femoral bleeding and the lethal triad of hypothermia, coagulopathy, and acidosis.[30,32] As such, it has become the first-line treatment of life-threatening hemorrhage caused by combat wounds, hence its name.[30] One disadvantage is that manual pressure must be applied in conjunction with QuikClot gauze for it to be effective.

Stasilon, manufactured and distributed by Entegrion (Durham, NC), is a woven textile composed of allergen-free fibers of continuous filament texturized E-glass yarn as the warp, and bamboo rayon fibers as the weft.[31,33] The fiberglass activates the coagulation cascade while the bamboo rayon fibers absorb the surrounding fluid, thus allowing for aggregation and binding of red blood cells.[31,34] The materials were selected for their thrombogenicity as measured by acceleration of platelet-dependent turnover within the coagulation cascade and subsequent generation of thrombin.[33,34] The nonadherent nature of this product makes it easy to remove from tissue without disrupting clot formation.[33] However, Stasilon has demonstrated poor performance in animal models and further investigation is needed to better delineate the role of this agent in clinical practice.[30]

Dry fibrin sealant dressing (DFSD) is a composite of 15 mg/cm² of human fibrinogen, 37.5 U/m² of purified human thrombin, and 72 μg/cm² CaCl₂ freeze-dried onto an absorbable polyglactin mesh backing Vicryl.[31,35,36] It is a three-layer sandwich formation consisting of two fibrinogen layers and one thrombin layer forming the continuous middle layer.[35–37] In a swine model simulating hypothermic coagulopathy, there was an 83% survival rate at 1 hour compared with 0% when plain gauze or gauze containing IgG were used.[36] This was attributed to the rapid achievement of hemostasis despite severe dilutional and hypothermic coagulopathy.[37] The very high concentrations of fibrinogen and thrombin supplied by DFSD seemed to offset the effects of dilutional and hypothermic coagulopathy because the conversion of fibrinogen to fibrin clot is an enzymatic reaction involving thrombin in the final pathway of coagulation.[36–38] With ballistic injuries, DFSD was demonstrated to reduce blood loss and maintenance of blood pressure when compared with gauze wound dressings.[38] Unfortunately, DFSD is expensive.[31] Another product that functions in a similar way is TachoSil (Baxter Healthcare). TachoSil is an equine collagen patch impregnated with pooled human plasma containing fibrinogen and thrombin.[39,40]

Pro or urgent QR Powder

Urgent QR Powder (Biolife, Sarasota, FL) consists of hydrophilic polymers with potassium salts. They function by concentrating the larger components of blood and binding blood to form an overlying, artificial eschar to stop bleeding. Urgent QR Powder is not able to be metabolized by the body and is consequently only able to be applied to wounds that will heal by second intention. One significant benefit of this product is that it is significantly lower cost than many other hemostatic agents.[41]

Active

Thrombin

Thrombin-based hemostatic agents are active in that they are biologically involved in the coagulation cascade.[1,2,31,42] Thrombin, also known as activated factor II, is a procoagulant and anticoagulant.[42,43] In its procoagulant state, it activates platelets, and cleaves fibrinogen to fibrin.[31,42,43] It also upregulates its own production by activating factors V, VIII, and XI.[1,43] Topical thrombin occurs in the forms of "bovine" thrombin (Thrombin-JMI, GenTrac, Inc, Middleton, WI), "human" thrombin (Evithrom, Johnson & Johnson, Brunswick, NJ), and "recombinant" thrombin (Recothrom, ZymoGenetics, Seattle, WA).[1,2,31] The differences in these topical forms are their reactivity, and associated risks. The bovine thrombin has a range of mild to severe coagulopathies associated with it related to antibodies against bovine thrombin and/or factor V that cross-reacts with human coagulation factors.[1] This risk of antibody reactivity increases with re-exposure to bovine thrombin.[1,2] It occurs as a powder in vial form that is used dry or reconstituted in sterile saline to be used within 3 hours of reconstitution.[42] Evithrom, which is a Food and Drug Administration–approved pooled human plasma thrombin, carries a risk of viral transmission even though the final product undergoes viral inactivation treatment to ensure the safety of the product.[2,42] Evithrom is stored frozen and needs to be thawed before use. At this point, it can then be used immediately, kept at room temperature for up to 24 hours, or refrigerated for up to 30 days.[2] It is not recommended for use in combination with human blood salvage or cardiopulmonary bypass systems.[1] Recothrom uses recombinant DNA; hence, it is called recombinant topical thrombin. It does not have bovine or human plasma but was instead produced by using a Chinese hamster ovary host cell protein.[2,42] It exists in a lyophilized powder in vial form that can be stored at room temperature and needs to be used within 24 hours after it is reconstituted in sterile saline.[1]

Combination Agents

Flowables

Flowable hemostatic agents use a combination of passive and active hemostatic agents as a single product application. The two commercially available products are FloSeal (Baxter Healthcare) and SurgiFlo (Johnson & Johnson). These products combine two hemostatic agents for a synergistic stemming of blood flow and leading to the conversion of fibrinogen in blood to fibrin at the bleeding site.[1] The active ingredient in both formulations is pooled human thrombin, whereas the passive agent is the gelatin. In FloSeal bovine gelatin is used, and in SurgiFlo porcine gelatin fills this role.[1,2] When combined and applied with a syringe applicator to a tissue surface, it starts to polymerize into a thick consistency and adheres to surfaces with high concentrations of fibrinogen, which includes blood.[1,44] They both are used in all surgical specialties except ophthalmic surgery.[1] The limitations to use include allergies or sensitivities to the composite materials, blood salvage and cardiopulmonary bypass systems, intravascular use, and use in absence of active blood flow in vessels because of potential for intravascular clotting.[1] In a multicenter trial of 93 cardiac surgery patients, FloSeal was found to be superior to Gelfoam plus thrombin at stopping bleeding within 10 minutes (94% compared with 60%).[1] In a multicenter, prospective, single-arm study, SurgiFlo was effective at hemostasis within 10 minutes of application during endoscopic sinus surgery.[1]

Fibrin sealants

Fibrin sealants form synthetic fibrin clot that acts as an adhesive and covering creating a fluid-impervious barrier that stops most liquids.[31,45] They are typically applied by means of a double syringe system.[45] They have high concentrations of fibrinogen, thrombin, calcium, and factor XIII, which in combination simulate the final stages of the coagulation cascade.[1,31] Tisseel made by Baxter, and Evicel (previously Crosseal) made by Ethicon are based on this mechanism.[1,31] Their drawback, however, is that the components need to be kept frozen, and the thawing and reconstitution process is time consuming, and requires warming with prolonged agitation. They also cannot be used in a significant venous and arterial bleed because the clot formed can be dislodged but do well in low-pressure bleeding and surface oozing.[46] In fact, the effort to address this brought about DFSD. Other products, such as Vitagel (Stryker, Kalamazoo, MI) and Costasis (Orthovita, Malvern, PA), are a combination of microfibrillar bovine collagen and bovine thrombin mixed with the patient's own plasma (obtained during surgery, centrifuged leaving only fibrin and platelets).[1,46,47] Unfortunately, they are expensive.[1,46]

Synthetic Agents/Adhesives

Synthetic agents and adhesives are agents that work by chemical reaction to form a strong seal and limit ongoing bleeding. These hemostatic adhesives exist as liquids that polymerize to form a solid film adhering to tissue surface.[45] Cyanoacrylate monomers polymerize through an exothermic reaction in the presence of local hydroxyl groups.[1,45,48] They form a barrier that is impervious to fluids and provides antimicrobial benefits.[45,48] Dermabond (Johnson & Johnson) is one such adhesive.[1,48]

Table 1
Mechanism of action, advantages/recommended use, and disadvantages/caution against use for topical hemostatic agents

Hemostatic Agent	Products	Mechanism of Action	Advantages/ Recommended Use	Disadvantages/Caution Against Use
Bone wax	Bone wax	Tamponade through occlusion of bleeding channels in bone	Can effectively control bleeding from bone surfaces (eg sternotomy)	Can impede bacterial clearance and act as a nidus for infection, therefore avoid use in a contaminated field May embolize Should not be used where bone fusion is critical, because it is not absorbed by the body
Ostene	Osiene (alkylene oxide copolymers)	Occlude bleeding channels in bone	Recommended for bleeding control on bone surfaces (eg sternotomy) Does not impede bone growth and is absorbed over time	Do not use at sites with active or latent infections Caution when using in areas which lend structural support to bone
Gelatin foams	Gelfoam, Gelfilm, Surgifoam	Provides physical matrix for clotting initiation	Effectively controls small-vessel bleeding May be used to control bleeding from bone Recommended as hemostatic plug wrapped in oxidized cellulose Absorbed by the body within 4–6 wk Nonantigenic Neutral pH allows use with biologic agents	Should not be used in closed spaces because significant swelling may compress nerves Use around brisk arterial bleeding can dislodge sponge May embolize if in an intravascular compartment

(continued on next page)

Table 1
(continued)

Hemostatic Agent	Products	Mechanism of Action	Advantages/ Recommended Use	Disadvantages/Caution Against Use
Oxidized cellulose	Surgicel	Provides physical matrix for clotting initiation, low pH contributes to coagulative necrosis	Low pH has antimicrobial effect Very good handling characteristics (cotton-like consistency, best when applied dry) Does not stick to instruments Typically dissolves in 2–6 wk	Must not be used with other biologic hemostatic agents (eg thrombin) because of low pH Low pH may increase inflammation of surrounding tissue Caution when using in close proximity of spinal cord because swelling and Surgicel fibers could pass through intervertebral foramen causing cord compression
Microfibrillar collagen	Avitene flour, Avitene Ultrafoam, Avitene Ultra wrap, Helistal, Helitene, Instat, Endoavitene	Platelet adherence and activation	No significant swelling Absorbed in less than 8 wk Can control wide areas of parenchymal bleeding Effective despite profound heparinization because of its mechanism of action	Less effective in patients with thrombocytopenia Sticks to operator's gloves May bind to neural structures Caution with blood scavenging systems, because microfibrillar collagen can pass through fillers
Thrombin	Thrombin-JM 1 (bovine) Evithrom (human plasma-derived), rh	Converts fibrinogen to fibrin to form clots, activation of clotting factors	Effectively controls minor bleeding from capillaries and small venules when pressure or ligature is	We discourage use of bovine thrombin because of immunologic response, and possible

Category	Product	Mechanism	Uses/Effects	Notes/Cautions
Thrombin with gelatin	ThrombinRecothrom (recombinant human)		insufficient Easy application Fast acting	increase in coagulopathy and thrombosis Do not use in individuals known to react to human blood products
	Floseal	Gelatin granules cross-linked into matrix and swell for tamponade effect; thrombin hemostatic effect	Better control of moderate arterial bleeding than fibrin sealants because of gelatin granule tamponade effect We recommend for use in cardiac surgery, and open and laparoscopic nephrectomies	Needs contact with blood as source of fibrinogen Can swell up to 20% in 10 min after application
Fibrin dressings	Dry fibrin sealant dressings	Freeze-dried (lyophilized) fibrinogen and thrombin on gauze dressing	Initial success with US forces with Iraq and Afghanistan under FDA investigational drag protocol Effectively stops bleeding from large surface abrasions Longer shelf-life than fibrin sealants and does not need mixing at site of application	Not FDA approved Needs strong packaging because of brittleness
Chitin dressings	Rapid Deployment Hemostat	Vasoconstriction, mechanical sealing, mobilization of RBCs, clotting factors, platelets	Intended for emergency field use by first responders Effective for minor wounds in animal model	Varied results for severe wounds, such as splenic lacerations in animal model
Chitosan dressings	HemCon	Deacylated form of chitin, similar mechanism	Intended for emergency field use by first responders	Success rate highly dependent on training of first responders (failure

(continued on next page)

Table 1
(continued)

Hemostatic Agent	Products	Mechanism of Action	Advantages/Recommended Use	Disadvantages/Caution Against Use
			Initial success with US forces with Iraq and Afghanistan Has antimicrobial properties	of bandage to adhere undermines effectiveness) Animal testing yields inconsistent results Contains chitosan from shellfish, so do not use in patients with shellfish allergies
Mineral zeolite dressings	QuikClot	Molecular sieves absorb water at site of wound to increase concentration of clotting factors, platelets, RBCs	Intended for emergency field use by first responders Powdered form effective for low-pressure bleeding Zeolite embedded in mesh for high-pressure bleeding Prehydration in newest products avoids exothermic burns of earlier versions	Caution with high-pressure bleeds because they can force powdered form out of wound Intracorporeal use generally effective, but foreign body reactions have been reported to contribute to scar tissue formation and associated complications
Fibrin sealants	Tisseel, Evicel, Crosseal	Thrombin and fibrinogen mixed at site of application; thrombin cleaves fibrinogen to fibrin that forms clots	Effective in heparinized patients; can be used for skin grafting, dural sealing, bone repair, splenic injuries, closure of colostomies, in reoperative cardiac	Before application, wounds must be cleaned of antiseptics containing alcohol, iodine, or heavy metal ions that can denature applied thrombin and fibrinogen

		surgery Recommended for controlling bleeding in urologic surgeries (see text for complete list) Tisseel and Eviceil good for venous oozing from raw surfaces	
Platelet sealants	Vitagel	Microfibrillar collagen and thrombin combined with patient's plasma-derived fibrinogen and platelets	Platelets from patients strengthen clot while proteins in gel facilitate tissue regeneration May be used in orthopedic, hepatic, reconstructive, and general surgical procedures	Need for centrifugation and preuse processing Caution when used in bypass or blood scavenging systems Do not use with methylmethacrylate or other acrylic adhesives because it may reduce their strength Caution when used near renal pelvis or ureters because foci can lead to calculus formation
Polyethylene glycol hydrogels	Coseal	Two synthetic polyethylene glycol polymers that mix and cross-link in wound site	Can prevent pericardial Good mechanical sealant for vascular reconstructions Is not exothermic, does not cause inflammation, and does not potentiate bacterial infection	Swelling up to 4 times initial volume after 1 d, and can continue swelling Does not perform well in partial nephrectomies
Cyanoacrylates	Dermabond	Liquid monomers form polymers in the presence	Use as a replacement for sutures (≤5–0) for wounds on the face,	Difficult to use in jagged lacerations Must not use for bites,

(continued on next page)

Table 1
(continued)

Hemostatic Agent	Products	Mechanism of Action	Advantages/Recommended Use	Disadvantages/Caution Against Use
		of water, and glue surfaces together	extremities, and torso Full binding strength within 2.5 min, attains strength of healed tissue after 7 d Forms waterproof barrier	puncture, or crush wounds Not recommended on mucosal surfaces, axilla, or perineum
Glutaraldehyde cross-linked albumin	Bioglue	Glutaraldehyde cross-links bovine albumin to cell proteins at wound site to form tough scaffold	Achieves 65% binding power in 20 s, full strength in 2 min regardless of temperature or whether in air or water Use for sealing holes around sutures or staple lines, good for arterial bleeding Most commonly used in complex cardiovascular procedures involving aortic aneurysms, valve replacements, and aortic dissections, and peripheral vascular procedures, such as carotid endarterectomy, and arteriovenous access	Do not apply circumferentially around developing structures because it can restrict growth Caution in proximity to nerves, because it may cause dysfunction Unreacted glutaraldehyde may have mutagenic effects Do not apply to valve leaflets or intracardiac structures May cause hypersensitivity reactions

A comprehensive review of topical hemostatic agents: efficacy and recommendations for use.
Abbreviations: FDA, Food and Drug Administration; RBC, red blood cell.

Achneck, Hardean E.; Sileshi, Bantayehu; Jamiolkowski, Ryan M.; Albala, David M.; Shapiro, Mark L.; Lawson, Jeffrey H. Annals of Surgery251(2):217-228, February 2010. https://doi.org/10.1097/SLA.0b013e3181c3bcca

Polyethylene glycol polymers (Coseal) made by Baxter is a composite of two biocompatible polyethylene glycols combined with dilute hydrogen chloride solution, rapidly forming a hydrogel that allows for adherence of synthetic graft materials to tissue.[1,49,50] It is used almost exclusively during vascular procedures to reinforce suture lines of graft anastomosis.[50] According to Baxter, it is said to fortify suture lines such that bleeding is decreased or prevented even with significant increases in blood pressure.[50] It remains intact for about 7 days as long as no antibiotic ointment or petroleum jelly is applied and is slowly resorbed by the body over a period of 30 days.[1,49,50] One potential disadvantage is the capacity for Coseal to swell more than four times its initial volume, so should be avoided around structures intolerant to compression.[1]

Another similar product is glutaraldehyde cross-link albumin (Bioglue, Cryolife Inc).[1] This is a semisynthetic form that uses albumin (a biologic agent) in its formulation to create a strong film that is effective at hemostasis in large vascular anastomosis and other thoracic and neurosurgical procedures.[1,45] Bioglue has excellent tensile and shear strength, polymerizes quickly, and is rapidly available.[48] These adhesives, however, do not adhere well to wet surfaces.[51] They are also inflammatory, and the inflammation persists until they are completely degraded.[48,51]

CLINICS CARE POINTS

- Caustic hemostats work best when applied topically for small amounts of bleeding during minor procedures. Avoid contact with surrounding healthy tissue because these products are damaging to surrounding tissues.

- Absorbable hemostats can be left in situ and the wound closed with the agents in place; the amount of inflammatory response and granuloma formation depends on the type of absorbable hemostat used.

- Oxidized regenerated cellulose-based hemostats depend on the presence of appropriate coagulation factors to develop clot and achieve hemostasis. Avoid these products in patients with coagulopathies.

- MFCs rely on platelet aggregation and the intrinsic pathway to achieve hemostasis and should be avoided in patients with thrombocytopenia, platelet dysfunction, or factor deficiencies within the intrinsic pathway.

- Absorbable hemostats often expand as they absorb blood and can compress surrounding structures including vessels and nerves. Use caution to avoid compression of important structures and remove excess product before wound closure.

- Gelatin-based products work well on their own but have a synergistic effect when combined with thrombin products.

- For bleeding from bony surfaces consider bone wax or Ostene, but keep in mind that bone wax can inhibit appropriate wound healing. Use only the minimum required amount to achieve hemostasis.

- MPH products help provide hemostasis over broad surface areas even in the setting of underlying coagulopathy. Their powder form makes them easy to apply over a large area even endoscopically.

- Hemostatic dressings, such as chitin, chitosan, combat gauze, QuikClot, Stasilon, and DFSD, are seldom used during operative intervention. However, these products effectively stop bleeding in first aid and combat situations.

- Thrombin products are potent hemostatic agents but require specific storage practices and time-intensive preparation before use. Thrombin is often combined with other hemostatic agents for a synergistic effect.

- Flowable agents combine gelatin and thrombin in formulations that is easily sprayed or spread over the area of bleeding to provide prompt hemostasis. These agents work rapidly and are easily applied endoscopically or during open procedures.
- Fibrin sealants develop artificial clot overlying the area of bleeding and are not dependent on the patient's physiology to aid in hemostasis. However, they are expensive compared with other products.
- See **Table 1** for a full summary of all listed agents.

FUTURE DIRECTIONS

Since their introduction in the 1880s, topical hemostatic agents have continued to develop as knowledge of coagulation physiology and pathophysiology has evolved. The agents commonly used in today's operating rooms, first aid scenes, and battlefields are increasingly effective. The addition of knowledge of hemostatic agents to a surgeon's armamentarium helps to push the boundaries of life-saving care. As understanding of the complex physiology of coagulation and hemorrhage improves, so will the potential for developing hemostatic agents that are safe, affordable, and readily available. Already, scientists, engineers, and surgeons are working to develop better agents to stop hemorrhage (some of which were not mentioned in this article). In today's operating rooms, it is essential to have a firm understanding of how and when to use various hemostatic agents to provide the highest quality care.

DISCLOSURE

No financial disclosures.

REFERENCES

1. Achneck HE, Sileshi B, Jamiolkowski RM, et al. A comprehensive review of topical hemostatic agents: efficacy and recommendations for use. Ann Surg 2010;251(2):217–28.
2. Fagan NL, Chau J, Malesker MA. Topical hemostats. Hematology Web Site. 2010. Available at: https://uspharmacist.com/article/topical-hemostats. Accessed February 17, 2021.
3. Tompeck AJ, Gajdhar AUR, Dowling M, et al. A comprehensive review of topical hemostatic agents: the good, the bad, and the novel. J Trauma Acute Care Surg 2020;88(1):e1–21.
4. Garrett AP, Wenham RM, Sheets EE. Monsel's solution: a brief history. J Low Genit Tract Dis 2002;6(4):225–7.
5. Shuhaiber JH, Lipnick S, Teresi M, et al. More on Monsel's solution. Surgery 2005; 137(2):263–4.
6. Chen CL, Wilson S, Afzalneia R, et al. Topical aluminum chloride and Monsel's solution block toluidine blue staining in Mohs frozen sections: mechanism and solution. Dermatol Surg 2019;45(8):1019–25.
7. Spitzer M, Chernys AE. Monsel's solution-induced artifact in the uterine cervix. Am J Obstet Gynecol 1996;175(5):1204–7.
8. Ho C, Argaez C. In: Topical silver nitrate for the management of hemostasis: a review of clinical effectiveness, cost-effectiveness, and guidelines. Ottawa (ON). 2018.

9. Howe N, Cherpelis B. Obtaining rapid and effective hemostasis: Part I. Update and review of topical hemostatic agents. J Am Acad Dermatol 2013;69(5): 659.e1–17.

10. Healthcare E. WoundClot gauze - advanced bleeding control. 2021. Available at: https://www.eboshealthcare.com.au/woundclot/#:~:text=WoundClot%C2%AE% 20is%20the%20world's,%2C%20moderate%2C%20and%20severe% 20bleeding. Accessed April 26, 2021.

11. Spangler D, Rothenburger S, Nguyen K, et al. In vitro antimicrobial activity of oxidized regenerated cellulose against antibiotic-resistant microorganisms. Surg Infect (Larchmt) 2003;4(3):255–62.

12. Zhang S, Li J, Chen S, et al. Oxidized cellulose-based hemostatic materials. Carbohydr Polym 2020;230:115585.

13. Ethicon. Featuring the latest innovation from the SURGICEL((R)) family of absorbable hemostats. SURGICEL((R)) Family of Absorbable Hemostats Web site. Available at: www.jnjmedicaldevices.com/en-US/product/surgicel-original-absorbable-hemostat. Accessed April 7, 2021.

14. Lewis KM, Spazierer D, Urban MD, et al. Comparison of regenerated and non-regenerated oxidized cellulose hemostatic agents. Eur Surg 2013;45:213–20.

15. MacDonald MH, Tasse L, Wang D, et al. Evaluation of the hemostatic efficacy of two powdered topical absorbable hemostats using a porcine liver abrasion model of mild to moderate bleeding. J Invest Surg 2020;1–9.

16. Parvulescu F, Sundar G, Shortri M. Surgicel on the post-operative CT: an old trap for radiologists. BJR Case Rep 2019;5(4):20190041.

17. Young ST, Paulson EK, McCann RL, et al. Appearance of oxidized cellulose (Surgicel) on postoperative CT scans: similarity to postoperative abscess. AJR Am J Roentgenol 1993;160(2):275–7.

18. BD. Avitene™ Microfibrillar Collagen Hemostat. In: Becton DaC, ed2018.

19. Wellisz T, Armstrong JK, Cambridge J, et al. Ostene, a new water-soluble bone hemostasis agent. J Craniofac Surg 2006;17(3):420–5.

20. BD. Arista™ AH Absorbable hemostat. Becton, Dickinson and Company. 2021. Available at: https://www.bd.com/en-us/offerings/capabilities/biosurgery/ hemostats/arista-ah-absorbable-hemostat. Accessed April 28, 2021.

21. BD. Arista™ AH Absorbable Hemostatic Particles: the latest generation in hemostasis from BD. In: Becton DaC, ed2018.

22. Alhan C, Ariturk C, Senay S, et al. Use of bone wax is related to increased postoperative sternal dehiscence. Kardiochir Torakochirurgia Pol 2014;11(4):385–90.

23. Bhatti F, Dunning J. Does liberal use of bone wax increase the risk of mediastinitis? Interact Cardiovasc Thorac Surg 2003;2(4):410–2.

24. Anitha A, Sowmya S, Sudheesh Kumar PT, et al. Chitin and chitosan in selected biomedical applications. Prog Polym Sci 2014;39(9):1644–67.

25. Muxika A, Etxabide A, Uranga J, et al. Chitosan as a bioactive polymer: processing, properties and applications. Int J Biol Macromol 2017;105(Pt 2):1358–68.

26. Wang YW, Liu CC, Cherng JH, et al. Biological effects of chitosan-based dressing on hemostasis mechanism. Polymers (Basel) 2019;11(11):1906.

27. Klokkevold PR, Fukayama H, Sung EC, et al. The effect of chitosan (poly-N-acetyl glucosamine) on lingual hemostasis in heparinized rabbits. J Oral Maxillofac Surg 1999;57(1):49–52.

28. Cripps MW, Cornelius CC, Nakonezny PA, et al. In vitro effects of a kaolin-coated hemostatic dressing on anticoagulated blood. J Trauma Acute Care Surg 2018; 85(3):485–90.

29. Trabattoni D, Montorsi P, Fabbiocchi F, et al. A new kaolin-based haemostatic bandage compared with manual compression for bleeding control after percutaneous coronary procedures. Eur Radiol 2011;21(8):1687–91.

30. Kheirabadi BS, Scherer MR, Estep JS, et al. Determination of efficacy of new hemostatic dressings in a model of extremity arterial hemorrhage in swine. J Trauma 2009;67(3):450–9 [discussion: 459-460].

31. Gajjar CR, McCord MG, King MW. Hemostatic wound dressings. In: King MW, Gupta BS, Guidoin R, editors. Biotextiles as Medical Implants. Woodhead Publishing Series in textiles: Woodhead Publishing; 2013. p. 563–89.

32. Causey MW, McVay DP, Miller S, et al. The efficacy of Combat Gauze in extreme physiologic conditions. J Surg Res 2012;177(2):301–5.

33. Rich PB, Douillet C, Buchholz V, et al. Use of the novel hemostatic textile Stasilon(R) to arrest refractory retroperitoneal hemorrhage: a case report. J Med Case Rep 2010;4:20.

34. Fischer TH, Vournakis JN, Manning JE, et al. The design and testing of a dual fiber textile matrix for accelerating surface hemostasis. J Biomed Mater Res B Appl Biomater 2009;91(1):381–9.

35. Pusateri AE, Kheirabadi BS, Delgado AV, et al. Structural design of the dry fibrin sealant dressing and its impact on the hemostatic efficacy of the product. J Biomed Mater Res B Appl Biomater 2004;70(1):114–21.

36. Holcomb JB, Pusateri AE, Harris RA, et al. Effect of dry fibrin sealant dressings versus gauze packing on blood loss in grade V liver injuries in resuscitated swine. J Trauma 1999;46(1):49–57.

37. Holcomb JB, Pusateri AE, Harris RA, et al. Dry fibrin sealant dressings reduce blood loss, resuscitation volume, and improve survival in hypothermic coagulopathic swine with grade V liver injuries. J Trauma 1999;47(2):233–40 [discussion: 240-232].

38. Holcomb J, MacPhee M, Hetz S, et al. Efficacy of a dry fibrin sealant dressing for hemorrhage control after ballistic injury. Arch Surg 1998;133(1):32–5.

39. Baxter. TachoSil Fibrin Sealant Patch. Informational pamphlet. In: Corporation BH, ed: Baxter International Inc.; 2016.

40. Genyk Y, Kato T, Pomposelli JJ, et al. Fibrin sealant patch (TachoSil) vs oxidized regenerated cellulose patch (Surgicel original) for the secondary treatment of local bleeding in patients undergoing hepatic resection: a randomized controlled trial. J Am Coll Surg 2016;222(3):261–8.

41. Ho J, Hruza G. Hydrophilic polymers with potassium salt and microporous polysaccharides for use as hemostatic agents. Dermatol Surg 2007;33(12):1430–3.

42. Lomax C, Traub O. Topical thrombins: benefits and risks. Pharmacotherapy 2009;29(7 Pt 2):8S–12S.

43. Narayanan S. Multifunctional roles of thrombin. Ann Clin Lab Sci 1999;29(4):275–80.

44. Sileshi B, Achneck HE, Lawson JH. Management of surgical hemostasis: topical agents. Vascular 2008;16(Suppl 1):S22–8.

45. Emilia M, Luca S, Francesca B, et al. Topical hemostatic agents in surgical practice. Transfus Apher Sci 2011;45(3):305–11.

46. Pereira BM, Bortoto JB, Fraga GP. Topical hemostatic agents in surgery: review and prospects. Rev Col Bras Cir 2018;45(5):e1900.

47. Prior JJ, Wallace DG, Harner A, et al. A sprayable hemostat containing fibrillar collagen, bovine thrombin, and autologous plasma. Ann Thorac Surg 1999;68(2):479–85.

48. Bao Z, Gao M, Sun Y, et al. The recent progress of tissue adhesives in design strategies, adhesive mechanism and applications. Mater Sci Eng C Mater Biol Appl 2020;111:110796.

49. Baxter. Advanced Surgery- Coseal. Informational pamphlet. In: Baxter, ed2016.

50. Baxter. Coseal Surgical Sealant. Informational pamphlet. In: Incorporated BI, ed2016.

51. Jakob H, Campbell CD, Stemberger A, et al. Combined application of heterologous collagen and fibrin sealant for liver injuries. J Surg Res 1984;36(6):571–7.

52. Lew WK, Weaver FA. Clinical use of topical thrombin as a surgical hemostat. Biologics 2008;2(4):593–9.

Critical Care Management of Surgical Patients with Heart Failure or Left Ventricular Assist Devices: A Brief Overview

Mohsin A. Zaidi, MD[a],*, Carl R. Christenson, MD[b]

KEYWORDS

- Heart failure • LVAD (left ventricular assist device) • Noncardiac surgery
- Mechanical circulatory support

KEY POINTS

- The surgical patient with heart failure introduces unique challenges to effective care.
- Volume management and avoidance of acute decompensation are the main therapeutic goals.
- Patients with left ventricular assist devices (LVAD) are increasingly prevalent, and surgical intensivists must be prepared to manage these patients.
- LVADs require adequate preload and avoiding excessive afterload.

HEART FAILURE

Introduction

Heart failure (HF) is defined as the reduction of the heart's ability to either generate force for forward flow or adequately fill with blood. Physiologically, HF is the mismatch of cardiac output (CO) to systemic demands.[1]

Subtypes of HF include heart failure with reduced ejection fraction (HFrEF) previously named *systolic HF* and heart failure with preserved ejection fraction previously named *diastolic HF*. By describing the primary site of impairment, HF can be identified as left ventricular (LV), right ventricular (RV), or biventricular. Chronicity further subdivides HF into acute versus chronic.

[a] Anesthesiology and Critical Care Medicine, Department of Anesthesiology, University of Cincinnati College of Medicine, 231 Albert Sabin Way, Cincinnati, OH 45267, USA;
[b] Department of Anesthesiology, University of Cincinnati College of Medicine, 231 Albert Sabin Way, M.L. 0531, Cincinnati, OH 45267, USA
* Corresponding author.
E-mail address: Mohsin.zaidi@uc.edu

Surg Clin N Am 102 (2022) 85–104
https://doi.org/10.1016/j.suc.2021.09.002
0039-6109/22/© 2021 Elsevier Inc. All rights reserved.

Prevalence

It is estimated that more than 26 million people worldwide have HF. In the United States, nearly 6 million people have HF with more than 8 million projected to have HF by 2030, a 46% increase in prevalence.[1]

Causes

There are multiple causes of HF. These are summarized in **Table 1**.

Biomarkers

Biomarker testing can be beneficial in evaluating HF exacerbation. See **Table 2** for common tests used for diagnosis and trending.

MANAGEMENT OF THE SURGICAL PATIENT WITH HEART FAILURE
Volume Management

The same principles of HF management apply to both surgical and nonsurgical patients. Avoidance of acute decompensation is of paramount importance, and volume management is the foundation of this goal.[2] There are various modalities to assess volume status including clinical examination, Swan-Ganz catheter, and point-of-care ultrasonography; details of these are beyond the scope of this review.

Volume overload can be avoided by resumption of the patient's home diuretic regimen and fluid and salt restriction. In critically ill patients with postoperative HF, although routine use is not recommended, a Swan-Ganz catheter can be used for goal-directed therapy, targeting a central venous pressure (CVP) less than 8 mm Hg and pulmonary capillary wedge pressure less than 16 mm Hg.[3]

Hypotension

Treatment of hypotension in patients with HF varies depending on the specific cause. Before considering hypovolemia or vasodilation, a primary cardiogenic cause should be excluded. In the authors' experience, in the latter scenario, diuresis and optimization of the patient's Frank-Starling curve, not administration of fluid or vasopressor, often improves hemodynamics. Inotropes can be considered if parameters do not improve.

Contradictory evidence exists regarding vasopressor effects on some surgical repairs, including intestinal anastomoses, free flaps for reconstruction, and pancreatectomy.[4–6] However, fluid administration can be more detrimental to these patients' hemodynamics, which also subsequently affects the integrity of their surgical repair.

If a primary cardiogenic cause is excluded, we recommend the following:

- Test fluid responsiveness with passive leg raise or small fluid bolus (250 mL).
  - If indicated, slow transfusion of blood products can be substituted.
- Repeat judicious fluid boluses.
- If refractory hypotension, initiate vasopressor infusion.
  - Norepinephrine is preferred, given its modest augmentation of contractility and less deleterious effect on splanchnic circulation compared with vasopressin.[7]
- Titrate to appropriate markers and signs of end-organ perfusion.

Afterload Reduction

Vasodilators are often a mainstay of therapy in patients with HFrEF to reduce the work of the weakened LV. Oral nitrates or hydralazine are often used for chronic HF management. In acute decompensated HF, parenteral afterload reducers like nitroglycerin

Table 1
Causes of heart failure

Ischemic cardiomyopathy	Nonischemic Cardiomyopathy	Nonmyocardial
Coronary disease with active ischemia	Dilated cardiomyopathy • Idiopathic • Drug induced • Peripartum • Infection (viral, parasitic, etc) • Sepsis • Takotsubo (stress induced)	Congenital defects
Past myocardial infarctions	Restrictive cardiomyopathy • Infiltrative disease (amyloidosis, sarcoidosis)	Valvular • Stenosis leading to chamber hypertrophy • Regurgitation leading to dilated chambers
	Hypertrophic cardiomyopathy	Pericardial

Data from Herzog E. Herzog's CCUBook. Philadelphia: Wolters Kluwer; 2018.

and nitroprusside are often required to control filling pressures and afterload; this often requires titration via pulmonary artery catheter and/or echocardiography.[3]

Resumption of Chronic Medications

In the absence of hemodynamic instability, these patients should have their home HF medications restarted postoperatively; this includes β-blockers (BB), antiarrhythmics, diuretics, angiotensin-converting enzyme inhibitors (ACEi) or angiotensin receptor blockers (ARB), and mineralocorticoid receptor antagonists (MRA).[8] Conversion to intravenous forms or administration via feeding tube may be required.

Home BB should be restarted immediately to avoid observed increases in mortality in patients with HF whose BB were not restarted during hospitalization.[9] Although often arbitrarily held postoperatively, ACEi or ARB should be resumed postoperatively unless hypotension, acute kidney injury, or electrolyte imbalance develops. Prolonged withholding of ACEi or ARB has been shown to increase 30-day mortality in postoperative patients with HF.[10,11] Finally MRA, such as spironolactone, should be resumed postoperatively with careful monitoring of renal function and potassium levels.

Monitoring

Patients with HF require close monitoring while hospitalized. Some of the more common monitors are summarized in **Table 3**.

Acute Decompensated Heart Failure

Acute decompensation is particularly problematic in the postoperative patient with HF. Goals include achieving euvolemia, maintenance of perfusion to vital organs, afterload reduction, and direct myocardial support. Diuresis with loop diuretic boluses or infusion is often needed, and renal replacement therapy may be required in the setting of renal dysfunction or poor response to diuresis. Inotropes and vasopressors can be used for direct myocardial augmentation and to maintain systemic perfusion pressure, respectively. Afterload reduction can be achieved with parenteral vasodilators. Consider temporary mechanical circulatory support (MCS) in refractory cases.

Table 2		
Biomarkers in heart failure		
Biomarker (Serum)	**Source or Definition**	**Interpretation**
BNP[a]	Released secondary to LV wall stress	In acute decompensated HF(>100 pg/mL)
NT-proBNP[a]	Terminal amino acid equivalent to BNP. Released secondary to LV wall stress	In acute decompensated HF (>900 pg/mL)
Serum creatinine[a] and BUN	Elevated in renal dysfunction	Independent markers of hospital mortality
Liver function tests	Transaminases, serum albumin, bilirubin	Suggestive of hepatic congestion due to RV failure
Hemoglobin/haematocrit	Anemia	Anemia is an independent predictor of mortality in HF
Troponin	Released from cardiac myocytes	Myocardial necrosis from infarction
Lactate	Excessive anaerobic metabolism	Poor prognostic indicator in acute HF decompensation

Abbreviations: BNP, brain natriuretic peptide; BUN, blood urea nitrogen.
[a] Patients with chronic kidney disease have higher baseline due to reduced filtration of these markers.
Data from Ibrahim NE, Januzzi JL. Established and emerging roles of biomarkers in heart failure. Circ Res. 2018;123(5):614–29; Fonarow GC, Adams KF, Abraham WT, et al. Risk stratification for in-hospital mortality in acutely decompensated heart failure: classification and regression tree analysis. JAMA. 2005;293(5):572–80.

Inotropes and Pressors

Some important considerations:

- In decompensated HF, dobutamine and milrinone are the most commonly used inotropes.
- Inotropes increase myocardial demand and can cause myocardial ischemia.
- Use vasoconstrictors with caution due to increases in systemic vascular resistance (SVR) and pulmonary vascular resistance (PVR), and consequently LV and RV afterload, respectively.
- Perform frequent assessment of ventricular function (echocardiography or biomarker trends) while on inotropes.

See **Table 4** for a summary of the commonly used agents in HF.

Clinics Care Points for Heart Failure

- Avoid acute decompensated heart failure (ADHF) by resuming home HF medications as soon as safely possible and avoiding volume overload.
- Consider the underlying cause of your patient's HF when managing hemodynamic instability.
- Consider the risks and benefits when choosing between fluid resuscitation and use of vasopressors postoperatively.
- ADHF may require parenteral inotrope and vasodilator therapy guided by Swan-Ganz catheter, or even temporary mechanical support. We recommend cardiology consultation in this scenario.

Table 3
Common monitors used for patients with heart failure or mechanical circulatory support

Monitor Type	Common Uses	Advantages	Disadvantages
Arterial line	• Active, or high risk of hemodynamic instability • Patient with LVAD/MCS: beneficial where frequent Doppler measurement is impractical	• Provides accurate determination of BP in real time • Ideal for patients with MCS/LVAD with continuous, rather than pulsatile, flow	• May be difficult to place due to artery sclerosis from repeated cannulations • Readings can be affected by patient movement • Invasive: can cause rare arterial thrombosis
Oscillometric cuff	• Automated BP monitor; ubiquitous in the inpatient and operating room setting	• Inexpensive • Noninvasive • No special training required	• Limited use in patients with LVAD and MCS due to lack of pulsatile blood flow • Accuracy affected by cuff size and location, and movement
FloTrac (Edwards Lifesciences, Irvine CA, USA) or similar devices using SVV and pulse contour tracing	• May guide volume management and hemodynamic support • Can be used to show trends in hemodynamics • Developed to replace Swan-Ganz	• Can estimate parameters such as CO, SV, and SVR • Invasive (requires arterial line) and noninvasive options (finger probe)	• Conflicting studies concerning accuracy Criteria to use SVV include: • Controlled mechanical ventilated with low PEEP • Tidal volumes 8 mL/kg • Normal sinus rhythm or paced • Pulsatile blood flow • No vasoactive medications that alter vascular tone
Pulmonary artery catheter (Swan-Ganz)	• Remains the gold standard • Directly measures filling pressures and mixed-venous oxygen saturation	• Multiple parameters can be calculated, including CO, SVR, SV, etc • Can guide interventions to reduce filling pressures and/or augment contractility	• Accuracy depends on operator and physician experience • Routine use is not recommended • Rare, but catastrophic adverse events (ie, pulmonary artery rupture, pulmonary embolism)

(continued on next page)

Table 3
(continued)

Monitor Type	Common Uses	Advantages	Disadvantages
TTE or TEE	• Determination of volume status • Can determine EF, CO, and altered wall motion	• Real-time evaluation of structure and function • TTE: Noninvasive. Can be done at the bedside • TEE: Superb views of nearly all cardiac structures	• Interpretation requires training and is operator dependent • TTE: Views can be obscured by patient habitus, recent thoracic surgery, and implanted devices • TEE: Invasive and requires sedation

Abbreviations: BP, blood pressure; EF, ejection fraction; MCS, mechanical circulatory support; PEEP, positive end-expiratory pressure; SV, stroke volume; SVR, systemic vascular resistance; SVV; TEE, transesophageal echocardiography; TTE, transthoracic echocardiography.

Data from Lancellotti P, Price S, Edvardsen T, et al. The use of echocardiography in acute cardiovascular care: recommendations of the European Association of Cardiovascular Imaging and the Acute Cardiovascular Care Association. Eur Heart J Acute Cardiovasc Care. 2015;4(1):3–5; Li C, Lin FQ, Fu SK, et al. Stroke volume variation for prediction of fluid responsiveness in patients undergoing gastrointestinal surgery. Int J Med Sci. 2013;10(2):148–55; Binanay C, Califf RM, Hasselblad V, et al. Evaluation study of congestive heart failure and pulmonary artery catheterization effectiveness: the ESCAPE trial. JAMA. 2005;294(13):1625–33; Lewis PS, British and Irish Hypertension Society's Blood Pressure Measurement Working Party. Oscillometric measurement of blood pressure: a simplified explanation. A technical note on behalf of the British and Irish Hypertension Society. J Hum Hypertens. 2019;33(5):349–51.

Table 4
Common vasoactive drugs used in decompensated heart failure

Medication	Mechanism of Action	Considerations	Adverse effects
Dopamine	• Alpha-1 and beta-1 receptor agonist • Dopamine receptor agonist	Dose-dependent effects: • Low dose: vasodilation of renal vasculature (dopamine receptor agonism) • Medium dose: inotropy and chronotropy (beta agonism). • High dose: vasoconstriction (alpha agonism)	• Arrhythmogenic • Rarely used in HF due to lack of evidence for benefit and better alternatives
Dobutamine	• Synthetic analogue of dopamine with beta-1 and beta-2 adrenergic agonist effects • Used primarily as an inotrope, but also increases chronotropy	• Typical doses increase inotropy with mild peripheral vasodilation that may cause hypotension • Tolerance can develop, necessitating higher doses over time • Short half-life	• Arrhythmogenic • Hypotension • Increases myocardial O_2 demand • Rare eosinophilic myocarditis
Norepinephrine	• Alpha-1 and beta-1 adrenergic receptor agonist. • Potent vasoconstrictor with modest inotropic and chronotropic effects	• First-line vasopressor for hypotensive patients in cardiogenic or septic shock • Used to offset hypotension of inodilators • Less splanchnic vasoconstriction than vasopressin	• Increased myocardial O_2 demand • Can be arrhythmogenic
Epinephrine	• Alpha-1 and beta-1 and beta-2 adrenergic agonist • Potent vasoconstrictor, inotrope, and chronotrope	• Vasoconstricts both systemic and pulmonary circulations • Increased mortality in cardiogenic shock, therefore rarely used except short-term use in cardiac arrest or refractory shock	• Lactic acidosis • Arrhythmogenic • Splanchnic and myocardial hypoperfusion
Milrinone	• Inodilator • Phosphodiesterase-3 inhibitor (nonadrenergic)	• Ideal for patients on chronic β-blockers • Decreases pulmonary vascular resistance	• Hypotension • Arrhythmogenic • Decreased clearance in renal dysfunction

(continued on next page)

Table 4 (continued)			
Medication	**Mechanism of Action**	**Considerations**	**Adverse effects**
		• Often requires pairing with a vasoconstrictor like norepinephrine	
Vasopressin	• V-1 and V-2 receptors • Vasoconstriction via V-1 receptors • Free water resorption via V-2 receptors	• May allow catecholamine sparing in catecholamine-depleted states • May allow reduction in dose of norepinephrine for inotrope-induced vasodilation • No direct myocardial effect	• Cardiac ischemia • Splanchnic vasoconstriction • Increases afterload without compensatory inotropic effect

Data from Bistola V, Arfaras-Melainis A, Polyzogopoulou E, et al. Inotropes in acute heart failure: from guidelines to practical use: therapeutic options and clinical practice. Card Fail Rev. 2019;5(3):133–39; Overgaard CB, Dzavik V. Inotropes and vasopressors: review of physiology and clinical use in cardiovascular disease. Circulation. 2008;118(10):1047–56; Farmakis D, Agostoni P, Baholli L, et al. A pragmatic approach to the use of inotropes for the management of acute and advanced heart failure: an expert panel consensus. Int J Cardiol. 2019;297:83–90.

MECHANICAL CIRCULATORY SUPPORT
Introduction

Although heart transplant remains the gold standard treatment for end-stage HF, less than 5% of patients with end-stage HF qualify, and therefore alternatives are required.[3] MCS provides temporary or permanent support for the failing heart. Devices include venoarterial extracorporeal membrane oxygenation (VA-ECMO), Impella (Abiomed Inc, Danvers, MA, USA), TandemHeart (LivaNova,PLC; Boston, MA, USA), Total Artificial Heart (SynCardia, Tucson, AZ, USA), right ventricular assist devices (RVAD), and implantable LVADs.

Left Ventricular Assist Devices

LVADs assist and functionally replace the native LV by providing continuous blood flow from the LV to the aorta, thereby decreasing the work of the LV. The device is surgically implanted, usually via midline sternotomy, and less commonly via left thoracotomy.

The earliest ventricular assist devices were used by DeBakey and Liotta in the 1960s. In the early 2000s, the US Food and Drug Administration approved the first LVAD for long-term use, and from 2006 to the time of this review, more than 18,000 LVADs have been implanted worldwide.[12] At present, there are 3 indications for LVAD implantation: bridge to recovery of native cardiac function, bridge to heart transplant, and destination therapy.[13]

Use of durable implantable devices for circulatory support has increased exponentially over the last 2 decades. Today, LVAD patients will likely have one of the following devices: Heartmate II (Abbott; Abbott Park, IL, USA), which uses an axial flow pump (**Fig. 1**); the HeartWare HVAD (Medtronic; Minneapolis, MN, USA); or the Heartmate 3 (HM3; Abbott; Abbott Park, IL, USA), the last two using centrifugal flow pumps

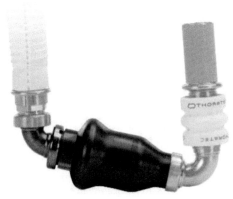

Fig. 1. Heartmate II: (*From* https://www.cardiovascular.abbott/us/en/hcp/products/heart-failure/left-ventricular-assist[1]devices/heartmate-2/about.htm. HeartMate II, HeartMate 3, and Thoratec are trademarks of Abbott or its related companies. Reproduced with permission of Abbott, © 2021. All rights reserved.)

(**Figs. 2 and 3**). These devices have been approved for destination therapy and bridging to transplant or recovery. At the time of this review the HM3 is the newest generation model of LVAD and has shown similar 2-year survival compared to heart transplant (87% HM3 vs 85% transplant).[14] Centrifugal flow pumps, specifically the HM3, are now the most common LVADs being implanted.[15] See **Table 5** for a comparison of the currently used LVADs. Of note, an alert from the U.S. Food and Drug Administration in June 2021 instructed providers to no longer implant the HVAD system due to new evidence showing increased complications, including pump failure, stroke, and mortality.

Left Ventricular Assist Device Components

- Driveline: Wire that connects external components to the internal pump. Usually tunneled under the skin of the abdomen.
- Controller/console: Used to adjust speed and monitor parameters. Delivers power to the pump via batteries or AC power.
- Pump: Internal motor with an impeller.
- Inflow cannula: Sewn into the LV apex to drain blood from the LV and deliver it to the pump.
- Outflow cannula: Sewn into the aorta and delivers blood from the pump to the systemic circulation.

See **Figs. 4 and 5** to see a complete LVAD system.

LEFT VENTRICULAR ASSIST DEVICE PARAMETERS
Pump Speed

Pump speed is the only variable that can be directly adjusted by the operator. All other parameters described here are measured. The range of speeds that can be set vary depending on the specific model. The ideal pump speed unloads the LV and consequently decreases RV workload, without causing significant hemolysis or suction events.[16] A visual assessment via echocardiography of the interventricular septum can help determine optimal speed.[16] Newer-generation LVADs attempt to simulate pulsatile flow by automated intermittent modulation of their pump speed.[17,18]

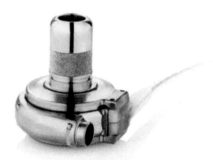

Fig. 2. HeartWare HVAD: https://www.medtronic.com/us-en/healthcare-professionals/products/cardiac-rhythm/ventricular-assist-devices/hvad-system.html.

Pump Power

Pump power, measured in watts, is the power output required to drive blood forward at the set pump speed. Observed gradual or abrupt increases in power consumption can be a diagnostic indicator of increased resistance to flow within the pump.

Pump Flow

Pump flow, measured in liters per minute, is estimated by the controller. Pump flow is a function of power consumption at the set pump speed and corresponds to the "cardiac output" of the device.[17] The actual flow rate is determined by the pressure gradient across the device, defined as the difference between outflow pressure and inflow pressure, analogous to the aortic and LV pressures, respectively.[19]

Pulsatility Index

The pulsatility index (PI) is the representation of the flow through the pump due to the patient's native contractility. Changes in the PI can represent changes in the patient's native cardiac function or volume status and are also helpful in diagnosing complications.[20]

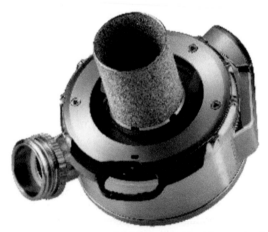

Fig. 3. Heartmate 3: (*From* https://www.cardiovascular.abbott/us/en/hcp/products/heart-failure/left[1]ventricular-assist-devices/heartmate-3/about.html. HeartMate 3 is a trademark of Abbott or its related companies. Reproduced with permission of Abbott, © 2021. All rights reserved.)

Table 5
Comparison of current left ventricular assist device models

Device Model	Pump Type	Model-Specific Information	Normal Parameters
HVAD	Centrifugal	First LVAD to be approved for implantation via less-invasive thoracotomy	Speed (rpm): 2400–3200 Power (W): 3–7 PI: 2–4 Flow (lpm): 4–6
Heartmate II	Axial	Most common device found in patients with existing LVAD[a] Less commonly implanted now with advent of the Heartmate 3	Speed (rpm): 8000–10,000 Power (W): 5–8 PI: 5–8 Flow (lpm): 4–7
Heartmate 3	Centrifugal via magnetic levitation	Newest device[b] Simulates pulsatile flow Less likely to cause pump thrombosis than Heartmate II	Speed (rpm): 5000–6000 Power (W): 4.5–6.5 PI: 3.5–5.5 Flow (lpm): 4–6

Abbreviation: PI, pulsatility index.
[a] At the time of this review.
[b] Most common LVAD being newly implanted in the United States at the time of this review.
Data from DeVore AD, Patel PA, Patel CB. Medical management of patients with a left ventricular assist device for the non-left ventricular assist device specialist. JACC Heart Fail. 2017;5(9):621–31.

LEFT VENTRICULAR ASSIST DEVICE MANAGEMENT

LVAD management is best performed at facilities where these devices are implanted.[21] However, given their increasing prevalence, patients may present for surgical care at facilities without LVAD-specific resources. A cohort study of more than 8000 LVAD patients revealed that 16.3% underwent noncardiac surgery (NCS) after implantation in a 5-year period, 75% of which were urgent/emergent procedures. Perioperative major adverse cardiac events occurred in nearly 30% undergoing NCS.[22] In a retrospective case series, acute kidney injury, hypotension, elevated lactate dehydrogenase, and bleeding were the most common major complications after NCS, with a 30-day postoperative mortality rate of 5.3%.[23] These studies illustrate the significant risk taken when performing procedures on the LVAD population.

Although ideally these patients should be transferred to an appropriate facility for specialized care, surgical intensivists must be prepared to manage common device issues. Management principles are similar among all the currently used LVADs, but device-specific strategies do exist. Consultation with cardiologists or the device manufacturer may be warranted.

Hemodynamic Monitoring in Patients with Left Ventricular Assist Devices

Special considerations in patients with LVADs:

- Given the lack of normal pulsatile flow, mean arterial pressure (MAP) is the primary hemodynamic variable used.
- Automated blood pressure (BP) cuff measurement may not be accurate due to lack of normal pulsatile flow.
- Manual BP measurement using bedside Doppler can be performed.
- Arterial line placement should be strongly considered in any critically ill LVAD patients.

Refer to **Table 2** for a summary of the commonly used monitors.

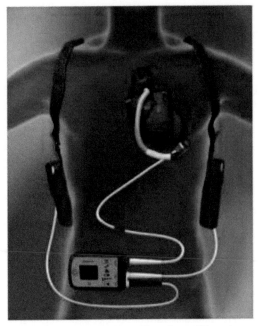

Fig. 4. Heartmate 3 system. (HeartMate II, HeartMate 3, and Thoratec are trademarks of Abbott or its related companies. Reproduced with permission of Abbott, © 2021. All rights reserved).

Preload

LVADs are preload dependent. The device will only pump what it receives from the RV, assuming adequate RV function, which in turn depends on venous return. Impedance of venous return, such as with hypovolemia, venodilation, or increased intrathoracic pressure, will lead to decreased preload. Furthermore, situations that impede flow from the RV to the LV, such as pulmonary embolism or RV failure, will lead to poor

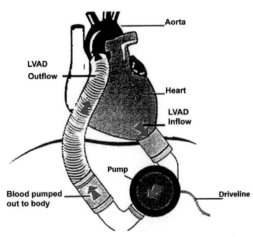

Fig. 5. Schematic of LVAD components. (*Adapted, with alterations, from* Helmy SM, Albinali A, Hajar R. Echocardiography in left ventricular assist device. Heart Views 2010;11:74–6.)

filling of the LV and LVAD. If the LVAD has poor preload at a given speed, flow will decrease.

Afterload

LVADs are also afterload sensitive. Changes in SVR or afterload will directly affect LVAD pump flow. High afterload (MAP >90 mm Hg) will decrease pump output and can lead to such resistance to flow that thrombus can form within the pump. Conversely, hypotension (low afterload) with MAP less than 65 mmHg, while increasing LVAD flow at a given pump speed, can lead to organ malperfusion. Some recommendations state that the MAP should be maintained less than 80 mm Hg.[16,20,24] A goal MAP range of 65 to 85 mm Hg is more practical. Any MAP greater than 90 mm Hg should warrant immediate treatment because the current devices have limited capability to adapt to significant increases in afterload.[25]

Right Ventricular Function

The LVAD does not provide direct support to the RV and in fact depends on a working RV to deliver preload to the device. It is imperative to protect RV function by avoiding volume overload and using similar principles of volume management previously discussed in patients with HF. In addition, PVR must be minimized by avoiding hypoxia, hypercarbia, acidosis, and high airway pressures. Assessment of RV function can include PA catheterization, CVP monitoring, and echocardiography. If the RV is failing, judicious diuresis, pulmonary vasodilators, and inotropes should be used to augment function and additional mechanical support should be considered (ie, VA-ECMO or RVAD).[24]

Anticoagulation

LVAD patients must be anticoagulated to avoid catastrophic thrombosis of the device. The mainstay of therapy is warfarin combined with an antiplatelet agent, usually aspirin. The currently recommended goal international normalized ratio (INR) is 2.0 to 3.0.[24] Heparin bridging is recommended when warfarin therapy must be temporarily stopped.[24] If discontinued for surgery, anticoagulation must be restarted as soon as safely possible to prevent pump thrombosis.[26]

TROUBLESHOOTING ABNORMAL LEFT VENTRICULAR ASSIST DEVICE PARAMETERS

Changes in parameters displayed on the controller can reveal patient or device complications; these are summarized in **Table 6**.

Low Flow

Low flow occurs secondary to numerous physiologic and mechanical conditions. Decreased intravascular volume, RV failure leading to decreased LV preload, sustained systemic hypertension (high afterload), tamponade, device thrombus, and mechanical obstruction of the inflow cannula can all lead to a decreased output from the device.[20] Management of low flow depends on determining the underlying cause and treating accordingly.

Suction Events

Suction events usually result from an abrupt decrease in preload at a set pump speed where negative pressure forces a portion of the LV wall against the pump inlet[16]; this decreases flow and can result in hypotension and ventricular arrhythmias.[20] The controller will usually sound an alarm and compensate by automatically reducing

Table 6
Changes in left ventricular assist device parameters

Issue	Differential diagnosis	Management
Low flows	• Hypovolemia • Tamponade • Pulmonary embolism • RV failure • Arrhythmia	• Small-volume bolus • Relieve obstruction based on specific cause • Inotropes • Pharmacologic or electrical cardioversion
High flows with hypotension (MAP<60 mm Hg)	• Vasodilation • Septic shock	• Vasopressors • Cultures and antibiotics
Low power	• Device malfunction	• Check driveline and power supply or battery
High power	• Pump thrombosis, until proven otherwise • Resistance to flow	• Anticoagulation • Immediate cardiac surgery consult for possible pump exchange
Low PI	• Hypovolemia • Too much support • Worsening native LV function	• Small-volume bolus • Decrease pump speed • Consider inotropes
High PI	• Improving native LV function • Device malfunction	• Potential for discontinuation of LVAD support • Check connections, contact manufacturer

Adapted from Feldman D, Pamboukian SV, Teuteberg JJ, et al. The 2013 International Society for Heart and Lung Transplantation Guidelines for mechanical circulatory support: executive summary. J Heart Lung Transplant. 2013;32(2):157 to 187, with permission.

pump speed enough to release the suction. Increasing preload with fluid administration as well as decreasing the set pump speed will usually address this issue.[20]

COMPLICATIONS AND TREATMENT STRATEGIES

Common complications and their management are summarized in **Table 7**

Bleeding

LVAD patients require anticoagulation to avoid thrombosis. Furthermore, most patients develop an acquired, reversible von Willebrand factor deficiency due to the sheer forces created by the pump. These factors lead to hemorrhage being the most common adverse event in LVAD patients.[27]

The gastrointestinal tract is the most common site of bleeding in these patients.[28] The increased incidence of gastrointestinal bleeding is hypothesized to be related to the formation of arteriovenous malformations and increased vessel friability from the absence of normal pulsatile blood flow.[16] Workup should start with upper and lower endoscopy, which also allows treatment at the site of hemorrhage.

During the acute phase of bleeding, anticoagulation therapies should be held but must be promptly restarted after hemostasis is obtained to decrease the risk of LVAD thrombus.[16] Platelet transfusion can help mitigate the effects of antiplatelet agents, whereas fresh frozen plasma and vitamin K can be given to reverse warfarin anticoagulation.[20] If hemorrhage is not controlled by the aforementioned measures,

Table 7
Left ventricular assist device complications

Issue	Common Causes	Diagnosis	Management
Bleeding	• GI tract • Brain • Uterine	• Upper and lower endoscopy • Imaging • Clinical examination	• Hold anticoagulation • Consider reversal of anticoagulants • Treat site of bleeding if possible
Thrombosis	• Inadequate anticoagulation • Persistent low flows • Cannula malposition • High afterload (MAP >90) leading to stasis within the pump	• Check hemolysis markers (LDH, plasma-free hemoglobin) • Signs of cardiogenic shock • High-power Echo findings • LV dilation • ↑ Mitral regurgitation • ↑ Aortic valve opening (reduced flow through the pump)	• Anticoagulation • Optimize preload and afterload • Fibrinolytics • Immediate cardiac surgery consultation for possible pump exchange
Mechanical malfunction	• Power disconnected • Battery drained • Driveline damage	• Device will alarm • Check connections	• Restore power or connections immediately • Support patient by alternative means (inotropes, alternative MCS) • Immediate cardiac surgery consult
Neurologic change	• Ischemic stroke • Embolic stroke • Hemorrhagic stroke	• Noncontrast head CT • Frequent neurologic checks	*If hemorrhagic:* • Hold anticoagulation • Neurosurgical consultation *If ischemic:* • Start IV heparin • Consider thrombolytics or mechanical thrombectomy • Rule out LVAD thrombus
Infection	• Usually driveline, rarely the pump itself	• Pan-culture • Echocardiography to rule out endocarditis	• IV antimicrobials • Driveline debridement • Refractory cases may warrant device exchange

Abbreviations: ↑, increase; CT, computed tomography; GI, gastrointestinal; IV, intravenous; LDH, lactate dehydrogenase.
Data from Refs.[16,20,24,28] and Stainback RF, Estep JD, Agler DA, et al. Echocardiography in the management of patients with left ventricular assist devices: recommendations from the American Society of Echocardiography. J Am Soc Echocardiogr. 2015;28(8):853–909.

prothrombin complex concentrate and recombinant factor VII have been used; however, their use will significantly increase the risk of pump thrombosis.[20]

Thrombosis

Pump thrombosis occurs at a rate of 8% per year.[20]
    Signs of thrombosis may include:

- Clinical manifestations: hypotension, cardiogenic shock, and hematuria (secondary to hemolysis). Some are asymptomatic.
- Device manifestations: increased power and low flow.

Intravenous heparin drip is the initial treatment. An increased target INR or an additional antiplatelet agent may also be warranted.[24] Pump exchange can be performed in cases of refractory thrombus. If the patient is a poor candidate for pump exchange, intravenous thrombolysis can be considered in discussion with cardiology or cardiac surgery.[24] Fortunately, the MOMENTUM3 trial showed that patients now receiving the HM3 device are far less likely to develop thrombus than its axial pump predecessor.[29]

Mechanical Malfunction

The driveline, controller, or pump can rarely be the cause of instability. A spare controller and batteries should be quickly available. Infection or external damage to the driveline can result in pump malfunction or even failure. Radiographic examination may demonstrate kinking, fraying, or interruption of the driveline internally.[20] We recommend the driveline be imaged and marked on the skin to avoid inadvertent damage from incisions, paracentesis, or drain insertion.

Stroke

Although the incidence of stroke has decreased with the newest generation of LVAD, it remains a devastating complication in these patients. Any neurologic change in a LVAD patients warrants high suspicion for cerebrovascular accident. Head computed tomographic imaging must be obtained to determine the type of stroke, because this will determine whether to adjust or hold anticoagulation. Poststroke management is similar to that in non-LVAD patients.[24]

Infection

Infection is the fourth leading cause of death in LVAD patients.[30] The most common site of infection is the driveline, because it is a direct conduit between the external environment and internal device components. Signs of infection in a LVAD patients warrant immediate evaluation of the driveline insertion site and pump. A 2-week course of antibiotics is adequate for driveline infection; however, if bacteremia is present extended therapy may be indicated.[20] For refractory cases, surgical debridement of the driveline may be necessary. In rare instances of pump infection, urgent replacement may be required.

Cardiac Arrhythmias

Atrial arrhythmias, especially atrial fibrillation, occur in nearly 50% of LVAD patients and are associated with increased morbidity and mortality.[31] Ventricular arrhythmias occur in 22% to 59% of patients with LVAD.[32] Depending on native cardiac function, some LVAD patients may be asymptomatic during ventricular arrhythmias; others will become unstable. The approach to management is similar to that of patients without MCS.

Initial steps include:

- Confirm stable hemodynamics.
- Obtain an electrocardiogram.
- Correct electrolyte derangements.
- Discontinue QT-prolonging drugs.
- Interrogate controller for abnormal parameters that suggest suction events or low flows.
- Echocardiography

The goal of treatment is to restore normal sinus rhythm, or in the case of atrial fibrillation, at least establish rate control. BB and amiodarone can be used for atrial and ventricular arrhythmias; lidocaine can also be used short term for the latter.[32]

If an arrhythmia is leading to hemodynamic instability or shock, immediate electrical cardioversion should be performed. Electrical cardioversion/defibrillation is safe in LVAD patients; however, external defibrillator pads should not be placed directly over the pump. Note that most LVAD patients have an automatic implantable cardioverter-defibrillator (AICD) that may discharge.[33] Electrophysiology experts should be consulted for any arrhythmias or AICD shocks in LVAD patients. If unstable arrhythmias are refractory to the aforementioned interventions, temporary biventricular MCS such as VA-ECMO should be considered.

Cardiac Arrest in the Patient with Left Ventricular Assist Device

For patients with cardiovascular collapse and subsequent shock, modified Advanced Cardiac Life Support (ACLS) procedures are recommended. These procedures are summarized in **Fig. 6**.

Previously, during ACLS for LVAD patients, there was hesitation to perform chest compressions, because they theoretically risked pump dislodgement. Expert consensus now recommends chest compressions in the event of cardiac arrest,

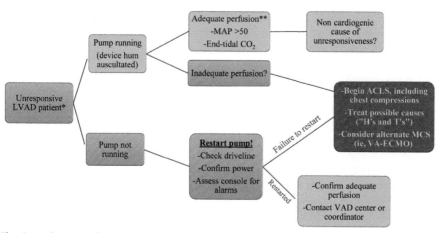

Fig. 6. – Algorithm for unresponsive patient with LVAD. *Manage airway and breathing as needed per usual ACLS recommendations. **Doppler ultrasonography and arterial line are indicated for assessment of patient hemodynamics. VAD, ventricular assist device. (*Data from* Peberdy MA, Gluck JA, Ornato JP, et al. Cardiopulmonary resuscitation in adults and children with mechanical circulatory support: a scientific statement from the American Heart Association. Circulation. 2017;135(24):e1115–34.)

provided reversible pump malfunction has been ruled out.[33,34] If flow is interrupted for any length of time, the risk of thrombosis increases and restarting the device can result in embolic phenomena.[13] If unable to restart the LVAD and the patient remains unstable, alternative means of MCS, such as VA-ECMO, may be needed.

Clinics Care Points for Left Ventricular Assist Devices

- LVAD patients requiring NCS are at high risk for perioperative complications.
- Maintain preload to the pump by ensuring adequate intravascular volume and RV function.
- Control afterload to maintain MAP at 65 to 85 mm Hg.
- Vigilant monitoring is essential to diagnose common issues in patients with LVADs patient, such as bleeding, infection, thrombosis, and stroke.
- Become familiar with the LVAD models being used today, including console interface, normal parameter ranges, and alarms. For updated information, see manufacturer Web sites.

DISCLOSURE

The authors have nothing to disclose.

REFERENCES

1. Savarese G, Lund LH. Global Public Health Burden of Heart Failure. Card Fail Rev 2017;3(1):7–11.
2. Inamdar AA, Inamdar AC. Heart Failure: Diagnosis, Management and Utilization. J Clin Med 2016;5(7). https://doi.org/10.3390/jcm5070062.
3. Nohria A, Lewis E, Stevenson LW. Medical management of advanced heart failure. JAMA 2002;287(5):628–40.
4. van Rooijen SJ, Huisman D, Stuijvenberg M, et al. Intraoperative modifiable risk factors of colorectal anastomotic leakage: Why surgeons and anesthesiologists should act together. Int J Surg 2016;36(Pt A):183–200.
5. Al Saied G, Almutairi HM, Alharbi Y, et al. Comparison Between the Impact of Vasopressors and Goal-Directed Fluid Therapy on the Management of Free Flap Reconstruction of Head and Neck and Monitoring in ICU. Cureus 2020;12(12): e12108.
6. Laks S, Isaak RS, Strassle PD, et al. Increased Intraoperative Vasopressor Use as Part of an Enhanced Recovery After Surgery Pathway for Pancreatectomy Does Not Increase Risk of Pancreatic Fistula. J Pancreat Cancer 2018;4(1):33–40.
7. Harper D, Chandler B. Splanchnic circulation. BJA Education 2016;16(2):66–71.
8. Kristensen SD, Knuuti J, Saraste A, et al. 2014 ESC/ESA Guidelines on non-cardiac surgery: cardiovascular assessment and management: The Joint Task Force on non-cardiac surgery: cardiovascular assessment and management of the European Society of Cardiology (ESC) and the European Society of Anaesthesiology (ESA). Eur J Anaesthesiol 2014;31(10):517–73.
9. Fonarow GC, Abraham WT, Albert NM, et al. Influence of beta-blocker continuation or withdrawal on outcomes in patients hospitalized with heart failure: findings from the OPTIMIZE-HF program. J Am Coll Cardiol 2008;52(3):190–9.
10. Mudumbai SC, Takemoto S, Cason BA, et al. Thirty-day mortality risk associated with the postoperative nonresumption of angiotensin-converting enzyme inhibitors: a retrospective study of the Veterans Affairs Healthcare System. J Hosp Med 2014;9(5):289–96.

11. Lee SM, Takemoto S, Wallace AW. Association between Withholding Angiotensin Receptor Blockers in the Early Postoperative Period and 30-day Mortality: A Cohort Study of the Veterans Affairs Healthcare System. Anesthesiology 2015; 123(2):288–306.

12. Kormos RL, Cowger J, Pagani FD, et al. The Society of Thoracic Surgeons Intermacs Database Annual Report: Evolving Indications, Outcomes, and Scientific Partnerships. Ann Thorac Surg 2019;107(2):341–53.

13. Peura JL, Colvin-Adams M, Grady KL, et al. Recommendations for the use of mechanical circulatory support: device strategies and patient selection: a scientific statement from the American Heart Association. Circulation 2012;126(22): 2648–67.

14. Lim S, Shaw S, Venkateswaran R, et al. HeartMate 3 Compared to Heart Transplant Outcomes in England. J Heart Lung Transplant 2020;39(4, Supplement): S15–6.

15. Teuteberg JJ, Cleveland JC, Cowger J, et al. The Society of Thoracic Surgeons Intermacs 2019 Annual Report: The Changing Landscape of Devices and Indications. Ann Thorac Surg 2020;109(3):649–60.

16. Birati EY, Rame JE. Left Ventricular Assist Device Management and Complications. Crit Care Clin 2014;30(3):607–27.

17. DeVore AD, Patel PA, Patel CB. Medical Management of Patients With a Left Ventricular Assist Device for the Non-Left Ventricular Assist Device Specialist. JACC Heart Fail 2017;5(9):621–31.

18. Mehra MR, Naka Y, Uriel N, et al. A Fully Magnetically Levitated Circulatory Pump for Advanced Heart Failure. N Engl J Med 2017;376(5):440–50.

19. Chung M. Perioperative Management of the Patient With a Left Ventricular Assist Device for Noncardiac Surgery. Anesth Analg 2018;126(6):1839–50.

20. Sen A, Larson JS, Kashani KB, et al. Mechanical circulatory assist devices: a primer for critical care and emergency physicians. Crit Care 2016;20(1). https://doi.org/10.1186/s13054-016-1328-z.

21. Singhvi A, Trachtenberg B. Left Ventricular Assist Devices 101: Shared Care for General Cardiologists and Primary Care. J Clin Med 2019;8(10). https://doi.org/10.3390/jcm8101720.

22. Mentias A, Briasoulis A, Vaughan Sarrazin MS, et al. Trends, Perioperative Adverse Events, and Survival of Patients With Left Ventricular Assist Devices Undergoing Noncardiac Surgery. JAMA Netw Open 2020;3(11):e2025118.

23. Mathis M, Sathishkumar S, Kheterpal S, et al. Complications, Risk Factors, and Staffing Patterns for Noncardiac Surgery in Patients with Left Ventricular Assist Devices. Anesthesiology (Philadelphia) 2017;126(3):450–60.

24. Feldman D, Pamboukian SV, Teuteberg JJ, et al. The 2013 International Society for Heart and Lung Transplantation Guidelines for mechanical circulatory support: executive summary. J Heart Lung Transpl 2013;32(2):157–87.

25. Slininger KA, Haddadin AS, Mangi AA. Perioperative management of patients with left ventricular assist devices undergoing noncardiac surgery. J Cardiothorac Vasc Anesth 2013;27(4):752–9.

26. Dalia AA, Cronin B, Stone ME, et al. Anesthetic Management of Patients With Continuous-Flow Left Ventricular Assist Devices Undergoing Noncardiac Surgery: An Update for Anesthesiologists. J Cardiothorac Vasc Anesth 2018;32(2): 1001–12.

27. Kirklin JK, Pagani FD, Kormos RL, et al. Eighth annual INTERMACS report: Special focus on framing the impact of adverse events. J Heart Lung Transpl 2017; 36(10):1080–6.

28. Eisen HJ. Left Ventricular Assist Devices (LVADS): History, Clinical Application and Complications. Korean Circ J 2019;49(7):568–85.
29. Mehra MR, Uriel N, Naka Y, et al. A Fully Magnetically Levitated Left Ventricular Assist Device — Final Report. New Engl J Med 2019;380(17):1618–27.
30. McIlvennan CK, Grady KL, Matlock DD, et al. End of life for patients with left ventricular assist devices: Insights from INTERMACS. J Heart Lung Transpl 2019; 38(4):374–81.
31. Enriquez AD, Calenda B, Gandhi PU, et al. Clinical impact of atrial fibrillation in patients with the HeartMateII left ventricular assist device. J Am Coll Cardiol 2014;64(18):1883–90.
32. Nakahara S, Chien C, Gelow J, et al. Ventricular arrhythmias after left ventricular assist device. Circ Arrhythm Electrophysiol 2013;6(3):648–54.
33. Peberdy MA, Gluck JA, Ornato JP, et al. Cardiopulmonary Resuscitation in Adults and Children With Mechanical Circulatory Support: A Scientific Statement From the American Heart Association. Circulation 2017;135(24):e1115–34.
34. Vierecke J, Schweiger M, Feldman D, et al. Emergency procedures for patients with a continuous flow left ventricular assist device. Emerg Med J 2017;34(12): 831–41.

Multimodal Analgesia in the Era of the Opioid Epidemic

Thomas Arthur Nicholas IV*, Raime Robinson

KEYWORDS

- Multimodal analgesia • Appropriate opioid use • Acute pain
- Acute postsurgical pain

INTRODUCTION

A long introduction exposing the origins of the opioid crisis with its associated dismal mortality and morbidity rate should not be needed to encourage providers to adopt new analgesic strategies with less reliance on opioid medications. Unfortunately, we are in the midst of this crisis due to an overreliance on opioids. The thought that better pain control can be achieved with just adding more opioids was clearly wrong. It should be profoundly evident to all providers that a new paradigm is needed in order to curb this opioid crisis. Achieving good pain control with less or no opioid medications while minimizing complications should be our new goal. Multimodal analgesic regimens can achieve this new goal of reducing opioids while providing improved pain control. These regimens that should incorporate a more holistic approach to pain control are explored and discussed.

PATIENT EVALUATION OVERVIEW

There is no silver bullet for good postoperative pain control. Historically, analgesic regimens focused on the postoperative period. However, contemporary pain control begins as soon as the preoperative period. Using strategies of enhanced recovery after surgery (ERAS) encapsulate the ideas of focusing on the patient's total perioperative timeline in order to affect positive outcomes for the surgical intervention. ERAS pathways have identified not only improved pain control and opioid reduction[1,2] but also other parameters such as decreasing length of stay and postoperative complications.[3,4] These pathways do not rely on one component but rather attempt to use evidence-based interventions to improve surgical outcomes including pain control. This multifaceted approach attempts to improve areas that may have not been directly linked to pain control but could certainly affect patient analgesia in a downstream manner. For instance, postoperative complications such as vomiting are associated with poor pain control.[5] Specific strategies used by ERAS pathways that may have

Anesthesiology, University of Nebraska Medical Center, 984455 Nebraska Medical Center, Omaha, NE, 68198-4455, USA
* Corresponding author.
E-mail address: tnicholasiv@gmail.com

Surg Clin N Am 102 (2022) 105–115
https://doi.org/10.1016/j.suc.2021.09.003
0039-6109/22/© 2021 Elsevier Inc. All rights reserved.

direct or downstream effects on pain control include patient and family preoperative education, minimally invasive surgical techniques, standardized anesthesia regimens, goal directed fluid administration, use of postoperative regional anesthesia techniques, restrictive use of surgical site drains, and multimodal approach to opioid sparing pain control.[6] Even though these strategies were conceived for elective surgery, they can certainly be used in a nonelective setting when appropriate.

PATIENT AND FAMILY PREOPERATIVE EDUCATION

It is helpful to identify patients at risk for poor postoperative pain control so that interventions may be tailored to the patient's individual needs. Several patient characteristics have been described as contributing to poor postoperative pain control: psychiatric illnesses such as depression, anxiety, catastrophizing,[7–10] younger age,[8,11] elevated preoperative pain scores,[8–11] longer operative times,[11] sole use of general anesthesia,[9] and chronic opioid use.[12] Many of these factors can be modified, for example, presurgical planning to include anesthesiology input to maximize the use of regional anesthetic techniques. Preoperative psychosocial interventions, especially patient education and relaxation techniques, have contributed to improved postoperative pain control.[13] Chronic opioid use will need to be addressed by consultation with the patient's chronic pain physician. Patient-specific opioid regimens may be determined or other helpful information such as identification of a provider narcotic agreement. Buprenorphine-containing products necessitate particular attention. Several regimens have been developed to address this unique medication that has become quite common for the treatment of chronic pain or opioid use disorder. The adoption of a buprenorphine management algorithm by all key providers will help prevent perioperative complications or surgical delays. A novel management pathway was reported by Acampora and colleagues.[14] This pathway allows for the continuation or titration down to 8 mg of buprenorphine twice daily, which does not interfere with full agonist opioids that will likely be required following a major surgery.

STANDARDIZED ANESTHESIA REGIMENS

The anesthetic care that a patient receives can greatly affect postoperative analgesia. Regular consultation with your anesthesiologist will help ensure that anesthesia therapy is being delivered in a manner that maximizes analgesia and reduces opioid exposure; this can be achieved by developing expectations for optimization of regional anesthesia, minimizing agents such as remifentanil that have been associated with hyperalgesia,[15] and increasing the utilization of agents such as ketamine,[16] which can improve analgesia and reduce opioid use. Indiscriminate use of intraoperative opioids should be avoided because it will not achieve improved postoperative pain but will certainly worsen postoperative complications.[17] Using the tenants of ERAS is an effective way of conducting an anesthetic in order to improve analgesia and reduce complications. However, these may be difficult to achieve in emergent surgical cases.

APPROPRIATE USE OF OPIOIDS

Opioids have been used for centuries to treat acute pain, and unfortunately, they still play an important role in the management of acute pain. However, physicians must understand the many caveats that exist with this drug class in order to use opioids in an appropriate manner while being sensitive to the potential pitfalls. Namely, physicians must understand that all opioids are addictive, which is contrary to prior false assumptions contributing to the current opioid epidemic.[18] Historically, the pharmaceutical industry has at times developed synthetic opioids or opioidlike drugs that are touted as less addictive or nonaddictive. One such drug is tramadol. It was approved by the US Food and Drug Administration (FDA) in 1995 as the only nonscheduled opioid available. The drug's use continued to increase since that time due to physicians' belief that it was less addictive and safer for patients. Tramadol ranked second in the total US opioid market sales in 2013.[19] Unfortunately, it became apparent that tramadol was addictive and was assigned to schedule IV by the Drug Enforcement Agency in 2014.[20] This oversight was likely because it was not well understood that there exists many genetic polymorphisms modulating CYP enzyme activity that are responsible for the ultimate activity of this prodrug. Patients with the gene CYP2D6 ultrametabolizers (UM) are most at risk of opioid addiction as well as other opioid side effects.[19] Tramadol is efficiently converted to the more active M1 metabolite in patients who are UM. Several factors make it a less attractive first-line opioid analgesic aside from its unpredictable analgesic response. Namely, tramadol has serotonin reuptake inhibition that can result in serotonin syndrome in patients already receiving serotonergic antidepressants, antipsychotics, anticonvulsants, antiparkinsonian agents, or monoamine oxidase inhibitors.[21] Seizure is another limiting potential side effect because this drug can lower the seizure threshold.[22] Clearly, this drug lacks reliable analgesic response and has numerous potential nonopioid side effects. Therefore, tramadol does not meet the basic requirements for a first-line opioid analgesic in postoperative pain control, which is reliable analgesia with minimal drug side effects or interactions.

One must follow a few simple opioid-prescribing tenants that will help provide consistency, safety, and efficacy. These tenants are as follows: (1) select opioids with reliable analgesia and limited medication interactions. Understand the pharmacodynamics and pharmacogenomics related to these individual medications. (2) Reduce a patient's opioid exposure by providing the most effective individualized dose at the shortest duration. A reduction of overall opioid exposure throughout the entirety of a patient's surgical experience should be a goal. (3) Avoid range dosing orders. Many times providers place these types of orders to reduce nurse phone calls; however, range dosing makes it difficult for the provider to accurately determine dose responses if the patient is receiving variable doses at variable times. (4) Avoid long-acting agents or basal rates for acute pain issues. There are no long-acting agents that have indications for acute pain. These agents do have higher risk of opioid toxicity. (5) Avoid therapeutic duplication of opioids, which can be confusing for ancillary staff as well as a potential Joint Commission violation. An appropriate example would be to provide oxycodone, 5 mg, orally (PO) every 4 hours as needed for severe or moderate pain. Hydromorphone, 0.5 mg, intravenous (IV) every 2 hours as needed for breakthrough pain or physical therapy. This regimen will avoid a duplicate therapy citation but will also be effective by providing the patient with an IV drug (onset of 8–10 minutes) that will provide analgesia faster so that they can participate in physical therapy. (6) Avoid combined opioid analgesics. The combination of acetaminophen or nonsteroidal antiinflammatory drugs (NSAIDs) to opioids makes it confusing and difficult for patients or nurses to safely maximize nonopioid medications. (7) Attempt to maximize oral administration when appropriate. Oral opioid immediate release medications typically last 3–4 hours, whereas IV medication lasts on average 90 minutes. Oral medications are less costly and require far less work for nurses to administer. A patient moves much closer to disposition when they are not reliant on IV medications. However, oral opioids should not be used when enteric absorption is in question. (8) Consider patient-controlled analgesia (PCA) when the patient is requiring frequent IV administration due to poor absorption or severe pain. PCA has been shown to be safer and provides better patient and nurse satisfaction.[23,24] (9) Consider increasing doses by 50% to 100% when a patient is not experiencing analgesia at the current dose. An increase of less than 50% will likely not be appreciated by the patient. (10) Always monitor for signs of opioid toxicity before escalation of opioid regimen. Less overt signs of toxicity can include slurred speech, heavy eyelids, or drowsiness. (11) Consider switching from a prodrug opioid such as oxycodone to a parent compound opioid such as hydromorphone. The patient may have improved response to a lower equianalgesic dose when changing to a parent compound because specific cytochrome conversion is not required to obtain analgesic activity. Parent and prodrug opioids are listed in (**Table 1**). (12) Use equianalgesic dosing calculation to switch between different opioid formulations and classes. (13) Chronic opioid use requires more complex dosing regimens. One cannot simply place a patient on home dose of opioids and expect adequate pain control. Although opioid dosing for patients on chronic opioids can be quite complex and is outside of the focus of this manuscript, there are some simple guidelines that can be used to temporize care until further consultation with the pain service is obtained: continue long-acting opioids at the home dosing schedule. Immediate release opioids should be increased by 50% to 100%. For instance, a patient is consuming 5 mg of oral oxycodone every 4 hours and subsequently undergoes a total knee arthroplasty then a reasonable oxycodone dose would be 10 mg every 4 hours as needed. Breakthrough pain dosing is typically 10% to 15% of total 24-hour morphine equivalents.[25] These are general guidelines and should be tailored with the patient clinical response and in conjunction with the addition of multimodal regimens.

Deescalation of an opioid should always be considered and plans set in place to facilitate safe opioid titration; this can be achieved through numerous regimens including prepared discharge opioid titrated prescriptions, patient discharge education, pain service opioid titration clinics, counseling during follow-up surgical visits, and pharmacist-led deescalation.[26] The basis for timely reduction of opioid use without exacerbating pain can be achieved by a 25% weekly (or daily if tolerated) reduction of individual doses. The speed of deescalation should be based on the patient's motivation and clinical condition. A provider must be aware of local legislation dictating the total amount of opioids that can be prescribed on discharge so deescalation may need to occur within this time frame. Assistance on determining the amount of opioids prescribed may also be obtained from expert panel guidelines.[27] Difficulties with deescalation may require referral to psychiatric evaluation if there are signs of opioid use disorder.

Table 1 Opioid compounds	
Parent Compounds	**Prodrug Compounds**
Morphine	Tramadol
Oxymorphone	Hydrocodone
Hydromorphone	Oxycodone
Methadone	Codeine
Tapentadol	-
Fentanyl and analogues	-

MULTIMODAL THERAPY

"Aggregation of marginal gains in cardiac surgery" was coined by Dr Fleming and colleagues[28] in his study, which embodies the intent of multimodal therapy, which is to provide improved outcomes while reducing complications. There is currently no "silver bullet" for postoperative analgesia; therefore, a provider must use therapies that reduce pain but do not cause undue side effects. For instance, prescribing high-dose gabapentin in the hopes of improved analgesia may result in oversedation of the patient. More is not necessarily better. Several medications and treatment options commonly identified as multimodal nonopioid therapies are explored in this article. This list is not all encompassing because there are other nonopioid medications that have been tried with variable results and evidence.

Acetaminophen and Nonsteroidal Antiinflammatory Drugs

Acetaminophen and NSAIDs have provided worldwide safe and effective analgesia for decades. However, these medications, as with any analgesic, have a therapeutic ceiling that may not be sufficient for some serious postsurgical pain issues. Regardless, these medications are appropriate for most analgesic regimens unless a medication contraindication exists. At the authors' institutions, most analgesic regimens include scheduled doses of acetaminophen ± NSAIDsm, which has helped ensure that the patient receives a maximized dose and if further analgesia is required then an opioid may be offered. They have found that this has reduced patient bias, which may include the belief that only opioids will be effective for pain control. Analgesia has improved since patients started receiving adequate acetaminophen ± NSAIDs, which likely was improved by sole use or other augmented modalities. As well, patients no longer had to wait for a nurse reassessment to receive another class of medication if acetaminophen or NSAIDs were ineffective.

Typically, these medications are delivered and easily absorbed enterally. This mode of delivery is cost-effective. There is much evidence demonstrating no improved efficacy of IV delivery of these medications versus enteral delivery.[29–33] However, it may be imperative to use an IV route when poor enteral absorption states exist or oral intake is contraindicated.

Acetaminophen has been generally accepted as safe with limited side effects. Yet, providers are more hesitant to use concomitant NSAIDs for fear of potential side effects such as bleeding, acute renal failure, cardiovascular events, or bone regeneration impairment. However, these potential side effects can be ameliorated by using the lowest effective dose at a short duration, careful patient selection, coadministration of proton pump inhibitor, and renal function monitoring in at-risk patients. At the institution, the authors use celecoxib when the patient is receiving thoracic epidural analgesia with concomitant heparin or enoxaparin thromboprophylaxis. Celecoxib as a cyclooxygenase-2 selective NSAID has theoretically less risk of bleeding and platelet dysfunction. Although this drug was assigned a black box warning for increased cardiovascular events (stroke and myocardial infarction), subsequent trials have identified that there is no increased risk with respect to nonselective NSAIDs.[34] Providers as with any drug therapy should always conduct a risk/benefit analysis when prescribing any NSAID.

Gabapentenoids

Gabapentenoids (gabapentin and pregabalin) have been used for decades to treat chronic neuropathic pain. Over the past decade, these medications have gained attention as opioid sparing analgesics. A wide range of dosing has occurred with variable evidence of analgesia effect. Unfortunately, this medication is limited by sedation and central nervous system (CNS) effects especially in elderly patients. A research trend seems to be developing identifying no benefit of this drug class for postoperative pain.[35–37] However, the validity of the body of past work conducted on this topic can be questioned.[38] If a provider chooses to administer this drug for postoperative pain then the lowest effective dose for this medication should be used. The medication should also be avoided in patients at risk for CNS side effects such as the frail and elderly.

Ketamine

This N-methyl-D-aspartate receptor antagonist has gained significant interest as an opioid sparing analgesic. Consensus guidelines developed by the American Academy of Pain Medicine (AAPM) support the use of subanesthetic doses for acute pain therapy. Because ketamine subanesthetic versus anesthetic dosing differs significantly, the AAPM guidelines were also developed to help providers administer this medication in an appropriate manner for acute pain control. Recent randomized, double-blind, placebo-controlled trials have demonstrated significant reduction in pain scores and opioid consumption.[39,40] Postoperative subanesthetic ketamine infusions were used in these trials, which is likely more beneficial for providing sustained opioid sparing analgesia rather than intermittent bolus dosing. Although the benefits of ketamine have been demonstrated, its safe use requires knowledge of subanesthetic dosing regimens. As well, local restrictions on administration of this dissociative drug may impede widespread hospital use. Local hospital guidelines with combined nursing education should be established and executed in order to safely administer this medication.

Lidocaine

Lidocaine infusion for acute pain is another modality of nonopioid analgesia that is gaining popularity. Unfortunately, the evidence for its benefits have been equivocal at best due to poor methodology of prior studies.[41] Safety concerns for the potential of local anesthetic systemic toxicity have not been clearly defined because lidocaine dosing has varied widely and serum lidocaine levels are inconsistently monitored. Further investigation of this regimen should be conducted before its acceptance as a safe opioid alternative.

Skeletal Muscle Relaxants

This drug class has surprisingly not received significant scrutiny is skeletal muscle relaxants. These agents were introduced in the United States as early as 1957. Carisoprodol, chlorzoxazone, metaxalone, and methocarbamol were all approved by the FDA before the Kefauver-Harris Amendment of 1962. This amendment required manufacturers to document safety and efficacy before allowing medication approval to enter the market place. Many of these medications would likely not achieve the market under current FDA standards. As well, most of these medications have mechanism of action that are unknown but they all consistently cause CNS depression. CNS depression can be potentiated with the identified risk of opioid overdose.[42] To date there is only one study in younger adults suffering rib fractures that identified some opioid reduction with methocarbamol use.[42] However, these findings must be taken cautiously because this was a limited retrospective study (n = 50) with low evidence methodology. Routine use of these medications should be discouraged due to potential medication interactions, side effects, and lack of evidence especially in a critical care or postsurgical setting.

INTERVENTIONAL TREATMENT OPTIONS
Regional Anesthesia

Regional anesthesia represents 2 distinct categories: peripheral and neuroaxial anesthesia. Both of these techniques can be introduced into a multimodal regimen. Historically, thoracic or lumbar epidural analgesia has been considered the gold-standard regional analgesia. However, this standard is quickly changing with the improvement of technology namely ultrasound technology, and this has allowed the expanded use of peripheral nerve blocks as well as improved the safety of this technique. The list of effective ultrasound-guided peripheral nerve blocks (**Box 1**) has grown significantly in the past decade. Peripheral nerve blocks have surpassed or replaced neuroaxial techniques that have been contraindicated due to a patient coagulation status, cardiovascular instability, or traumatic spinal cord injury; this is particularly evident in the critical care arena in which patients may not be candidates for epidural analgesia yet are suffering from significant painful injuries. Peripheral nerve blocks in critically ill patients typically do not affect central sympathetic tone similar to thoracic epidural analgesia; therefore, hypotension likely will not occur. As well, a peripheral nerve block technique is not necessarily contraindicated in patients suffering coagulopathy or who are receiving aggressive thromboprophylaxis.[43] All peripheral nerve blocks can be performed using single shot or continuous catheter techniques. A continuous catheter can provide extended pain relief for up to 7 days. Regional anesthesia has demonstrated robust evidence of its opioid sparing effects and should be maximized in all multimodal regimens.

MULTIDISCIPLINARY APPROACH

Providing a multidisciplinary approach to complex acute pain issues may be necessary in many patients. An evidence-based approach such as ERAS protocols can incorporate a multidisciplinary approach to patient care in the setting of surgery. Similarly, utilization of guidelines such the American College of Critical Care Medicine's pain, agitation, and delirium guidelines in an intensive care setting may facilitate optimized analgesic care in a critically injured patient.[44] These guidelines take into account the downstream effects of poor pain control on other entities such as delirium. As well, incorporating these guidelines with ventilator weaning, early mobility, and sleep hygiene protocols may provide improved outcomes.[45] The local development of guidelines to facilitate treatment options is important to effectively use a systems resource such as physical therapy, psychiatric services, or medical

---

Box 1
Peripheral nerve blocks

Peripheral nerve block and coverage areas

Truncal Blocks:
  Transversus thoracis plane, serratus anterior plane, erector spinae, parasternal

Abdominal Blocks:
  Transversus abdominis, rectus sheath, erector spinae

Upper Extremities:
  Supraclavicular, infraclavicular, interscalene, axillary

Lower Extremites:
  Subgluteal sciatic, popliteal sciatic, adductor canal, femoral, fascia iliacus

comanagement teams. These guidelines can incorporate a more broad approach to pain management because a strong relationship exists between effective pain management and a patient's ultimate outcome.

NONPHARMACEUTICAL THERAPY

These treatment options are often times overlooked due to lack of evidence or reimbursement issues. They can range from simple measures such as warm and cold compresses that require little effort but may safely provide analgesia.[46,47] Distraction therapies such as guided imagery, meditation,[48] and music[49] have also shown benefits in improving analgesia. Nurse education can include training for instituting these types of techniques. Transcutaneous electrical nerve stimulation is another modality with some evidence of improved analgesia in various pain syndromes including postsurgical pain from inguinal herniorrhaphy.[50] Although TENS units are relatively inexpensive, in a hospital setting utilization of TENS therapy can be cost prohibitive. Even though evidence is lacking in many of these modalities, they do represent a devotion to the patient to "do everything possible" to treat pain that certainly will not go unappreciated by a suffering patient or family.

SUMMARY

The opioid crisis has certainly brought attention to the use of opioids to treat pain. This crisis has helped reveal that analgesic regimens should not be heavily relied on opioids to deliver pain control. The potential risk of overutilization of opioids has been self-evident. Unfortunately, until a new class of drug is discovered these medications will still play an important role in analgesia especially in critically injured patients. Even though these medications are still used, they should be used in an adjunct fashion in conjunction with other evidence-based multimodal therapies. Scrutiny and caution should be applied when introducing nonopioid analgesics to a regimen because these medications may have an unintended delirious impact on patient care. There may be increased time and costs to achieve a robust opioid-minimized or opioid-free multimodal regimen but as providers we must accept this cost in order to prevent further negative impacts on the current opioid crisis.

REFERENCES

1. Razi SS, Stephens McDonnough JA, Haq S, et al. Significant reduction of postoperative pain and opioid analgesics requirement with an enhanced recovery after thoracic surgery protocol. J Thorac Cardiovasc Surg 2020;161(5):1689–701.

2. Rice D, Rodriguez-Restrepo A, Mena G, et al. Matched pairs comparison of an enhanced recovery pathway versus conventional management on opioid exposure and pain control in patients undergoing lung surgery. Ann Surg 2020.

3. Memtsoudis SG, Fiasconaro M, Soffin EM, et al. Enhanced recovery after surgery components and perioperative outcomes: a nationwide observational study. Br J Anaesth 2020;124:638–47.

4. Noba L, Rodgers S, Chandler C, et al. Enhanced recovery after surgery (ERAS) reduces hospital costs and improve clinical outcomes in liver surgery: a systematic review and meta-analysis. J Gastrointest Surg 2020;24:918–32.

5. Van Boekel RL, Warlé MC, Nielen RG, et al. Relationship between postoperative pain and overall 30-day complications in a broad surgical population: an observational study. Ann Surg 2019;269:856–65.

6. Ljungqvist O, Scott M, Fearon KC. Enhanced recovery after surgery: a review. JAMA Surg 2017;152:292–8.
7. Bierke S, Petersen W. Influence of anxiety and pain catastrophizing on the course of pain within the first year after uncomplicated total knee replacement: a prospective study. Arch Orthop Trauma Surg 2017;137:1735–42.
8. Coppes OJM, Yong RJ, Kaye AD, et al. Patient and surgery-related predictors of acute postoperative pain. Curr Pain Headache Rep 2020;24:1–8.
9. Arefayne NR, Tegegne SS, Gebregzi AH, et al. Incidence and associated factors of post-operative pain after emergency orthopedic surgery: a multi-centered prospective observational cohort study. Int J Surg 2020;27:103–13.
10. Dunn L, Durieux M, Fernández L, et al. Influence of catastrophizing, anxiety, and depression on in-hospital opioid consumption, pain, and quality of recovery after adult spine surgery. J Neurosurg Spine 2017;28:119–26.
11. Jenkins NW, Parrish JM, Mayo BC, et al. The identification of risk factors for increased postoperative pain following minimally invasive transforaminal lumbar interbody fusion. Eur Spine J 2020;29(6):1304–10.
12. Jain N, Phillips FM, Weaver T, et al. Preoperative chronic opioid therapy: a risk factor for complications, readmission, continued opioid use and increased costs after one-and two-level posterior lumbar fusion. Spine 2018;43:1331–8.
13. Szeverenyi C, Kekecs Z, Johnson A, et al. The use of adjunct psychosocial interventions can decrease postoperative pain and improve the quality of clinical care in orthopedic surgery: a systematic review and meta-analysis of randomized controlled trials. J Pain 2018;19:1231–52.
14. Acampora GA, Nisavic M, Zhang Y. Perioperative buprenorphine continuous maintenance and administration simultaneous with full opioid agonist: patient priority at the interface between medical disciplines. J Clin Psychiatry 2020;81(1). 19com12810.
15. Santonocito C, Noto A, Crimi C, et al. Remifentanil-induced postoperative hyperalgesia: current perspectives on mechanisms and therapeutic strategies. Local Reg Anesth 2018;11:15.
16. Schwenk ES, Viscusi ER, Buvanendran A, et al. Consensus guidelines on the use of intravenous ketamine infusions for acute pain management from the American Society of regional anesthesia and pain medicine, the American Academy of pain medicine, and the American Society of Anesthesiologists. 2018;43(5):456–66.
17. Frauenknecht J, Kirkham K, Jacot-Guillarmod A, et al. Analgesic impact of intraoperative opioids vs. opioid-free anaesthesia: a systematic review and meta-analysis 2019.
18. Jones MR, Viswanath O, Peck J, et al. A brief history of the opioid epidemic and strategies for pain medicine. Pain 2018;7:13–21.
19. Miotto K, Cho AK, Khalil MA, et al. Trends in tramadol: pharmacology, metabolism, and misuse. Anesth Analgesia 2017;124:44–51.
20. Drug Enforcement Administration DoJ. Schedule of controlled substances: placement of tramadol into schedule IV. Final rule. J Fed Regist 2014;79:37623–30.
21. Park SH, Wackernah RC, Stimmel GL. Serotonin syndrome: is it a reason to avoid the use of tramadol with antidepressants? J Pharm Pract 2014;27:71–8.
22. Sansone RA, Sansone LA. Tramadol: seizures, serotonin syndrome, and coadministered antidepressants. Psychiatry 2009;6:17.
23. Macintyre P. Safety and efficacy of patient-controlled analgesia. J Br J Anaesth 2001;87:36–46.
24. Sidebotham D, Dijkhuizen MR, Schug SA. The safety and utilization of patient-controlled analgesia. J Pain Symptom Management 1997;14:202–9.

25. American Society of Health-System Pharmacists, McPherson ML. Demystifying opioid conversion calculations: a guide for effective dosing. ASHP; 2014.

26. Bui T, Grygiel R, Konstantatos A, et al. The impact of an innovative pharmacist-led inpatient opioid de-escalation intervention in post-operative orthopedic patients. J Opioid Manag 2020;16:167–76.

27. Overton HN, Hanna MN, Bruhn WE, et al. Opioid-prescribing guidelines for common surgical procedures: an expert panel consensus. J Am Coll Surg 2018;227: 411–8.

28. Fleming IO, Garratt C, Guha R, et al. Aggregation of marginal gains in cardiac surgery: feasibility of a perioperative care bundle for enhanced recovery in cardiac surgical patients. J Cardiothorac Vasc Anesth 2016;30:665–70.

29. Bhoja R, Ryan MW, Klein K, et al. Intravenous vs oral acetaminophen in sinus surgery: a randomized clinical trial. Laryngoscope Invest Otolaryngol 2020;5: 348–53.

30. Cain KE, Iniesta MD, Fellman BM, et al. Effect of preoperative intravenous vs oral acetaminophen on postoperative opioid consumption in an enhanced recovery after surgery (ERAS) program in patients undergoing open gynecologic oncology surgery. Gynecol Oncol 2021;160:464–8.

31. Patel A, BH PP, Diskina D, et al. Comparison of clinical outcomes of acetaminophen IV vs PO in the peri-operative setting for laparoscopic inguinal hernia repair surgeries: a triple-blinded, randomized controlled trial. J Clin Anesth 2020;61: 109628.

32. Teng Y, Zhang Y, Li B. Intravenous versus oral acetaminophen as an adjunct on pain and recovery after total knee arthroplasty: a systematic review and meta-analysis. J Med 2020;99:e23515.

33. Arora S, Wagner JG, Herbert M. Myth: parenteral ketorolac provides more effective analgesia than oral ibuprofen. J Can J Emerg Med 2007;9:30–2.

34. Nissen SE, Yeomans ND, Solomon DH, et al. Cardiovascular safety of celecoxib, naproxen, or ibuprofen for arthritis. N Engl J Med 2016;375:2519–29.

35. Verret M, Lauzier F, Zarychanski R, et al. Perioperative use of gabapentinoids for the management of postoperative acute pain: a systematic review and meta-analysis. J Anesthesiol 2020;133:265–79.

36. Liu B, Liu R, Wang L. A meta-analysis of the preoperative use of gabapentinoids for the treatment of acute postoperative pain following spinal surgery. J Med 2017;96:e8031.

37. Hamilton TW, Strickland LH, Pandit HG. A meta-analysis on the use of gabapentinoids for the treatment of acute postoperative pain following total knee arthroplasty. J Bone Joint Surg Am 2016;98:1340–50.

38. Joshi GP, Kehlet H. Meta-analyses of gabapentinoids for pain management after knee arthroplasty-a caveat emptor? A narrative review. Acta Anaesthesiol Scand 2021;65:865–9.

39. Murphy GS, Avram MJ, Greenberg SB, et al. Perioperative methadone and ketamine for postoperative pain control in spinal surgical patients: a randomized, double-blind, placebo-controlled trial. Anesthesiology 2021;134:697–708.

40. Ricciardelli RM, Walters NM, Pomerantz M, et al. The efficacy of ketamine for postoperative pain control in adolescent patients undergoing spinal fusion surgery for idiopathic scoliosis. Spine Deform 2020;8:433–40.

41. Masic D, Liang E, Long C, et al. Intravenous lidocaine for acute pain: a systematic review. Pharmacother J Hum Pharmacol Drug Ther 2018;38:1250–9.

42. Li Y, Delcher C, Wei YJJ, et al. Risk of opioid overdose associated with concomitant use of opioids and skeletal muscle relaxants: a population-based cohort study. Clin Pharmacol Ther 2020;108:81–9.
43. Horlocker TT, Vandermeuelen E, Kopp SL, et al. Regional anesthesia in the patient receiving antithrombotic or thrombolytic therapy: American Society of regional anesthesia and pain medicine evidence-based guidelines. Obstet Anesth Dig 2019;39:28–9.
44. Barr J, Fraser GL, Puntillo K, et al. Clinical practice guidelines for the management of pain, agitation, and delirium in adult patients in the intensive care unit: executive summary. Am J Health Syst Pharm 2013;70:53–8.
45. Barr J, Pandharipande PP. The pain, agitation, and delirium care bundle: synergistic benefits of implementing the 2013 Pain, Agitation, and Delirium Guidelines in an integrated and interdisciplinary fashion. Crit Care Med 2013;41:S99–115.
46. Klintberg IH, Larsson ME. Shall we use cryotherapy in the treatment after surgical procedures, after acute pain or injury, or in long term pain or dysfunction?-a systematic review. J Bodyw Mov Ther 2021;27:368–87.
47. Chabal C, Dunbar PJ, Painter I, et al. Properties of thermal analgesia in a human chronic low back pain model. J Pain Res 2020;13:2083.
48. Miller-Matero LR, Coleman JP, Smith-Mason CE, et al. A brief mindfulness intervention for medically hospitalized patients with acute pain: a pilot randomized clinical trial 2019;20:2149–54.
49. Cepeda MS, Carr DB, Lau J, et al. Music for pain relief. Cochrane Database Syst Rev 2006:CD004843.
50. Parseliunas A, Paskauskas S, Kubiliute E, et al. Transcutaneous Electric Nerve Stimulation reduces acute postoperative pain and analgesic use after open inguinal hernia surgery: a randomized, double-blind, placebo-controlled trial. J Pain 2021;22(5):533–44.

Management of Decompensated Cirrhosis and Associated Syndromes

Shaun Chandna, DO[1], Eduardo Rodríguez Zarate, MD[1],
Juan F. Gallegos-Orozco, MD*

KEYWORDS

- Decompensated cirrhosis • Acute-on-chronic liver failure • Variceal hemorrhage
- Hepatorenal syndrome • Hepatic encephalopathy • Pulmonary hypertension
- Hepatopulmonary syndrome

KEY POINTS

- Patients with cirrhosis account for around 3% of intensive care unit admissions and have a poor prognosis, with hospital mortality exceeding 50%.
- Significant improvements in survival among patients with acutely decompensated cirrhosis and organ failure have been described when treated in specialized liver transplant centers
- Acute-on-chronic liver failure is a distinct clinical syndrome in patients with cirrhosis characterized by decompensated state associated with the development of one or more organ failures resulting in a significantly higher short-term mortality.
- Common life-threatening complications in patients with cirrhosis which require intensive care management include hepatic encephalopathy, hypovolemic, and/or distributive shock, pulmonary complications (portopulmonary hypertension and hepatopulmonary syndrome), and renal complications (hepatorenal syndrome).
- Selected patients with acute-on-chronic liver failure can benefit from liver transplantation with very good posttransplant survival.

INTRODUCTION

Cirrhosis is the final common pathway of sustained injury to the liver from a multitude of different etiologies, including most commonly nonalcoholic fatty liver disease (NAFLD), alcohol use and chronic viral hepatitis. The number of people around the

Division of Gastroenterology and Hepatology, Department of Medicine, University of Utah School of Medicine, 30 N 1900 E, SOM-4R118, Salt Lake City, UT 84106, USA
[1] These authors contributed equally to this work.
* Corresponding author.
E-mail address: Juan.gallegos@hsc.utah.edu
Twitter: @JuanGallegosMD (J.F.G.-O.)

Surg Clin N Am 102 (2022) 117–137
https://doi.org/10.1016/j.suc.2021.09.005
0039-6109/22/Published by Elsevier Inc.

surgical.theclinics.com

world with cirrhosis is increasing, mostly due to a rising number of patients with NAFLD associated with increasing incidence and prevalence of obesity and associated metabolic complications. In the United States, there is a concerning rise in the number of young men and women developing alcohol-induced liver disease, with increasing mortality disproportionally affecting young men.[1-3] Similarly, there has been an increase in the proportion of patients listed for transplant that have alcohol liver disease.[4,5]

Although patients with compensated cirrhosis can have a good prognosis, with median survival exceeding 12 years, patients with decompensated disease (characterized by the development of ascites, variceal hemorrhage, and/or hepatic encephalopathy (HE)) have a significantly worse prognosis with a median survival of only 2 or 3 years. These are typically the patients that are seen in the medical wards of our hospitals and frequently in our intensive care units.

Patients with cirrhosis account for around 3% of intensive care unit admissions.[6,7] These patients have a poor prognosis, with hospital mortality exceeding 50%.[8-10] Mortality is closely tied to the number of organ failures present, such that patients with 2 or more organ failures by the third day of ICU admission have a greater than 80% risk of succumbing before hospital discharge.[11] However, significant improvements in survival among patients with acutely decompensated cirrhosis and organ failure have been described when treated in specialized liver transplant centers.[12,13] Even among patients with cirrhosis treated in nonspecialized medical ICUs, there has been an improvement in survival. In a large database from Australia and New Zealand, the hospital mortality of 17,000 patients with cirrhosis who had a nonelective admission to the medical ICU declined from 44% in 2000% to 29% in 2015.[14] In a similar study from the United Kingdom, among 33,000 patients with cirrhosis admitted to an ICU, the hospital mortality decreased from 58% in 1998% to 46% in 2012.[15]

In the last decade, we have come to recognize a distinct clinical syndrome in patients with cirrhosis that is characterized by decompensated state associated with the development of one or more organ failures resulting in a significantly higher short-term mortality. This syndrome is termed "acute-on-chronic liver failure" (ACLF).[16,17] Many patients with cirrhosis who develop this syndrome will require management in a critical care unit.

Data from the United States suggest that a quarter of patients admitted to the hospital with decompensated cirrhosis meet the criteria for ACLF. Most have 1 or 2 organ failures, with a smaller proportion of patients with 3 or more organ failures (**Table 1**).

Table 1
Classification and grades of acute-on-chronic liver failure (ACLF)

ACLF Grade	Clinical Characteristics
No ACLF	No organ failure, or single non-kidney organ failure, creatinine <1.5 mg/dL, no HE
ACLF Ia	Single renal failure
ACLF Ib	Single non-kidney organ failure, creatinine 1.5–1.9 mg/dL *and/or* HE grade 1–2
ACLF II	Two organ failures
ACLF III	Three or more organ failures

Abbreviations: ACLF, acute-on-chronic liver failure; HE, hepatic encephalopathy.
adapted with permission from EASL, J Hepatology 2018[56].

The overall mortality for patients with ACLF was 26% at 28 days and 40% at 90 days; however, mortality was significantly higher among patients with 3 or more organ failures (53% at 28 days and 69% at 90 days).[18] In this study, care at a liver transplant center was associated with improved short-term survival in patients with ACLF.

In a recent meta-analysis, 35% of patients with decompensated cirrhosis had ACLF, with a global 90-day mortality of 58%. Alcohol was the most common etiology of cirrhosis (45%), infection was the most frequent trigger of ACLF (35%), and kidney dysfunction was the most common organ failure (49%).[19]

This review will focus on relevant aspects of the management of patients with decompensated liver disease and ACLF, as they are likely to require management in a critical care unit. Whereby appropriate, we will provide recommendations from recently published guidelines on the ICU management of patients with ACLF.[20]

HEPATIC ENCEPHALOPATHY

HE is the most common cause of altered mental status in patients with decompensated cirrhosis. It is thought to be caused by astrocyte swelling and cerebral edema due to synergistic effects of excess ammonia and inflammation, although the precise mechanism remains unclear.[21] It encompasses a spectrum of neuropsychological manifestations of impaired brain function which are the result of worsening liver disease or of precipitating events such as infections, gastrointestinal bleeding (GIB), renal, and/or electrolyte disorders or constipation.[22] A clear precipitant cannot be determined in up to 20%–30% of patients.[23,24] The West Haven Criteria classifies HE in four grades: 1 to 4 (**Table 2**).[25] Evaluating the severity of HE should be approached as a continuum,[26] ranging from unimpaired cognitive function and intact consciousness through coma, which is often present in critically ill patients with cirrhosis.[22]

The initial evaluation of a patient with cirrhosis and neurologic dysfunction should aim at assessing the response to ammonia-lowering agents. In patients failing these therapies or in those deteriorating rapidly, further investigation is recommended, such as imaging of the brain, electroencephalogram, or lumbar puncture.[27] Serum

Table 2	
Clinical stages of hepatic encephalopathy according to the West Haven criteria	
Grade	**Distinguishing Features**
0	No abnormality
1	Trivial lack of awareness Euphoria or anxiety Shortened attention span Impairment of addition or subtraction
2	Lethargy or apathy Disorientation for a time Obvious personality change Inappropriate behavior
3	Somnolence to semi-stupor Responsive to stimuli Confused Gross disorientation Bizarre behavior
4	Coma, unable to test mental state

ammonia may aid in differentiating HE from other neurologic conditions but does not actually establish a diagnosis of HE nor does the level correlate with the severity of HE.[22,28]

Patients with severe HE (grade 3 or 4) should be transferred to the ICU for the consideration of endotracheal intubation for airway protection (**Fig. 1**).[29] In patients with concurrent upper GIB, the threshold for airway intubation should be even lower.[30] In patients intubated only for depressed mental status, avoidance of sedation is recommended to allow for frequent neurocognitive evaluation. If concomitant respiratory impairment is present, it is preferred to use short-acting agents such as fentanyl (25–200 µg/h) or propofol (50–150 µg/Kg/min) over agents such as benzodiazepines.[31]

After addressing possible triggering events, lactulose remains the cornerstone of pharmacologic therapy for HE. This nonabsorbable disaccharide is metabolized by colonic bacterial flora into lactic acid, creating an acidic environment in the gut, helping in the conversion of ammonia (NH_3) to ionic ammonium (NH_4+) which is then discarded via fecal excretion.[21] Therapy consists of 20 g administered orally or via nasogastric tube each hour until the passage of bowel movement, followed by the titration of the dose to achieve 2 to 3 bowel movements per day with improvement in mentation. If unable to administer orally, 200 g via enema can be considered. Careful administration is recommended as hypovolemia and electrolyte disturbances could worsen HE.[32]

Another option is the use of oral polyethylene glycol (PEG-3350). When compared with lactulose in patients hospitalized with HE, a 4-L purge with PEG-3350 demonstrated shorter time to improvement and a trend toward shorter hospital stay.[33] An advantage of PEG-3350 over lactulose is that it does not ferment, decreasing the risk of bowel distention and ileus.[31] The other commonly used medication is rifaximin, an oral nonabsorbable antibiotic with broad-spectrum activity against aerobic and

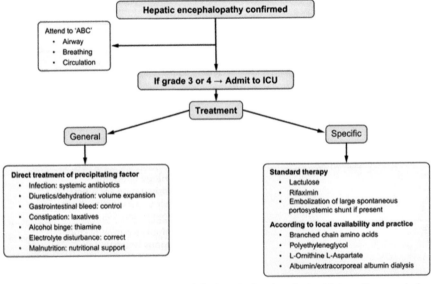

Fig. 1. Algorithm for the management of the hospitalized patient with hepatic encephalopathy. (*Reproduced with permission from* Rose CF, et al. J Hepatology 2020[29]).

anaerobic enteric flora. Given at a dose of 550 mg twice a day, it has demonstrated the prevention of HE-related events including hospital admissions.[34] Compared with lactulose alone, the combination of lactulose and rifaximin demonstrated a significant decrease in mortality and hospital length of stay.[35] Thus, it is our practice to add rifaximin to hospitalized patients with HE not responding to lactulose alone. In selected patients (MELD <11) with persistent neurologic deterioration, there might be a role for spontaneous portosystemic shunt embolization.[36] Other less commonly used therapies include L-ornithine/L-aspartate which aids in the reduction of ammonia and results in clinical improvement of HE,[37] however without enough evidence to support its routine use.

Extracorporeal liver devices have been designed to preserve hepatic function and to limit the progression of the disease while allowing hepatic recovery or liver transplantation to occur.[31] The main difference among them is the type of membranes used in the filtering process. Although some biochemical improvements have been described in patients with HE,[23] overall survival benefit has not been demonstrated.[38,39]

CARDIOVASCULAR COMPLICATIONS

Cardiac and circulatory abnormalities are often present in patients with cirrhosis. Portal hypertension induces sustained systemic and splanchnic vasodilatation mediated by nitric oxide and other vasoactive molecules. This, in turn, leads to a hyperdynamic state characterized by increased cardiac output and decreased systemic vascular resistance. Due to the pooling of blood within the splanchnic vascular bed, effective blood volume decreases, leading to compensatory mechanisms such as the activation of the neurohormonal axis resulting in water and sodium retention.[31,40] Similarly, morphologic and functional cardiac changes known collectively as cirrhotic cardiomyopathy develop in up to 50% of these patients. Cirrhotic cardiomyopathy is a syndrome characterized by both systolic and diastolic dysfunction, as well as QT interval prolongation that can lead to an increased risk of ventricular arrhythmias and sudden cardiac death.[41] Cirrhotic cardiomyopathy tends to be subclinical, with clinical manifestations generally only apparent during periods of physiologic stress, such as active infections conditioning a high output hypotensive state, shunting of portal flow into the systemic circulation after transjugular intrahepatic portosystemic shunt (TIPS) placement, and after liver transplantation.[42]

A thorough assessment of the volume status should be carried out with adequate correction in an effort to prevent hypotension and end-organ damage. A specific blood pressure goal has not been established in this population; however, a mean arterial pressure (MAP) >65 mm Hg in patients with end-organ hypoperfusion as described by the Surviving Sepsis guidelines, is frequently used.[43] Trying to correct and monitor the hemodynamics in these patients is challenging, as they often present with volume overload in the form of ascites and peripheral edema. Objective assessment with central venous access and central venous saturation and echocardiography can aid in the initial evaluation; however, data should be cautiously interpreted, as their use has not been validated in patients with cirrhosis.[44] Similarly, lactate-guided resuscitation has not been validated and while an elevated lactic acid can indicate tissue hypoperfusion in the general population, in patients with advanced cirrhosis it can reflect defective lactate clearance by the impaired liver.[45]

Volume resuscitation is indicated in patients with hemodynamic instability. In cases with decompensated cirrhosis along with other complications such as hypoalbuminemia and specific clinical conditions such as spontaneous bacterial peritonitis (SBP), after large-volume paracentesis and hepatorenal syndrome (HRS-AKI), concentrated albumin (100 mL of 20% or 25% albumin as needed) is recommended.[46] Of note, cautious administration is advised to prevent cardiac overload in patients with underlying cardiomyopathy.[45] In those with persistent shock after appropriate volume repletion, vasopressor therapy is recommended. The first-line agent in this scenario is norepinephrine at a dose of 0.01 to 0.3/kg/min, due to its better side effect profile compared with other vasopressors.[47] Vasopressin and terlipressin have also demonstrated hemodynamic improvement in this population.[48] In patients not appropriately responding to therapy, adrenal insufficiency should be considered as a possible contributing factor[49,50] and intravenous hydrocortisone at a dose of 50 mg every 6 hours should be considered.[51,52]

In case of large volume paracentesis (>5 L), plasma volume expansion with albumin (8 g/L of ascites removed) has been associated with a reduction in paracentesis-induced circulatory dysfunction (PICD).[53,54] PICD has been described as a state with reduced effective blood volume, associated with acute kidney injury (AKI), hyponatremia, HE, and decreased survival.[55] In patients undergoing removal <5 L of ascites, the risk of PICD is lower but it is still generally agreed that patients be treated with albumin due to poor safety profile of alternative plasma expanders.[56]

Nonselective beta-blockers (NSBBs) are routinely used as pharmacologic prophylaxis against esophageal variceal bleeding. The overall effect suggests a direct relationship between portal pressure and complications of cirrhosis.[57] In patients with refractory ascites and in those with SBP, the use of NSBBs has been associated with an increased mortality risk.[58,59] It is our practice to discontinue NSBBs in patients with decompensated cirrhosis and hemodynamic instability and/or AKI admitted to the critical care unit.

ACUTE VARICEAL HEMORRHAGE

GIB in patients with cirrhosis requires prompt management which is critical to improved outcomes (**Fig. 2**).[60] Patients with cirrhosis and GIB are commonly treated in the ICU and in 1 study accounted for 14% of medical ICU admissions.[8] Most GIB is due to portal hypertension, frequently presenting as esophageal variceal hemorrhage, which is responsible for 50%–90% of upper GIB episodes. Variceal hemorrhage has a short-term mortality of 15%–30%.[61] ICU management should focus on the rapid

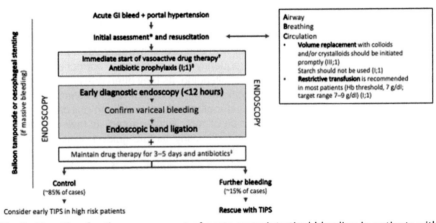

Fig. 2. Algorithm for the management of acute gastrointestinal bleeding in patients with cirrhosis. (*reproduced with permission from EASL, J Hepatology 2018[56]*).

correction of volume deficits from blood loss and on hemostasis.[61] A restrictive transfusion strategy with a hemoglobin threshold of 7 g/dL and a posttransfusion target of 7 to 9 g/dL improved short-term survival, decreased risk of rebleeding, and did not increase the portal pressure gradient.[62] Early intubation for airway protection should be considered in those at high risk for aspiration, including patients with pulmonary disease, severe encephalopathy, and/or large hematemesis.[31]

Vasoactive medications (vasopressin, octreotide, and terlipressin) are essential to hemostasis efforts and should be started as early as possible. Their use in acute variceal bleeding is associated with improved hemostasis, lower transfusion needs, shorter hospitalization, and lower risk of 7-day mortality.[63] There is no significant difference in hemostasis between terlipressin, somatostatin, and octreotide.[64] The most commonly used vasoactive agent in the United States is octreotide; vasopressin is rarely used for this indication and terlipressin is not yet available in North America. These medications should be used for 2 to 5 days.[60] Upper endoscopy with band ligation should be performed within 12 hours of presentation, which provides ample time to stabilize the hemodynamically compromised patient before endoscopic management.[60]

Patients with cirrhosis and GIB are at increased risk of infections, hence short-term prophylactic antibiotic use (such as ceftriaxone 1 g IV daily for 7 days) is recommended.[60] Bacterial infections (SBP, pneumonia, etc.) can occur in up to 50% of these patients.[65] A meta-analysis of 12 trials showed that antibiotic prophylaxis in this setting was associated with a reduction in mortality, bacterial infections, and rebleeding rates.[66]

Combination pharmacologic and endoscopic treatment can fail in up to 20% of patients with variceal bleed. In these cases, placement of a TIPS can be considered as rescue therapy.[60] It is important to monitor liver function and symptoms post-TIPS, as the procedure has a risk of precipitating liver failure and HE, the latter of which can develop in up to 40% of patients.[67] Absolute contraindications to TIPS include heart failure, polycystic liver disease, severe pulmonary hypertension, untreated biliary obstruction, and uncontrolled infection.[68]

Balloon tamponade can be used if needed as a bridge to definitive therapy such as TIPS, though it has a high risk of serious adverse events and mortality and should not be used for more than 24 hours.[60] Endoscopic esophageal stents may be a potential alternative to balloon tamponade, as they can result in improved bleeding control (short-term success 87% vs 65%), reduce adverse events, and improve short-term mortality compared to balloon tamponade.[69]

Preemptive (early TIPS) may be considered in select patients following standard therapy for variceal hemorrhage.[60] TIPS within 72 hours has been proposed based on an early randomized controlled trial for patients with cirrhosis and Child-Pugh class B with active bleeding or Child-Pugh class C regardless of endoscopic findings.[70] More recently, a large multicenter study demonstrated that Child-Pugh B patients had reduced mortality with standard therapy than Child-Pugh C patients, suggesting that they may not benefit from early TIPS, while those with Child-Pugh C and/or MELD $\geq$19 had the highest mortality.[71] While additional refinement of the criteria for early TIPS is needed, those with Child-Pugh C should be considered for early TIPS and involving gastroenterology, hepatology, and interventional radiology early on is likely beneficial.[56,72]

Although variceal bleeding is more commonly due to esophageal varices, gastric varices are present in 20% of patients with cirrhosis and when they bleed, it tends to be in a more severe fashion and with higher mortality than bleeding from esophageal varices.[73] Initial stabilization, use of vasoactive drugs, and prophylactic antibiotics are similar to the treatment of esophageal varices.[60] Gastroesophageal varices type 1 (GOV-1) are contiguous esophageal varices extending along the lesser curvature and account for 75% of gastric varices.[73] Treatment of GOV-1 hemorrhage should include band ligation if the varices are small or cyanoacrylate injection if available, with secondary prevention using endoscopic treatment and NSBBs, and TIPS being reserved for patients who fail first-line therapy.[60] The American Association for the Study of Liver Diseases (AASLD) guidelines recommend TIPS as the preferred treatment modality for hemorrhage from gastroesophageal type 2 (GOV-2) and isolated gastric varices type 1 (IGV-1) fundal varices, which have an increased early rebleed rate, and often will also need collateral variceal embolization.[60] TIPS or balloon-occluded retrograde transvenous obliteration (BRTO) are recommended in those who have recovered from GOV-2 or IGV-1 hemorrhage to prevent further episodes.[60]

TIPS was more effective in preventing rebleeding from gastric varices than endoscopic cyanoacrylate injection (11% vs 38%).[74] BRTO, which involves the occlusion of gastrorenal or splenorenal shunts, may be an option for those with decreased hepatic reserve or with HE, though it can worsen portal hypertension.[75] BRTO has high success rates and should be considered in those with contraindications to TIPS.[76,77] The decision to proceed with one of these treatment options must include multidisciplinary conversations between the critical care team and the consulting gastroenterology, hepatology, and interventional radiology teams.

PULMONARY COMPLICATIONS

The most common pulmonary vascular complications in patients with chronic liver disease are portopulmonary hypertension (PoPH) and hepatopulmonary syndrome (HPS).[78]

PoPH is pulmonary arterial hypertension that occurs in the setting of portal hypertension in the absence of other etiologies.[79] The diagnosis of PoPH requires confirmation by right heart catheterization demonstrating a mean pulmonary arterial pressure (mPAP) >25 mm Hg and pulmonary vascular resistance (PVR) >3 wood units (240 dyn*sec*cm-5) with a normal wedge pressure less than 15 mm Hg.[79,80] Severity is categorized by mPAP into mild (25 to <35 mm Hg), moderate (35 to <45 mm Hg), and severe ($\geq$45 mm Hg).[80] PoPH is present in 3%–10% of patients evaluated for liver transplant.[56] The most common symptom is dyspnea and signs of right heart failure can also occur.[81] The risk of mortality is high, with one study showing 54% mortality at 1 year without treatment[82] and the US REVEAL study showed worse 5-year survival of 40% than 64% in those with idiopathic or familial pulmonary arterial hypertension.[83] Transthoracic echocardiography is commonly used for screening and is supported by the International Liver Transplant Society and the European Association for the Study of the Liver in patients being considered for TIPS or liver transplant.[56,79] A pulmonary artery systolic pressure greater than 50 mm Hg had a positive predictive value of 38% and negative predictive value of 92% to identify clinically significant pulmonary hypertension.[84] The AASLD recommends echocardiography in transplant candidates followed by right heart catheterization for those with a right ventricular systolic pressure (RVSP) $\geq$45 mm Hg.[85]

The pharmacologic management of PoPH is similar to that of other forms of pulmonary arterial hypertension and can include prostacyclin analogues, phosphodiesterase subtype 5 inhibitors, and endothelin receptor antagonists, though the latter should be used with caution given concerns in patients with hepatic impairment.[56,79] Beta-blockers in moderate to severe PoPH have been associated with worsening exercise capacity and pulmonary hemodynamics and should be avoided in these patients.[86]

Moderate and severe pulmonary hypertension are relative and absolute contraindications to TIPS, respectively.[68] Severe PoPH should be considered an absolute contraindication to liver transplantation.[56,79] Liver transplant can be considered in those with mild disease or in patients with moderate and severe PoPH who have improved with medical management to an mPAP less than 35 mm Hg and PVR less than 400 dyn*sec*cm-5.[56,79,85] In a retrospective review of the French PAH cohort, overall 5-year survival was 51% with medical therapy, whereas the 5-year survival increased to 81% among patients who underwent liver transplant.[87]

HPS is defined by the presence of liver disease, intravascular pulmonary dilations, and abnormal arterial oxygenation with an alveolar-arterial oxygen gradient $\geq$15 mm Hg or $\geq$20 mm Hg if older than 64 years (**Fig. 3**).[80] The prevalence of HPS is 5%–32%, it can occur with acute or chronic liver disease, and is frequently seen with portal hypertension though this is not required for diagnosis, and is not related to the severity of liver disease.[88] Symptoms can include dyspnea and low oxygenation, and platypnea and orthodeoxia may be seen.[88] The 5-year survival is poor, especially among patients with the more severe forms of HPS, with one study showing 23% survival without liver transplantation.[89]

Pulse oximetry can be used for the screening of HPS; however, room air ABG is required to establish the diagnosis and assess severity.[56,79,85] An SpO2 less than 96% on room air has a sensitivity of 100% and specificity of 88% to detect a Pao$_2$ less than 60 mm Hg.[90] Contrast-enhanced transthoracic echocardiography is recommended to detect intravascular pulmonary dilations and is considered positive with the appearance of microbubbles in the left heart after 3 cardiac cycles. The severity of HPS is stratified based on the partial pressure of oxygenation at room air, mild: Pao$_2$ $\geq$80 mm Hg, moderate: 60 to 79 mm Hg, severe 50 to 59 mm Hg and very severe less than 50 mm Hg.[80] Other diagnostic modalities can be considered if needed, including transesophageal echocardiography to assess for intracardiac shunts or Tc99m macroaggregated albumin scan to assess the contribution of HPS in the presence of other comorbid lung conditions.[79,88] Supplemental oxygen is recommended for supportive care, though there is no effective treatment of HPS other than liver

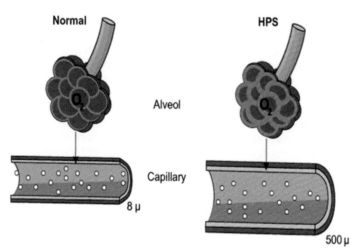

Fig. 3. The pathophysiology of hepatopulmonary syndrome (HPS) resulting in intrapulmonary vasodilation and a widened alveolar-arterial oxygen gradient. (*reproduced with permission from* EASL, J Hepatology 2018[56]).

transplantation.[79] In one study, 5-year postliver transplant survival was shown to be improved at 88% since UNOS MELD exceptions began in 2002 versus a 67% 5-year posttransplant survival before this.[91] Patients with HPS and a Pao_2 less than 60 mm Hg should be referred for liver transplantation.[79,85]

ACUTE KIDNEY INJURY AND HEPATORENAL SYNDROME

Renal dysfunction is a common complication of patients with advanced cirrhosis. This manifests as AKI, defined as an abrupt decline in renal function, marked by rising serum creatinine and/or reduction in urine output. AKI occurs in 19%–26% of hospitalized patients with cirrhosis and in up to a third of patients with severe alcoholic hepatitis.[92,93] Other than the typical classification of AKI into prerenal, intrinsic, and postrenal; patients with cirrhosis can suffer from a specific type of renal dysfunction known as HRS.[94] This "functional" AKI occurs in the setting of decompensated cirrhosis with ascites and is thought to be a direct consequence of severely reduced renal arterial perfusion resulting from hemodynamic derangements in arterial circulation observed in patients with advanced cirrhosis, as well as the dysregulation of endogenous vasoactive systems which lead to splanchnic vasodilation, increased portal vein inflow, and reduced renal perfusion.[95]

Following the Kidney Disease Improving Global Outcome (KDIGO) guidelines, AKI is defined as an increase in serum creatinine of at least 0.3 mg/dL within 48 hours, an increase in serum creatinine of at least 1.5 times baseline within the previous 7 days, or a urine output of less than 0.5 mL/kg/h for 6 hours.[96] Similar criteria are currently used to diagnose HRS-AKI (previously called type 1 HRS). By adopting these diagnostic criteria, patients with AKI can be identified earlier which can lead to improvements in short-term inpatient outcomes and even 90-day mortality.[97–100] Although the International Club of Ascites (group of experts who defined HRS) does not use the urine volume as a diagnostic criterion, a recent study in ICU patients demonstrated that those with AKI and reduction in urine volume less than 0.5 mL/kg/h for at least 6 hours had higher mortality than did patients who only met the creatinine criteria for AKI.[101] Therefore, urine output can be used in the ICU for diagnosis and staging of AKI.[95]

The current definition of HRS-AKI includes not only the changes in serum creatinine but also the criteria listed in **Box 1**.[94]

The most common cause of AKI in cirrhosis is prerenal azotemia (46%-66%), and is typically differentiated from HRS-AKI and intrinsic AKI by clinical presentation and prompt response to IV fluids.[102,103] That leaves the differential diagnosis of AKI not responsive to fluids as either HRS-AKI or intrinsic AKI, namely acute tubular necrosis (ATN). The treatment of these conditions is generally quite different, so it is important to distinguish them and this is not always straightforward on clinical grounds alone. Urine microscopy, urinary sodium, fractional excretion of sodium (FeNa), and urine osmolality can be helpful in differentiating ATN from HRS-AKI; however, there is still overlap and these parameters may not allow for a clear diagnosis. In patients with cirrhosis, the urinary excretion of sodium may be elevated due to diuretic use, which can limit the usefulness of FeNa as a diagnostic marker for HRS-AKI. To circumvent this limitation, the fractional excretion of urea can be used in these patients to better distinguish ATN from HRS-AKI.[104] More recently, novel biomarkers of tubular injury have been evaluated in an effort to distinguish HRS-AKI from ATN. Although not yet ready for widespread use, urinary neutrophil gelatinase-associated lipocalin (NGAL) has demonstrated the greatest diagnostic accuracy in differentiating between ATN and HRS-AKI.[105–107]

Box 1
Current definition of hepatorenal syndrome-acute kidney injury (HRS-AKI) as per the International Club of Ascites

Diagnostic criteria HRS-AKI:

Increase in serum creatinine ≥0.3 mg/dL within 48 hours

or

Increase in serum creatinine ≥1.5 times from baseline (creatinine value within 3 months, when available, may be used as a baseline, and value closest to the presentation should be used)

No response to diuretic withdrawal and a 2-day fluid challenge with 1 g/kg/d 20%–25% IV albumin.

Cirrhosis with ascites

Absence of shock

No current or recent use of nephrotoxic drugs (NSAIDs, contrast dye, etc.)

No signs of structural kidney injury:

  Absence of proteinuria (>500 mg/d),

  Absence of hematuria (>50 RBCs per high power field)

  Normal renal sonogram

reproduced with permission from Angeli P, et al. J Hepatology 2015[94]

Once the diagnosis of AKI is made, it is important to stage its severity (**Box 2**) as this not only impacts prognosis, it also guides management (**Fig. 4**). Stage 1A (AKI with serum creatinine <1.5 mg/dL) is generally due to hypovolemia and commonly resolves with discontinuation of diuretics and albumin fluid challenge. However, only about 50% of patients with stage 1B (serum creatinine ≥1.5 mg/dL) will respond to a 2-day IV albumin challenge and a significant proportion will go on to more advanced stages of AKI.[94,95] For this reason, the EASL guidelines recommend starting vasopressors at this stage (see **Fig. 4**).[56] In this setting, vasopressors result in splanchnic vasoconstriction, reduction in portal pressure, increased effective arterial

---

Box 2
Staging of acute kidney injury in patients with cirrhosis according to the International Club of Ascites

Stage 1
  Increase in Cr ≥0.3 mg/dL within 48 hours *or* Cr ≥1.5 to 2 times from baseline
    Stage 1a: Cr <1.5 mg/dL
    Stage 1b: Cr ≥1.5 mg/dL

Stage 2
  Increase in Cr of 2 to 3 times from the baseline

Stage 3
  Increase in Cr ≥ 3 times from baseline *or* Cr ≥ 4 mg/dL *or* initiation of renal replacement therapy

Abbreviation: Cr, serum creatinine.

reproduced with permission of Angeli P, et al. J Hepatology 2015[94]

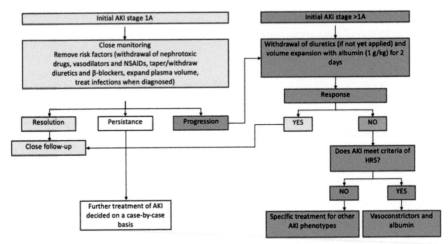

Fig. 4. Algorithm for the management of acute kidney injury in patients with cirrhosis. (reproduced with permission from EASL, J Hepatology 2018[56]).

blood volume and arterial flow through the kidneys, especially when used in combination with IV albumin.[108] Renal perfusion directly correlates with changes in MAP, such that a significant increase in MAP is associated with a greater likelihood of HRS-AKI reversal.[109]

Several randomized trials have confirmed the efficacy of vasoconstrictors in combination with IV albumin in reversing HRS-AKI.[110] The most common one used throughout the world is terlipressin; however, this is not yet available in North America, even though a recent trial demonstrated significantly higher reversal of HRS-AKI when compared with albumin and placebo (32% vs 17%, $P = .006$), although with a higher rate of respiratory complications.[111] Interestingly, among patients with systemic inflammatory response including those with severe alcoholic hepatitis, terlipressin shows greater efficacy in reversing HRS-AKI.[111,112]

Alternatives to terlipressin include the combination of midodrine and octreotide (in the non-ICU setting) or norepinephrine for patients in the ICU. However, their efficacy in reversing HRS-AKI is limited than that of terlipressin with albumin,[113–115] especially among patients with decompensated cirrhosis and ACLF.[116]

The best treatment of patients with HRS-AKI is liver transplant, as this addresses the underlying pathogenesis of this syndrome. Unfortunately, many patients with HRS-AKI are not liver transplant candidates, so their short-term mortality is quite high.

Patients with HRS-AKI who do not respond to medical therapy have few treatment options outside of liver transplant. Renal replacement therapy can be challenging in these patients, as they typically have significant hemodynamic compromise, limiting the role of intermittent hemodialysis. When renal replacement is used, it will typically come in the form of continuous veno-venous hemodialysis in the ICU. The prognosis of this group of patients is dismal. Among a group of 462 patients with cirrhosis and AKI (either HRS-AKI or ATN) who initiated renal replacement therapy, only 15% of those not listed for liver transplant were alive 6 months later. Median survival was 21 days for those with HRS-AKI and only 12 days for those with ATN. Among the patients listed for liver transplant, 48% went on to receive one, including a third of them who received a simultaneous liver and kidney transplant. In this retrospective study, the short-term mortality of patients with cirrhosis and AKI requiring renal replacement therapy was extremely high (especially among those not listed for liver transplant) and similar regardless of AKI etiology (HRS vs ATN).[117] For this reason, it might be futile to offer renal replacement therapy, especially in those patients who are not transplanted candidates. In concert with the consulting hepatology and nephrology teams, goals of care discussions with patient and family should be held.[118]

SUMMARY

Patients with cirrhosis account for approximately 3% of intensive care unit admissions and have a poor prognosis, with hospital mortality exceeding 50%. However, significant improvements in survival among patients with acutely decompensated cirrhosis and organ failure have been described recently. Common life-threatening complications in patients with cirrhosis that require intensive care management include HE, hypovolemic and/or distributive shock, cardiac, pulmonary, and renal complications. ACLF is a distinct clinical syndrome in patients with cirrhosis characterized by decompensated state associated with the development of one or more organ failures resulting in poor short-term survival. Select patients with ACLF liver failure will benefit from liver transplantation with excellent posttransplant survival.

CLINICS CARE POINTS

- Lactulose remains the cornerstone of pharmacologic therapy for HE in the patient with decompensated cirrhosis, followed by rifaximin in patient with inadequate response to lactulose.

- A specific blood pressure goal has not been established in patient with cirrhosis and shock; however, a MAP greater than 65 mm Hg in patients with end-organ hypoperfusion is generally recommended.

- In select patients with decompensated cirrhosis, albumin is the volume expander of choice.

- In patients with variceal hemorrhage with acute blood loss anemia, a restrictive blood transfusion strategy (hemoglobin <7 g/dL) decreases the risk of rebleeding and improves short-term survival.

- Antibiotic prophylaxis in patients with variceal bleeding is associated with a reduction in bacterial infections, rebleeding rates, and short-term mortality.

- Pharmacologic management of portopulmonary hypertension is similar to that of other forms of pulmonary arterial hypertension.

- Severe portopulmonary hypertension unresponsive to medical therapy is an absolute contraindication to liver transplant.

- Vasopressors in combination with albumin are the mainstay of pharmacologic therapy in hepatorenal syndrome.

DISCLOSURE

Dr J.F. Gallegos-Orozco was the principal investigator for the University of Utah site of the terlipressin and albumin in type 1 hepatorenal syndrome trial sponsored by Mallinckrodt Pharmaceuticals. Dr S. Chandna and Dr E. Rodriguez Zarate have nothing to disclose.

REFERENCES

1. Gallegos-Orozco JF. The growing challenge of advanced liver disease due to alcohol use in the United States. Am J Gastroenterol 2019;114(11):1712–3. https://doi.org/10.14309/ajg.0000000000000422.

2. Dang K, Hirode G, Singal AK, et al. Alcoholic liver disease epidemiology in the united states: a retrospective analysis of 3 US databases. Am J Gastroenterol 2020;115(1):96–104. https://doi.org/10.14309/ajg.0000000000000380.

3. Tapper EB, Parikh ND. Mortality due to cirrhosis and liver cancer in the United States, 1999-2016: observational study. BMJ 2018;362:k2817. https://doi.org/10.1136/bmj.k2817.

4. Goldberg D, Ditah IC, Saeian K, et al. Changes in the Prevalence of Hepatitis C virus infection, nonalcoholic steatohepatitis, and alcoholic liver disease among patients with cirrhosis or liver failure on the waitlist for liver transplantation. Gastroenterology 2017;152(5):1090–9.e1. https://doi.org/10.1053/j.gastro.2017.01.003.

5. Cholankeril G, Gadiparthi C, Yoo ER, et al. Temporal trends associated with the rise in alcoholic liver disease-related liver transplantation in the United States. Transplantation 2019;103(1):131–9. https://doi.org/10.1097/TP.0000000000002471.

6. Christiansen CF, Christensen S, Johansen MB, et al. The impact of pre-admission morbidity level on 3-year mortality after intensive care: a Danish cohort study. Acta Anaesthesiol Scand 2011;55(8):962–70. https://doi.org/10.1111/j.1399-6576.2011.02480.x.

7. O'Brien AJ, Welch CA, Singer M, et al. Prevalence and outcome of cirrhosis patients admitted to UK intensive care: a comparison against dialysis-dependent chronic renal failure patients. Intensive Care Med 2012;38(6):991–1000. https://doi.org/10.1007/s00134-012-2523-2.

8. Skurzak S, Carrara G, Rossi C, et al. Cirrhotic patients admitted to the ICU for medical reasons: Analysis of 5506 patients admitted to 286 ICUs in 8years. J Crit Care 2018;45:220–8. https://doi.org/10.1016/j.jcrc.2018.03.018.

9. Galbois A, Trompette ML, Das V, et al. Improvement in the prognosis of cirrhotic patients admitted to an intensive care unit, a retrospective study. Eur J Gastroenterol Hepatol 2012;24(8):897–904. https://doi.org/10.1097/MEG.0b013e3283544816.

10. Saliba F, Ichai P, Levesque E, et al. Cirrhotic patients in the ICU: prognostic markers and outcome. Curr Opin Crit Care 2013;19(2):154–60. https://doi.org/10.1097/MCC.0b013e32835f0c17.

11. Arabi Y, Ahmed QA, Haddad S, et al. Outcome predictors of cirrhosis patients admitted to the intensive care unit. Eur J Gastroenterol Hepatol 2004;16(3):333–9. https://doi.org/10.1097/00042737-200403000-00014.

12. Theocharidou E, Pieri G, Mohammad AO, et al. The Royal Free Hospital score: a calibrated prognostic model for patients with cirrhosis admitted to intensive care unit. Comparison with current models and CLIF-SOFA score. Am J Gastroenterol 2014;109(4):554–62. https://doi.org/10.1038/ajg.2013.466.

13. McPhail MJ, Shawcross DL, Abeles RD, et al. Increased survival for patients with cirrhosis and organ failure in liver intensive care and validation of the chronic liver failure-sequential organ failure scoring system. Clin Gastroenterol Hepatol 2015;13(7):1353–60.e8. https://doi.org/10.1016/j.cgh.2014.08.041.

14. Majumdar A, Bailey M, Kemp WM, et al. Declining mortality in critically ill patients with cirrhosis in Australia and New Zealand between 2000 and 2015. J Hepatol 2017;67(6):1185–93. https://doi.org/10.1016/j.jhep.2017.07.024.

15. McPhail MJW, Parrott F, Wendon JA, et al. Incidence and outcomes for patients with cirrhosis admitted to the United Kingdom critical care units. Crit Care Med 2018;46(5):705–12. https://doi.org/10.1097/CCM.0000000000002961.

16. Moreau R, Jalan R, Gines P, et al. Acute-on-chronic liver failure is a distinct syndrome that develops in patients with acute decompensation of cirrhosis. Gastroenterology 2013;144(7):1426–37. https://doi.org/10.1053/j.gastro.2013.02.042, 1437.e1–9.

17. Arroyo V, Moreau R, Jalan R. Acute-on-chronic liver failure. N Engl J Med 2020; 382(22):2137–45. https://doi.org/10.1056/NEJMra1914900.

18. Hernaez R, Kramer JR, Liu Y, et al. Prevalence and short-term mortality of acute-on-chronic liver failure: a national cohort study from the USA. J Hepatol 2019; 70(4):639–47. https://doi.org/10.1016/j.jhep.2018.12.018.

19. Mezzano G, Juanola A, Cardenas A, et al. Global burden of disease: acute-on-chronic liver failure, a systematic review and meta-analysis. Gut 2021. https://doi.org/10.1136/gutjnl-2020-322161.

20. Nanchal R, Subramanian R, Karvellas CJ, et al. Guidelines for the management of adult acute and acute-on-chronic liver failure in the ICU: cardiovascular, endocrine, hematologic, pulmonary, and renal considerations. Crit Care Med 2020;48(3):e173–91. https://doi.org/10.1097/CCM.0000000000004192.

21. DellaVolpe JD, Garavaglia JM, Huang DT. Management of complications of end-stage liver disease in the intensive care unit. J Intensive Care Med 2016;31(2): 94–103. https://doi.org/10.1177/0885066614551144.

22. Cordoba J, Ventura-Cots M, Simón-Talero M, et al. Characteristics, risk factors, and mortality of cirrhotic patients hospitalized for hepatic encephalopathy with and without acute-on-chronic liver failure (ACLF). J Hepatol 2014;60(2): 275–81. https://doi.org/10.1016/j.jhep.2013.10.004.

23. Hassanein TI, Tofteng F, Brown RS, et al. Randomized controlled study of extracorporeal albumin dialysis for hepatic encephalopathy in advanced cirrhosis. Hepatology 2007;46(6):1853–62. https://doi.org/10.1002/hep.21930.

24. Bajaj JS. Review article: the modern management of hepatic encephalopathy. Aliment Pharmacol Ther 2010;31(5):537–47. https://doi.org/10.1111/j.1365-2036.2009.04211.x.

25. Vilstrup H, Amodio P, Bajaj J, et al. Hepatic encephalopathy in chronic liver disease: 2014 Practice Guideline by the American Association for the Study of Liver Diseases and the European Association for the Study of the Liver. Hepatology 2014;60(2):715–35. https://doi.org/10.1002/hep.27210.

26. Bajaj JS, Wade JB, Sanyal AJ. Spectrum of neurocognitive impairment in cirrhosis: Implications for the assessment of hepatic encephalopathy. Hepatology 2009;50(6):2014–21. https://doi.org/10.1002/hep.23216.

27. Nadim MK, Durand F, Kellum JA, et al. Management of the critically ill patient with cirrhosis: a multidisciplinary perspective. J Hepatol 2016;64(3):717–35. https://doi.org/10.1016/j.jhep.2015.10.019.

28. Shawcross DL, Sharifi Y, Canavan JB, et al. Infection and systemic inflammation, not ammonia, are associated with Grade 3/4 hepatic encephalopathy, but not mortality in cirrhosis. J Hepatol 2011;54(4):640–9. https://doi.org/10.1016/j.jhep.2010.07.045.

29. Rose CF, Amodio P, Bajaj JS, et al. Hepatic encephalopathy: novel insights into classification, pathophysiology and therapy. J Hepatol 2020;73(6):1526–47. https://doi.org/10.1016/j.jhep.2020.07.013.

30. Ginès P, Fernández J, Durand F, et al. Management of critically-ill cirrhotic patients. J Hepatol 2012;56(Suppl 1):S13–24. https://doi.org/10.1016/S0168-8278(12)60003-8.

31. Olson JC, Karvellas CJ. Critical care management of the patient with cirrhosis awaiting liver transplant in the intensive care unit. Liver Transpl 2017;23(11): 1465–76. https://doi.org/10.1002/lt.24815.

32. MacDonald AJ, Olson J, Karvellas CJ. Critical care considerations in the management of acute-on-chronic liver failure. Curr Opin Crit Care 2020;26(2): 171–9. https://doi.org/10.1097/MCC.0000000000000698.

33. Rahimi RS, Singal AG, Cuthbert JA, et al. Lactulose vs polyethylene glycol 3350–electrolyte solution for treatment of overt hepatic encephalopathy: the HELP randomized clinical trial. JAMA Intern Med 2014;174(11):1727–33. https://doi.org/10.1001/jamainternmed.2014.4746.

34. Bass NM, Mullen KD, Sanyal A, et al. Rifaximin treatment in hepatic encephalopathy. N Engl J Med 2010;362(12):1071–81. https://doi.org/10.1056/NEJMoa0907893.

35. Sharma BC, Sharma P, Lunia MK, et al. A randomized, double-blind, controlled trial comparing rifaximin plus lactulose with lactulose alone in treatment of overt hepatic encephalopathy. Am J Gastroenterol 2013;108(9):1458–63. https://doi.org/10.1038/ajg.2013.219.

36. Laleman W, Simon-Talero M, Maleux G, et al. Embolization of large spontaneous portosystemic shunts for refractory hepatic encephalopathy: a multicenter survey on safety and efficacy. Hepatology 2013;57(6):2448–57. https://doi.org/10.1002/hep.26314.

37. Cash WJ, McConville P, McDermott E, et al. Current concepts in the assessment and treatment of hepatic encephalopathy. QJM 2010;103(1):9–16. https://doi.org/10.1093/qjmed/hcp152.

38. Bañares R, Nevens F, Larsen FS, et al. Extracorporeal albumin dialysis with the molecular adsorbent recirculating system in acute-on-chronic liver failure: the RELIEF trial. Hepatology 2013;57(3):1153–62. https://doi.org/10.1002/hep.26185.

39. Kribben A, Gerken G, Haag S, et al. Effects of fractionated plasma separation and adsorption on survival in patients with acute-on-chronic liver failure. Gastroenterology 2012;142(4):782–9.e3. https://doi.org/10.1053/j.gastro.2011.12.056.

40. Gustot T, Fernandez J, Garcia E, et al. Clinical Course of acute-on-chronic liver failure syndrome and effects on prognosis. Hepatology 2015;62(1):243–52. https://doi.org/10.1002/hep.27849.

41. Møller S, Hove JD, Dixen U, et al. New insights into cirrhotic cardiomyopathy. Int J Cardiol 2013;167(4):1101–8. https://doi.org/10.1016/j.ijcard.2012.09.089.

42. Thalheimer U, Burroughs AK. Bacterial translocation and cardiovascular complications of cirrhosis. Gut 2008;57(8):1181–2.

43. Rhodes A, Evans LE, Alhazzani W, et al. Surviving sepsis campaign: international guidelines for management of sepsis and septic shock: 2016. Crit Care Med 2017;45(3):486–552. https://doi.org/10.1097/CCM.0000000000002255.

44. Biancofiore G, Critchley LA, Lee A, et al. Evaluation of a new software version of the FloTrac/Vigileo (version 3.02) and a comparison with previous data in cirrhotic patients undergoing liver transplant surgery. Anesth Analg 2011; 113(3):515–22. https://doi.org/10.1213/ANE.0b013e31822401b2.

45. Paugam-Burtz C, Levesque E, Louvet A, et al. Management of liver failure in general intensive care unit. Anaesth Crit Care Pain Med 2020;39(1):143–61. https://doi.org/10.1016/j.accpm.2019.06.014.

46. Ortega R, Ginès P, Uriz J, et al. Terlipressin therapy with and without albumin for patients with hepatorenal syndrome: results of a prospective, nonrandomized

study. Hepatology 2002;36(4 Pt 1):941–8. https://doi.org/10.1053/jhep.2002. 35819.

47. De Backer D, Biston P, Devriendt J, et al. Comparison of dopamine and norepinephrine in the treatment of shock. N Engl J Med 2010;362(9):779–89. https://doi.org/10.1056/NEJMoa0907118.

48. Delmas A, Leone M, Rousseau S, et al. Clinical review: vasopressin and terlipressin in septic shock patients. Crit Care 2005;9(2):212–22. https://doi.org/10.1186/cc2945.

49. Annane D, Bellissant E, Sebille V, et al. Impaired pressor sensitivity to noradrenaline in septic shock patients with and without impaired adrenal function reserve. Br J Clin Pharmacol 1998;46(6):589–97. https://doi.org/10.1046/j.1365-2125.1998.00833.x.

50. Beishuizen A, Thijs LG. Relative adrenal failure in intensive care: an identifiable problem requiring treatment? Best Pract Res Clin Endocrinol Metab 2001;15(4): 513–31. https://doi.org/10.1053/beem.2001.0167.

51. Tsai MH, Peng YS, Chen YC, et al. Adrenal insufficiency in patients with cirrhosis, severe sepsis and septic shock. Hepatology 2006;43(4):673–81. https://doi.org/10.1002/hep.21101.

52. Fernández J, Escorsell A, Zabalza M, et al. Adrenal insufficiency in patients with cirrhosis and septic shock: Effect of treatment with hydrocortisone on survival. Hepatology 2006;44(5):1288–95. https://doi.org/10.1002/hep.21352.

53. Solà R, Vila MC, Andreu M, et al. Total paracentesis with dextran 40 vs diuretics in the treatment of ascites in cirrhosis: a randomized controlled study. J Hepatol 1994;20(2):282–8. https://doi.org/10.1016/s0168-8278(05)80070-4.

54. Bernardi M, Caraceni P, Navickis RJ, et al. Albumin infusion in patients undergoing large-volume paracentesis: a meta-analysis of randomized trials. Hepatology 2012;55(4):1172–81. https://doi.org/10.1002/hep.24786.

55. Ginès P, Titó L, Arroyo V, et al. Randomized comparative study of therapeutic paracentesis with and without intravenous albumin in cirrhosis. Gastroenterology 1988;94(6):1493–502. https://doi.org/10.1016/0016-5085(88)90691-9.

56. European Association for the Study of the Liver. EASL Clinical Practice Guidelines for the management of patients with decompensated cirrhosis. J Hepatol 2018;69(2):406–60. https://doi.org/10.1016/j.jhep.2018.03.024.

57. Abraldes JG, Tarantino I, Turnes J, et al. Hemodynamic response to pharmacological treatment of portal hypertension and long-term prognosis of cirrhosis. Hepatology 2003;37(4):902–8. https://doi.org/10.1053/jhep.2003.50133.

58. Mandorfer M, Bota S, Schwabl P, et al. Nonselective β blockers increase risk for hepatorenal syndrome and death in patients with cirrhosis and spontaneous bacterial peritonitis. Gastroenterology 2014;146(7):1680–90.e1. https://doi.org/10.1053/j.gastro.2014.03.005.

59. Sersté T, Melot C, Francoz C, et al. Deleterious effects of beta-blockers on survival in patients with cirrhosis and refractory ascites. Hepatology 2010;52(3): 1017–22. https://doi.org/10.1002/hep.23775.

60. Garcia-Tsao G, Abraldes JG, Berzigotti A, et al. Portal hypertensive bleeding in cirrhosis: Risk stratification, diagnosis, and management: 2016 practice guidance by the American Association for the study of liver diseases. Hepatology 2017;65(1):310–35. https://doi.org/10.1002/hep.28906.

61. Rajwani K, Fortune BE, Brown RS. Critical care management of gastrointestinal bleeding and ascites in liver failure. Semin Respir Crit Care Med 2018;39(5): 566–77. https://doi.org/10.1055/s-0038-1672200.

62. Villanueva C, Colomo A, Bosch A. Transfusion for acute upper gastrointestinal bleeding. N Engl J Med 2013;368(14):1362–3. https://doi.org/10.1056/NEJMc1301256.

63. Wells M, Chande N, Adams P, et al. Meta-analysis: vasoactive medications for the management of acute variceal bleeds. Aliment Pharmacol Ther 2012;35(11):1267–78. https://doi.org/10.1111/j.1365-2036.2012.05088.x.

64. Seo YS, Park SY, Kim MY, et al. Lack of difference among terlipressin, somatostatin, and octreotide in the control of acute gastroesophageal variceal hemorrhage. Hepatology 2014;60(3):954–63. https://doi.org/10.1002/hep.27006.

65. Simonetto DA, Liu M, Kamath PS. Portal hypertension and related complications: diagnosis and management. Mayo Clin Proc 2019;94(4):714–26. https://doi.org/10.1016/j.mayocp.2018.12.020.

66. Chavez-Tapia NC, Barrientos-Gutierrez T, Tellez-Avila F, et al. Meta-analysis: antibiotic prophylaxis for cirrhotic patients with upper gastrointestinal bleeding - an updated Cochrane review. Aliment Pharmacol Ther 2011;34(5):509–18. https://doi.org/10.1111/j.1365-2036.2011.04746.x.

67. Saab S, Kim NG, Lee EW. Practical tips on TIPS: when and when not to request it. Am J Gastroenterol 2020;115(6):797–800. https://doi.org/10.14309/ajg.0000000000000611.

68. Boyer TD, Haskal ZJ, Diseases AAftSoL. The role of transjugular intrahepatic portosystemic shunt in the management of portal hypertension. Hepatology 2005;41(2):386–400. https://doi.org/10.1002/hep.20559.

69. Rodrigues SG, Cárdenas A, Escorsell À, et al. Balloon tamponade and esophageal stenting for esophageal variceal bleeding in cirrhosis: a systematic review and meta-analysis. Semin Liver Dis 2019;39(2):178–94. https://doi.org/10.1055/s-0039-1678726.

70. Escorsell À, Pavel O, Cárdenas A, et al. Esophageal balloon tamponade versus esophageal stent in controlling acute refractory variceal bleeding: a multicenter randomized, controlled trial. Hepatology 2016;63(6):1957–67. https://doi.org/10.1002/hep.28360.

71. Conejo I, Guardascione MA, Tandon P, et al. Multicenter external validation of risk stratification criteria for patients with variceal bleeding. Clin Gastroenterol Hepatol 2018;16(1):132–9.e8. https://doi.org/10.1016/j.cgh.2017.04.042.

72. Garcia-Tsao G. Management of acute variceal hemorrhage as a model of individualized care for patients with cirrhosis. Clin Gastroenterol Hepatol 2018;16(1):24–6. https://doi.org/10.1016/j.cgh.2017.08.035.

73. Sarin SK, Lahoti D, Saxena SP, et al. Prevalence, classification and natural history of gastric varices: a long-term follow-up study in 568 portal hypertension patients. Hepatology 1992;16(6):1343–9. https://doi.org/10.1002/hep.1840160607.

74. Lo GH, Liang HL, Chen WC, et al. A prospective, randomized controlled trial of transjugular intrahepatic portosystemic shunt versus cyanoacrylate injection in the prevention of gastric variceal rebleeding. Endoscopy 2007;39(8):679–85. https://doi.org/10.1055/s-2007-966591.

75. Saad WE. Balloon-occluded retrograde transvenous obliteration of gastric varices: concept, basic techniques, and outcomes. Semin Intervent Radiol 2012;29(2):118–28. https://doi.org/10.1055/s-0032-1312573.

76. Park JK, Saab S, Kee ST, et al. Balloon-occluded retrograde transvenous obliteration (BRTO) for treatment of gastric varices: review and meta-analysis. Dig Dis Sci 2015;60(6):1543–53. https://doi.org/10.1007/s10620-014-3485-8.

77. Turon F, Casu S, Hernández-Gea V, et al. Variceal and other portal hypertension related bleeding. Best Pract Res Clin Gastroenterol 2013;27(5):649–64. https://doi.org/10.1016/j.bpg.2013.08.004.

78. Porres-Aguilar M, Gallegos-Orozco JF, Garcia H, et al. Pulmonary vascular complications in portal hypertension and liver disease: a concise review. Rev Gastroenterol Mex 2013;78(1):35–44. https://doi.org/10.1016/j.rgmx.2012.10.004.

79. Krowka MJ, Fallon MB, Kawut SM, et al. International liver transplant society practice guidelines: diagnosis and management of hepatopulmonary syndrome and portopulmonary hypertension. Transplantation 2016;100(7):1440–52. https://doi.org/10.1097/TP.0000000000001229.

80. Rodriguez-Roisin R, Krowka MJ, Herve P, et al. Pulmonary-hepatic vascular disorders (PHD). Eur Respir J 2004;5:861–80.

81. McLaughlin VV, Archer SL, Badesch DB, et al. ACCF/AHA 2009 expert consensus document on pulmonary hypertension a report of the American College of Cardiology Foundation Task Force on Expert Consensus Documents and the American Heart Association developed in collaboration with the American College of Chest Physicians; American Thoracic Society, Inc.; and the Pulmonary Hypertension Association. J Am Coll Cardiol 2009;53(17):1573–619. https://doi.org/10.1016/j.jacc.2009.01.004.

82. Swanson KL, Wiesner RH, Nyberg SL, et al. Survival in portopulmonary hypertension: Mayo Clinic experience categorized by treatment subgroups. Am J Transpl 2008;11:2445–53.

83. Krowka MJ, Miller DP, Barst RJ, et al. Portopulmonary hypertension: a report from the US-based REVEAL Registry. Chest 2012;4:906–15.

84. Cotton CL, Gandhi S, Vaitkus PT, et al. Role of echocardiography in detecting portopulmonary hypertension in liver transplant candidates. Liver Transpl 2002;11:1051–4.

85. Martin P, DiMartini A, Feng S, et al. Evaluation for liver transplantation in adults: 2013 practice guideline by the American Association for the Study of Liver Diseases and the American Society of Transplantation. Hepatology 2014;59(3): 1144–65. https://doi.org/10.1002/hep.26972.

86. Provencher S, Herve P, Jais X, et al. Deleterious effects of beta-blockers on exercise capacity and hemodynamics in patients with portopulmonary hypertension. Gastroenterology 2006;1:120–6.

87. Savale L, Guimas M, Ebstein N, et al. Portopulmonary hypertension in the current era of pulmonary hypertension management. J Hepatol 2020;73(1): 130–9. https://doi.org/10.1016/j.jhep.2020.02.021.

88. Rodriguez-Roisin R, Krowka MJ. Hepatopulmonary syndrome–a liver-induced lung vascular disorder. N Engl J Med 2008;22:2378–87.

89. Swanson KL, Wiesner RH, Krowka MJ. Natural history of hepatopulmonary syndrome: Impact of liver transplantation. Hepatology 2005;41(5):1122–9. https://doi.org/10.1002/hep.20658.

90. Arguedas MR, Singh H, Faulk DK, et al. Utility of pulse oximetry screening for hepatopulmonary syndrome. Clin Gastroenterol Hepatol 2007;6:749–54.

91. Iyer VN, Swanson KL, Cartin-Ceba R, et al. Hepatopulmonary syndrome: favorable outcomes in the MELD exception era. Hepatology 2013;57(6):2427–35. https://doi.org/10.1002/hep.26070.

92. Piano S, Rosi S, Maresio G, et al. Evaluation of the Acute Kidney Injury Network criteria in hospitalized patients with cirrhosis and ascites. J Hepatol 2013;59(3): 482–9. https://doi.org/10.1016/j.jhep.2013.03.039.

93. Sujan R, Cruz-Lemini M, Altamirano J, et al. A validated score predicts acute kidney injury and survival in patients with alcoholic hepatitis. Liver Transpl 2018;24(12):1655–64. https://doi.org/10.1002/lt.25328.

94. Angeli P, Ginès P, Wong F, et al. Diagnosis and management of acute kidney injury in patients with cirrhosis: revised consensus recommendations of the International Club of Ascites. J Hepatol 2015;62(4):968–74. https://doi.org/10.1016/j.jhep.2014.12.029.

95. Angeli P, Garcia-Tsao G, Nadim MK, et al. News in pathophysiology, definition and classification of hepatorenal syndrome: a step beyond the International Club of Ascites (ICA) consensus document. J Hepatol 2019;71(4):811–22. https://doi.org/10.1016/j.jhep.2019.07.002.

96. Summary of recommendation statements. Kidney Int Suppl 2012;2(1):8–12. https://doi.org/10.1038/kisup.2012.7.

97. Belcher JM, Garcia-Tsao G, Sanyal AJ, et al. Association of AKI with mortality and complications in hospitalized patients with cirrhosis. Hepatology 2013; 57(2):753–62. https://doi.org/10.1002/hep.25735.

98. Tsien CD, Rabie R, Wong F. Acute kidney injury in decompensated cirrhosis. Gut 2013;62(1):131–7. https://doi.org/10.1136/gutjnl-2011-301255.

99. Wong F, O'Leary JG, Reddy KR, et al. New consensus definition of acute kidney injury accurately predicts 30-day mortality in patients with cirrhosis and infection. Gastroenterology 2013;145(6):1280–8.e1. https://doi.org/10.1053/j.gastro.2013.08.051.

100. Altamirano J, Fagundes C, Dominguez M, et al. Acute kidney injury is an early predictor of mortality for patients with alcoholic hepatitis. Clin Gastroenterol Hepatol 2012;10(1):65–71.e3. https://doi.org/10.1016/j.cgh.2011.09.011.

101. Amathieu R, Al-Khafaji A, Sileanu FE, et al. Significance of oliguria in critically ill patients with chronic liver disease. Hepatology 2017;66(5):1592–600. https://doi.org/10.1002/hep.29303.

102. Garcia-Tsao G, Parikh CR, Viola A. Acute kidney injury in cirrhosis. Hepatology 2008;48(6):2064–77. https://doi.org/10.1002/hep.22605.

103. Huelin P, Piano S, Solà E, et al. Validation of a staging system for acute kidney injury in patients with cirrhosis and association with acute-on-chronic liver failure. Clin Gastroenterol Hepatol 03 2017;15(3):438–45.e5. https://doi.org/10.1016/j.cgh.2016.09.156.

104. Patidar KR, Kang L, Bajaj JS, et al. Fractional excretion of urea: a simple tool for the differential diagnosis of acute kidney injury in cirrhosis. Hepatology 2018; 68(1):224–33. https://doi.org/10.1002/hep.29772.

105. Allegretti AS, Solà E, Ginès P. Clinical application of kidney biomarkers in cirrhosis. Am J Kidney Dis 2020;76(5):710–9. https://doi.org/10.1053/j.ajkd.2020.03.016.

106. Belcher JM, Sanyal AJ, Peixoto AJ, et al. Kidney biomarkers and differential diagnosis of patients with cirrhosis and acute kidney injury. Hepatology 2014; 60(2):622–32. https://doi.org/10.1002/hep.26980.

107. Huelin P, Solà E, Elia C, et al. Neutrophil gelatinase-associated lipocalin for assessment of acute kidney injury in cirrhosis: a prospective study. Hepatology 2019;70(1):319–33. https://doi.org/10.1002/hep.30592.

108. Simonetto DA, Gines P, Kamath PS. Hepatorenal syndrome: pathophysiology, diagnosis, and management. BMJ 2020;370:m2687. https://doi.org/10.1136/bmj.m2687.

109. Velez JC, Nietert PJ. Therapeutic response to vasoconstrictors in hepatorenal syndrome parallels increase in mean arterial pressure: a pooled analysis of

clinical trials. Am J Kidney Dis 2011;58(6):928–38. https://doi.org/10.1053/j.ajkd. 2011.07.017.

110. Facciorusso A, Chandar AK, Murad MH, et al. Comparative efficacy of pharmacological strategies for management of type 1 hepatorenal syndrome: a systematic review and network meta-analysis. Lancet Gastroenterol Hepatol 2017;2(2): 94–102. https://doi.org/10.1016/S2468-1253(16)30157-1.

111. Wong F, Pappas SC, Curry MP, et al. Terlipressin plus albumin for the treatment of Type 1 hepatorenal syndrome. N Engl J Med 2021;384(9):818–28. https://doi. org/10.1056/NEJMoa2008290.

112. Wong F, Pappas SC, Boyer TD, et al. Terlipressin improves renal function and reverses hepatorenal syndrome in patients with systemic inflammatory response syndrome. Clin Gastroenterol Hepatol 2017;15(2):266–72.e1. https://doi.org/10. 1016/j.cgh.2016.07.016.

113. Moore K, Jamil K, Verleger K, et al. Real-world treatment patterns and outcomes using terlipressin in 203 patients with the hepatorenal syndrome. Aliment Pharmacol Ther 2020;52(2):351–8. https://doi.org/10.1111/apt.15836.

114. Allegretti AS, Israelsen M, Krag A, et al. Terlipressin versus placebo or no intervention for people with cirrhosis and hepatorenal syndrome. Cochrane Database Syst Rev 2017;6:CD005162. https://doi.org/10.1002/14651858. CD005162.pub4.

115. Israelsen M, Krag A, Allegretti AS, et al. Terlipressin versus other vasoactive drugs for hepatorenal syndrome. Cochrane Database Syst Rev 2017;9: CD011532. https://doi.org/10.1002/14651858.CD011532.pub2.

116. Arora V, Maiwall R, Rajan V, et al. Terlipressin is superior to noradrenaline in the management of acute kidney injury in acute on chronic liver failure. Hepatology 2020;71(2):600–10. https://doi.org/10.1002/hep.30208.

117. Allegretti AS, Parada XV, Eneanya ND, et al. Prognosis of patients with cirrhosis and AKI who initiate RRT. Clin J Am Soc Nephrol 2018;13(1):16–25. https://doi. org/10.2215/CJN.03610417.

118. Allegretti AS. Acute kidney injury treatment in decompensated cirrhosis: a focus on kidney replacement therapy. Kidney Med 2021;3(1):12–4. https://doi.org/10. 1016/j.xkme.2020.09.015.

Management of Delirium in the Intensive Care Unit

Dih-Dih Huang, MD*, Peter E. Fischer, MD

KEYWORDS

- Delirium • Intensive care unit • Elderly • Antipsychotics • Prevention

KEY POINTS

- Delirium in the intensive care unit is a widespread disease that often goes unrecognized.
- A high index of suspicion and the use of screening tools will increase the detection of delirium.
- Treatment requires addressing any underlying pathology in addition to behavioral interventions directed at risk factor reduction.
- Risk factor reduction with behavioral interventions is the only proven modality shown effective at delirium prevention.

INTRODUCTION/BACKGROUND

Delirium in the intensive care unit (ICU) is a major contributor to morbidity and mortality in patients. Although often underdiagnosed, delirium has been shown to increase mortality and length of stay with decreased functional outcomes.[1,2] It has been repeatedly shown that delirium in the ICU is an independent predictor of mortality, with as high as a 2-fold risk of mortality.[1,3–6] In addition to the short-term impact of delirium on a patient's outcome, some studies have shown the risk of dementia is elevated after experiencing delirium during a hospitalization.[7,8] The importance of recognizing and treating delirium has been highlighted, as the national cost to the health system has been estimated to be $152 billion annually.[5,9] Despite the prevalence of delirium in the ICU, it is estimated that 60% of patients with delirium go unrecognized.[5,10]

ASSESSMENT/EVALUATION

The diagnosis of delirium may be difficult to make with numerous confounding factors in the ICU. Although a high index of suspicion is required to diagnose

University of Tennessee Health Science Center, 910 Madison Avenue, Suite 220, Memphis, TN 38163, USA
* Corresponding author.
E-mail address: dhuang15@uthsc.edu

Surg Clin N Am 102 (2022) 139–148
https://doi.org/10.1016/j.suc.2021.09.006
0039-6109/22/© 2021 Elsevier Inc. All rights reserved.

delirium, it is crucial that other causes are excluded. These causes may include metabolic derangements, pain, medication toxicities, substance withdrawal, and neurologic pathology (**Fig. 1**). In addition, underlying conditions, such as dementia, Alzheimer disease, and other cognitive disorders, may cloud the diagnosis of delirium.

Delirium, as defined by the Diagnostic and Statistical Manual of Mental Disorders (DSM-V), is a disturbance in level of awareness and the reduced ability to direct, focus, sustain, or shift attention, marked by an acute onset and fluctuating course.[11] There are multiple phenotypes of delirium (**Fig. 2**). Hyperactive delirium manifests as hyperactive psychomotor activity accompanied by agitation, labile moods, and refusal to cooperate with care. The hypoactive variant presents with decreased level of psychomotor activity with sluggishness, lethargy, and near stupor. A third manifestation of delirium is mixed level of activity. Individuals have a normal level of psychomotor activity with disturbed attention and awareness.

However, application of the DSM-V definition is difficult by nonpsychiatric clinicians, and often in the ICU there are numerous confounding factors that make the diagnosis difficult. Because of the significant clinical impact of delirium and difficulty with recognition, there has been significant work put into creation of a recognition tool. The Confusion Assessment Method (CAM) was developed in 1990 as the first standardized, validated tool for any clinician to use for identification of delirium. When compared with trained psychiatric evaluators, the CAM had a sensitivity of 94% to 100% and specificity of 90% to 95%.[12] Although the development of the CAM was critical in the evaluation of delirium, the tool was not applicable to an intubated or sedated patient, which often comprise the patients in the ICU. Subsequently, the CAM tool was further adapted to create the CAM in the ICU (CAM-ICU).[13] Simple modification of the initial tool led to the CAM-ICU, initially published in 2001, which demonstrated a 97% sensitivity and 92% specificity when the 3 clinicians were averaged.[13] These clinicians were bedside nurses and intensivist physician. Subsequent

Trauma
Ischemia
Encephalopathy
Substance withdrawal
Drug toxicity
Thyroid disorder
Sepsis
Hypoxia
Hypercarbia
Cardiac shock
Hepatic failure
Hypoglycemia
Adrenal insufficiency
Uremia

Fig. 1. Other causes for altered mental status in the ICU.

Hyperactive	Agitation
	Labile moods
	Lack of cooperation
Hypoactive	Decreased activity
	Lethargy
	Stupor
Mixed	Normal activity level
	Disturbed attention
	Lack of awareness

Fig. 2. Types of delirium.

studies have proved the ease, speed, reliability, and validity of the CAM-ICU tool in delirium recognition.[14,15]

The use of the CAM-ICU, however, requires a patient to be arousable for examination. In the ICU, with patients frequently intubated and sedated, subsequent studies have demonstrated the use of arousal scores as adjuncts for the CAM-ICU.[16] The Richmond agitation and sedation scale and the Riker sedation-agitation scale screening tools have been shown to be equivalent with regard to assessment of level of consciousness,[16,17] assisting in determining whether a patient is appropriate for delirium assessment.

Although other scoring systems have been used in the diagnosis of delirium, the CAM-ICU is the most valid and reliable tool. Regardless of which tool is used, routine monitoring is strongly recommended in the ICU.[8]

TREATMENT OPTIONS

The initial management of delirium in the ICU has several priorities that all need to be managed simultaneously.[5]

1. Diagnose and treat physiologic causes
2. Manage symptoms (agitation)
3. Maintain safety

In the past, pharmacologic treatment (benzodiazepine, antipsychotics) were the main modalities of treatment. However, in recent years, there is increasing evidence that medications provide limited benefit. Currently, nonpharmacologic interventions remain the most effective in treating and preventing delirium.[10] Risk factors for development of delirium include advanced age, functional impairment, vision impairment, and underlying dementia.[5,10]

NONPHARMACOLOGIC TREATMENT

Nonpharmacologic strategies (**Fig. 3**) target risk factors for delirium as well as factors common in the ICU, including frequent alarms and prolonged bedrest. Reducing inciting factors is most effective in the treatment and prevention of delirium.[10] Frequent bedside reorientation of a patient with their location and circumstances in addition to the use of hearing and vision aids allows patients to recall and understand their surroundings. In addition, sleep deprivation has been known to increase delirium. The sleep and awake cycle in a patient can be restored with frequent mobilization, cognitive stimulation, and adequate lighting during the daytime followed by less frequent interruptions, darkness, and noise reduction at night. Reduction of these factors by all providers, aids, and therapists allows for decreased delirium in the ICU, resulting in decreased length of stay and improved functional outcomes.

Frequent orientation
Providing hearing and vision aids
Mobilization
Cognitive stimulation
Sleep restoration
Pain relief

Fig. 3. Therapy-based treatment of delirium.

PHARMACOLOGIC TREATMENT

Pharmacologic agents play a major role in the management of symptoms, predominantly agitation, and the maintenance of safety. Safety to the patient may include the prevention of dislodgement of supportive devices as well as safety to members of the care team. Although numerous classes of medications have been used in the past, there is no single treatment that has been proved to resolve and prevent delirium. Although often used to treat abrupt increases in agitation, benzodiazepines, antipsychotics, and cholinesterase inhibitors have not been proved to lead to resolution of delirium and thus decreased mortality and length of stay.[18,19] However, the priority of patient safety may require the use of pharmacologic treatment in abrupt changes in agitation and delirium.

BENZODIAZEPINES

Benzodiazepines, a class of sedatives and anxiolytics acting on gamma-aminobutyric acid receptors, are some of the most common medications used in the hospital. Although these medications have immediate sedative effects, reducing and controlling agitation, they are no longer recommended in the treatment of delirium[20–24] due to worsening delirium and is considered a risk factor for development of delirium.[8] The exception is the treatment of delirium secondary to alcohol withdrawal.[20,21]

ACETYLCHOLINESTERASE INHIBITORS

Acetylcholinesterase inhibitors, also known as cholinesterase inhibitors, inhibit the breakdown of acetylcholine, thus potentiating its effects. This class of medication is commonly used in the treatment of myasthenia gravis or cognitive disorders (such as Alzheimer disease or Lewy body dementia) or as reversal for neuromuscular blockage.[25] However, it is no longer recommended as treatment of delirium[5,8,23,24,26] due to lack of efficacy.

ANTIPSYCHOTICS (TYPICAL AND ATYPICAL)

Haloperidol (Haldol) is one of the longest used antipsychotics for the treatment of delirium. As a potent dopamine receptor antagonist, as other typical antipsychotics, haloperidol has a high risk of extrapyramidal symptoms.[27] Because of the risk of QT interval prolongation, monitoring with electrocardiograms is advised.[28] Although previously preferred as the antipsychotic in the treatment of delirium of critically ill patients, current guidelines from the Society of Critical Care Medicine in 2013 no longer advocate for haloperidol use, as no strong evidence shows reduction in duration of delirium in the ICU.[8,29,30]

Atypical antipsychotics (such as risperidone, olanzapine, quetiapine, ziprasidone, and aripiprazole) are a newer class of medications used to reduce and prevent delirium. With an overall lower risk of extrapyramidal symptoms, the off-label use for treatment of delirium may be better tolerated by patients.[27] This class of medications may reduce the duration of delirium in the ICU[8]; however, this recommendation comes from low level of evidence.[8,26,27,29,30]

ALPHA-2 RECEPTOR AGONISTS

Highly selective alpha-2 receptor agonists (commonly dexmedetomidine) have been found to decrease time to resolution and possibly reduce development of delirium.[23,31–33] Dexmedetomidine infusion is now recommended over benzodiazepine infusions for sedation to reduce the duration of delirium.[8] Addition benefits of dexmedetomidine include the lack of respiratory depression that allows for a wide application in the ICU. However, bradycardia, arrhythmias, and hypotension limit the use of dexmedetomidine in the ICU.

GERIATRIC PATIENTS

The geriatric patient is not a well-defined population, but often refers to patients aged 65 years and older. Regardless of the definition, the elderly patient requires special care and considerations in the ICU. In the United States, this population has been growing exponentially. It is estimated that the population older than 65 years will nearly double by the year 2030, from 39.6 million in 2009 to 77.0 million in 2034.[34] In addition to comorbidities and chronic illness leading to hospitalization in the ICU, elderly patients are also more susceptible to complications from trauma (including low energy mechanisms), requiring critical care. Elderly patients may have underlying decreased vision and hearing, slower reflexes, and impaired cognitive function that increase the risk of delirium in the ICU.[35] A higher level of vigilance to compensate for these decreased senses is critical in preventing and treating delirium in older patients. In addition to the physiologic decline in elderly patients, special attention to the continuation or cessation of preexisting medications is critical in reducing delirium in the ICU.

PREVENTION

An emerging area of research has been focused on pharmacologic intervention for prevention of delirium. Although studies of aripiprazole, an atypical antipsychotic,[36] and ramelteon,[37] a melatonin agonist, have been conducted with promising reduction in incidence of delirium, there still remains a lack of confirmatory evidence to recommend pharmacologic strategies for delirium prevention in the ICU.[5,8]

As with primary treatment of delirium, behavioral interventions directed toward risk factor reduction remain the most promising tools in the prevention of delirium. In 1999, a risk-factor based strategy was described, known as the Hospital Elder Life Program (HELP).[27,38] Trained interdisciplinary teams targeted 6 risk factors for delirium (**Fig. 4**) with a standardized protocol[38] and demonstrated a decrease in incidence of delirium.[27,39] Notably, the severity or risk of recurrence of delirium was unchanged, suggesting that primary prevention is critical in the way clinicians approach delirium.[38] Similar programs to HELP have been described that implement a multidisciplinary approach targeting risk factor modification with encouraging evidence of decreased

Cognitive impairment
Sleep deprivation
Immobility
Visual impairment
Hearing impairment
Dehydration

Fig. 4. Six risk factors of delirium targeted by HELP.[38].

length of stays and medication use.[40] The HELP program has also been shown to be cost-effective in patients with intermediate risk of delirium.[39]

LINK TO COGNITIVE DISORDERS

The association between delirium and dementia or cognitive impairment has been long recognized, however poorly understood.[41] Delirium has been shown to be a strong, independent predictor of subsequent cognitive impairment, with as much as a 3.5 increased risk of the development of dementia when compared to patients without delirium.[41,42] This decrease in cognitive function is seen in patients with and without preexisting dementia.[43–45] In addition, underlying cognitive disorder is one of the main risk factors for development of delirium,[46] and this suggests that delirium may cause injury to the brain in an independent fashion, leading to cognitive decline. In the setting of preexisting cognitive disease (dementia, Alzheimer disease, Lewy body dementia), delirium seems to accelerate the progression of cognitive decline when compared with patients without delirium.[42–44,47,48] Pathways of cholinergic deficiency leading to Lewy body dementia[47] and β-amyloid protein generation leading to Alzheimer disease[49] have been examined as potential pathogenesis of delirium. However, no causal relationship has been demonstrated between delirium and cognitive disorders. Proposed pathogenesis of delirium related brain injury and systemic stress, leading to reduced cerebral metabolism, alterations of cholinergic neurotransmitters, inflammation, and neuronal stress.[41,46] Regardless of the pathophysiology linking delirium to dementia and other cognitive disorders, their relationship is proved highlighting the importance of prevention and treatment of delirium.

SUMMARY

In the ICU, delirium is a major contributor to morbidity and mortality in adult patients. Patients with delirium have been shown to have increased length of stay, decreased functional outcomes, and increased risk for requiring placement at the time of discharge. Long-term patients suffering from delirium during hospitalization show decreased cognitive function after discharge and have been linked to dementia and other cognitive disorders. Although common in many critically ill patients, it goes unrecognized in most of the patients. Recognition and treatment of underlying causes for delirium in conjunction with supportive care is critical. The mainstay of treatment and prevention include therapy- and behavioral-based interventions that include frequent orientation, cognitive stimulation, mobilization, sleep restoration, and providing hearing and visual aids. When delirium still persists and requires treatment of patient safety, pharmacologic intervention with antipsychotics or alpha-2 agonists is recommended.

CLINICS CARE POINTS

- Delirium in the ICU is a widespread disease that often goes unrecognized, leading to increased morbidity and mortality in adult patients.

- high index of suspicion and the use of screening tools will increase the detection of delirium.

- Treatment requires addressing any underlying pathology in addition to behavioral interventions directed at risk factor reduction.

- Dexmedetomidine or antipsychotics are the preferred medication in treatment of delirium unable to be treated with behavior modification.

- Risk factor reduction with behavioral interventions is the only proved modality shown effective at delirium prevention.

DISCLOSURE

The authors have no disclosures.

REFERENCES

1. Siddiqi N, House AO, Holmes JD. Occurrence and outcome of delirium in medical in-patients: a systematic literature review. Age Ageing 2006;35(4): 350–64.
2. Pavone KJ, Jablonski J, Junker P, et al. Evaluating delirium outcomes among older adults in the surgical intensive care unit. Heart Lung 2020;49(5): 578–84.
3. Ely EW, Shintani A, Truman B, et al. Delirium as a predictor of mortality in mechanically ventilated patients in the intensive care unit. JAMA 2004;291(14):1753–62.
4. Lin SM, Liu CY, Wang CH, et al. The impact of delirium on the survival of mechanically ventilated patients. Crit Care Med 2004;32(11):2254–9.
5. Inouye SK, Westendorp RG, Saczynski JS. Delirium in elderly people. Lancet 2014;383(9920):911–22.
6. Sanchez D, Brennan K, Al Sayfe M, et al. Frailty, delirium and hospital mortality of older adults admitted to intensive care: the Delirium (Deli) in ICU study. Crit Care 2020;24(1):609.
7. Witlox J, Eurelings LS, de Jonghe JF, et al. Delirium in elderly patients and the risk of postdischarge mortality, institutionalization, and dementia: a meta-analysis. JAMA 2010;304(4):443–51.
8. Barr J, Fraser GL, Puntillo K, et al. Clinical practice guidelines for the management of pain, agitation, and delirium in adult patients in the intensive care unit. Crit Care Med 2013;41(1):263–306.
9. Leslie DL, Marcantonio ER, Zhang Y, et al. One-year health care costs associated with delirium in the elderly population. Arch Intern Med 2008;168(1):27–32.
10. Oh ES, Fong TG, Hshieh TT, et al. Delirium in older persons: advances in diagnosis and treatment. JAMA 2017;318(12):1161–74.
11. American Psychiatric Association. Diagnostic and Statistical Manual of mental disorders. 5th edition. Washington, DC: 2013.

12. Inouye SK, van Dyck CH, Alessi CA, et al. Clarifying confusion: the confusion assessment method. A new method for detection of delirium. Ann Intern Med 1990;113(12):941–8.

13. Ely EW, Margolin R, Francis J, et al. Evaluation of delirium in critically ill patients: validation of the Confusion Assessment Method for the Intensive Care Unit (CAM-ICU). Crit Care Med 2001;29(7):1370–9.

14. Wei LA, Fearing MA, Sternberg EJ, et al. The Confusion Assessment Method: a systematic review of current usage. J Am Geriatr Soc 2008; 56(5):823–30.

15. Chen TJ, Chung YW, Chang HR, et al. Diagnostic accuracy of the CAM-ICU and ICDSC in detecting intensive care unit delirium: a bivariate meta-analysis. Int J Nurs Stud 2021;113:103782.

16. Khan BA, Guzman O, Campbell NL, et al. Comparison and agreement between the Richmond Agitation-Sedation Scale and the Riker Sedation-Agitation Scale in evaluating patients' eligibility for delirium assessment in the ICU. Chest 2012; 142(1):48–54.

17. Grover S, Kate N. Assessment scales for delirium: A review. World J Psychiatr 2012;2(4):58–70.

18. Weaver CB, Kane-Gill SL, Gunn SR, et al. A retrospective analysis of the effectiveness of antipsychotics in the treatment of ICU delirium. J Crit Care 2017;41: 234–9.

19. Zayed Y, Barbarawi M, Kheiri B, et al. Haloperidol for the management of delirium in adult intensive care unit patients: A systematic review and meta-analysis of randomized controlled trials. J Crit Care 2019;50:280–6.

20. Lonergan E, Luxenberg J, Areosa Sastre A, et al. Benzodiazepines for delirium. Cochrane Database Syst Rev 2009;1:CD006379.

21. Hui D. Benzodiazepines for agitation in patients with delirium: selecting the right patient, right time, and right indication. Curr Opin Support Palliat Care 2018; 12(4):489–94.

22. Khan SH, Lindroth H, Hendrie K, et al. Time trends of delirium rates in the intensive care unit. Heart Lung 2020;49(5):572–7.

23. Reade MC, Finfer S. Sedation and delirium in the intensive care unit. N Engl J Med 2014;370(5):444–54.

24. Tahir TA. Delirium.Medicine. 2012;40(12):658–61.

25. von Arnim CAF, Bartsch T, Jacobs AH, et al. Diagnosis and treatment of cognitive impairment. Diagnose und Behandlung kognitiver Störungen. Z Gerontol Geriatr 2019;52(4):309–15.

26. Burry L, Hutton B, Williamson DR, et al. Pharmacological interventions for the treatment of delirium in critically ill adults. Cochrane Database Syst Rev 2019; 9(9):CD011749.

27. Marcantonio ER. Delirium in hospitalized older adults. N Engl J Med 2017; 377(15):1456–66.

28. Jacobi J, Fraser GL, Coursin DB, et al. Clinical practice guidelines for the sustained use of sedatives and analgesics in the critically ill adult [published correction appears in Crit Care Med 2002 Mar;30(3):726]. Crit Care Med 2002;30(1): 119–41.

29. Girard TD, Exline MC, Carson SS, et al. Haloperidol and Ziprasidone for Treatment of Delirium in Critical Illness. N Engl J Med 2018;379(26): 2506–16.

30. Schrijver EJ, de Graaf K, de Vries OJ, et al. Efficacy and safety of haloperidol for in-hospital delirium prevention and treatment: a systematic review of current evidence. Eur J Intern Med 2016;27:14–23.

31. Flükiger J, Hollinger A, Speich B, et al. Dexmedetomidine in prevention and treatment of postoperative and intensive care unit delirium: a systematic review and meta-analysis. Ann Intensive Care 2018;8(1):92.

32. Pieri M, De Simone A, Rose S, et al. Trials focusing on prevention and treatment of delirium after cardiac surgery: a systematic review of randomized evidence. J Cardiothorac Vasc Anesth 2020;34(6):1641–54.

33. Louis C, Godet T, Chanques G, et al. Effects of dexmedetomidine on delirium duration of non-intubated ICU patients (4D trial): study protocol for a randomized trial. Trials 2018;19(1):307.

34. Iriondo J. Older people projected to outnumber children for first time in U.S. History. United States Census Bureau website. Available at: https://www.census.gov/newsroom/press-releases/2018/cb18-41-population-projections.html. Accessed April 23, 2021.

35. Brooks SE, Peetz AB. Evidence-Based Care of Geriatric Trauma Patients. Surg Clin North Am 2017;97(5):1157–74.

36. Mokhtari M, Farasatinasab M, Jafarpour Machian M, et al. Aripiprazole for prevention of delirium in the neurosurgical intensive care unit: a double-blind, randomized, placebo-controlled study. Eur J Clin Pharmacol 2020; 76(4):491–9.

37. Hatta K, Kishi Y, Wada K, et al. Preventive effects of ramelteon on delirium: a randomized placebo-controlled trial. JAMA Psychiatry 2014;71(4):397–403.

38. Inouye SK, Bogardus ST Jr, Charpentier PA, et al. A multicomponent intervention to prevent delirium in hospitalized older patients. N Engl J Med 1999;340(9):669–76.

39. Rizzo JA, Bogardus ST Jr, Leo-Summers L, et al. Multicomponent targeted intervention to prevent delirium in hospitalized older patients: what is the economic value? Med Care 2001;39(7):740–52.

40. Friedman JI, Li L, Kirpalani S, et al. A multi-phase quality improvement initiative for the treatment of active delirium in older persons. J Am Geriatr Soc 2021; 69(1):216–24.

41. MacLullich AM, Beaglehole A, Hall RJ, et al. Delirium and long-term cognitive impairment. Int Rev Psychiatry 2009;21(1):30–42.

42. Davis DH, Muniz Terrera G, Keage H, et al. Delirium is a strong risk factor for dementia in the oldest-old: a population-based cohort study. Brain 2012;135(Pt 9):2809–16.

43. Maclullich AM, Anand A, Davis DH, et al. New horizons in the pathogenesis, assessment and management of delirium. Age Ageing 2013;42(6):667–74.

44. Davis DH, Muniz-Terrera G, Keage HA, et al. Association of delirium with cognitive decline in late life: a neuropathologic study of 3 population-based cohort studies. JAMA Psychiatry 2017;74(3):244–51.

45. McCusker J, Cole M, Dendukuri N, et al. Delirium in older medical inpatients and subsequent cognitive and functional status: a prospective study. CMAJ 2001; 165(5):575–83.

46. Eikelenboom P, Hoogendijk WJ. Do delirium and Alzheimer's dementia share specific pathogenetic mechanisms? Dement Geriatr Cogn Disord 1999;10(5):319–24.

47. Gore RL, Vardy ER, O'Brien JT. Delirium and dementia with Lewy bodies: distinct diagnoses or part of the same spectrum? J Neurol Neurosurg Psychiatr 2015; 86(1):50–9.
48. Fong TG, Jones RN, Shi P, et al. Delirium accelerates cognitive decline in Alzheimer disease. Neurology 2009;72(18):1570–5.
49. Xie Z, Dong Y, Maeda U, et al. Isoflurane-induced apoptosis: a potential pathogenic link between delirium and dementia. J Gerontol A Biol Sci Med Sci 2006; 61(12):1300–6.

Noninvasive Ventilation and Oxygenation Strategies

Patrycja Popowicz, MD, MS[a],*, Kenji Leonard, MD[b,1]

KEYWORDS

- Noninvasive ventilation • Surgery • Hypoxemia
- Low flow/variable performance devices • High flow/fixed performance devices
- Continuous positive airway pressure (CPAP)
- BPAP (Bi-level positive airway pressure)

KEY POINTS

- NIV does not bypass the upper airway.
- Contraindicated in patients who have facial trauma, GCS </10, inability to protect airway, or clear secretions, upper airway obstructions, severe upper gastrointestinal bleed, or requires urgent intubation.
- Different modalities can be used to deliver NIV: nasal cannula, simple mask, nonrebreather, high-flow nasal cannula, CPAP, and BPAP.
- NIV can be attempted in patients with acute COPD exacerbations, trauma, cardiogenic pulmonary edema, COVID-19, and in certain cases ARDS.

INTRODUCTION

It is not an uncommon clinical scenario in medicine and surgery whereby one encounters a hypoxemic patient due to a myriad of reasons. The ability to understand and use different noninvasive ventilation (NIV) modalities is a valuable tool to have in your armamentarium before transitioning to more invasive strategies. This article will review some essential noninvasive oxygenation and ventilation strategies most commonly used in the surgical arena, hoping that it will provide a good reference when deciding which modality to choose in a hypoxic patient.

In adults, hypoxemia is commonly defined as a Pao_2 less than 80 mm Hg on room air at sea level. As mentioned before, there are numerous reasons why a patient may become hypoxemic, including subambient $Fi0_2$, hypoventilation, V/Q mismatch, shunt, or diffusion defects which can manifests clinically as tachycardia, arrhythmias,

[a] Department of General Surgery, East Carolina University- Vidant Medical Center, 2100 Stantonsburg Road, Greenville, NC 27834, USA; [b] Division of Trauma, Surgical Critical Care, and Acute Care Surgery, Department of Surgery, East Carolina University- Vidant Medical Center, 2100 Stantonsburg Road, Greenville, NC 27834, USA
[1] Contributing Author.
* Corresponding author.
E-mail address: Popowiczp19@ecu.edu

Surg Clin N Am 102 (2022) 149–157
https://doi.org/10.1016/j.suc.2021.09.012
0039-6109/22/© 2021 Elsevier Inc. All rights reserved.

feeling short of breath, dyspnea, tachypnea, altered mental status, and use of accessory muscles and indicate the need for supplemental oxygen. Providing supplemental oxygen, whereas relatively free of complications, through noninvasive oxygenation and ventilation modalities are helpful as one investigates the underlying etiology for the patient's hypoxemia.[1]

NIV has gained more popularity as it provides ventilation to the patient without using an artificial airway and does not bypass the upper airway.[2] Invasive methods bypass the upper airway and include options such as an endotracheal tube, a laryngeal mask, or a tracheostomy.[3] Compared with invasive ventilation, NIV is more comfortable while preserving the patient's airway defense mechanism. Moreover, complications directly related to intubation and mechanical ventilation can be avoided, such as aspiration, trauma to surrounding structures, barotrauma, ventilator-associated pneumonia.[4] Of note, while supplemental oxygen is widely available, inexpensive, and safe, there are complications such as hyperoxemia that increases risk in mortality, nitrogen washout atelectasis, O2-induced hypoventilation, airway/nasal/oral dryness, gastric insufflation, and mechanical pressure wounds from the delivery source that need to have precautions taken to monitor and avoid them.[1,5,6]

There have been recent guidelines for the clinical use of NIV, including the 2017 European Respiratory Society (ERS) and American Thoracic Society (ATC) and the 2017 British Thoracic Society (BTS), an Intensive Care Society, which makes recommendations about when or when not to use NIV and offer technical and pragmatic advice on its use.[3,7–9] This is beyond the scope of this article, which will focus on the basic NIV strategies and modalities most commonly available with a discussion of their use in only some of the more common clinical scenarios.

NONINVASIVE VENTILATION/OXYGENATION MODALITIES

To begin the discussion of some NIV strategies, there are different categories of oxygen delivery/therapy systems, mainly low-flow (variable-performance) and high-flow (fixed-performance) devices. Examples of low-flow (variable-performance) delivery systems include a nasal cannula, simple mask, and nonrebreather. An example of a high-flow (fixed-performance) device would be Fisher Paykel Optiflow or AIRVO 2 devices, or Vapotherm (**Table 1**).

Low-flow nasal cannulas (NC) are a relatively old, simple, and commonly used method to deliver oxygen therapy.[10,11] Nasal cannula prongs come in a variety of sizes and styles to fit pediatric up to adult patients. Usually, the nasal cannula is secured using an elastic band over the head or loops of tubing that fit over the patients' ears. In theory, standard NC can deliver flows from 1L up to 6L with an expected delivery of Fio_2 of 0.22 to 0.24 at 1 L/min up to 0.4 at 5 to 6 L/min. Factors that affect inhaled volume such as flow, inspiratory flow and time, respiratory rate, and factors that affect O2 concentration or air dilution such as open or closed-mouth breathing

Table 1	
Indications and contraindications to NIV	
Indications	**Contraindications**
Tachypnea	Facial trauma ± deformity
Acute COPD exacerbation	Upper airway obstruction
Medically stable	Severe upper GI bleed
	Decreased GCS </10
	Inability to protect airway or clear secretions
	Reasons that would necessitate intubation

and anatomic factors that would act as a reservoir and dead space, the actual Fio_2 inspired is likely much less and variable between patients.[1,10,11] Other downsides to nasal cannula are the drying of the nasal mucosa with an inability to effectively humidify or heat the oxygen delivered and potential discomfort of the pressure of the prongs or tubing when used for a significant amount of time.

A simple mask can be used when a higher Fio_2 is needed. It also comes in a variety of sizes suitable for infants up to adults with a small O2 supply tubing that attaches to its base. The mask fits over the bridge of the nose and is held in place with an elastic band over the patient's head. The mask typically has an aluminum strip to help avoid leakage toward the eyes and covers the nose and mouth down to the chin. Exhaled air leaves through side boles and between the mask and face as there is no sealing device, allowing for the inhalation of room air around the mask interface. The mask acts differently than NC as it has approximately a 100 to 200 mL reservoir in an adult-sized mask that allows for an increase in inspired O2 concentration. The Fio_2 concentration delivered theoretically is approximately 0.3 to 0.8 with flows capable of ranging from 5 to 10 L/min, but given the design and ability to intake room air from around the mask, the actual delivered Fio_2 is variable and dependent on mask volume O2 flow and pattern of ventilation. The mask also allows for CO2 accumulation during exhalation, so O2 flow should be high enough to washout the mask and prevent rebreathing.[12]

A nonrebreather is essentially a simple mask with an attached 300 to 600 mL reservoir bag with a valve between the bag and the mask and one of the side exhalation ports. This valve prevents exhaled gas from flowing into the reservoir and flows out of the mask ports. During inhalation, the mask exhalation port valve closes, allowing minimal room air from being inhaled and allowing inhalation of the 300 to 600 mL reservoir bag. There is also no sealing device, so while Fio_2 concentrations of 0.6 to 0.9 are theorized it is variable. The flow rate for this mask allows up to 15 L/min.

The Venturi Mask is a facemask that allows the delivery of a predetermined Fio_2.[13] The mask operates using the Bernoulli principle, which allows a constant high flow of oxygen through a narrow tube that entrains room air through openings on the sides. This mode can deliver Fio_2 in a controlled and accurate manner between 24% and 60%.[14,15] Disadvantages include patient discomfort from the displacement of the mask in addition to a dry sensation from the delivery of nonhumidified oxygen.[13]

High-flow/fixed-performance devices such as Optiflow. High-flow/fixed-performance devices allow for blending of 100% O2 and room air to produce gas with the desired Fio_2 at a high enough flow, up to 60 L/min, to prevent dilution with room air while providing heated humidified air. The physiologic mechanisms that high flow provides are washout of physiologic dead space, decreased respiratory rate, increased tidal volume, increased end-expiratory volume, and some small degree of positive end-expiratory pressure.[16–19] High flow allows for the delivery of air volumes greater than what a patient ventilates physiologically and essentially washes out the pharyngeal dead space so that the Co2 is replaced by oxygen thus creating greater oxygen diffusion gradient allowing for improved breathing efficiency and patient oxygenation.[16,19] Mundel and colleagues provided several physiologic studies that showed HFNC could decrease respiratory rate and also increase tidal volume.[20] Parke and colleagues and Frat and colleagues have shown with closed mouth breathing high flow nasal cannula could approximate 1 mm Hg of PEEP for every 10 L/min of flow.[21,22]

Continuous positive airway pressure (CPAP) therapy continuously applies a constant level of positive end-expiratory pressure (PEEP) to a spontaneously breathing patient.[23] More specifically, this phenomenon occurs during both inspiration and expiration as PEEP is the pressure within the alveoli at the end of expiration.[24] The delivered PEEP increases the patient's functional residual capacity (FRC), opens underventilated alveoli, decreases atelectasis, and improves lung compliance. Oxygenation is also improved while decreasing the patient's work of breathing.[4] PEEP additionally has a positive effect on cardiac function. An increase in PEEP thereby increases intrathoracic pressure, simultaneously increasing intrapleural pressure. The difference between the left ventricle systolic pressure and intrapleural pressure determines the left ventricular afterload.[25] Thus, an increase in PEEP alternatively decreases left ventricular afterload and enhances cardiac output.[4,25]

Many commercial devices compatible with CPAP have an oronasal mask. However, not all patients can tolerate CPAP due to the discomfort from the mask and constant airflow. Thus, various face mask interfaces are available for better patient adherence. Recommended settings start at a level of 4 cm H2O and increase by 1 to 2 cm H2O intervals to a maximum of 20 cm H2O.[24] Fio_2 can be set starting at 21% to 100%.[26] If the patient does not have improved gas exchange or a reduced work of breathing at maximum settings, then alternative respiratory adjuncts should be considered.

Bilevel positive airway pressure (BPAP) therapy is another mode of delivering NIV and uses a pressure-cycling mode. The device alternates delivering inspiratory positive airway pressure (IPAP) and expiratory positive airway pressure (EPAP). The difference between the 2 preset pressures determines the tidal volume. If the respiratory rate is constant, a larger tidal volume increases alveolar ventilation.[24] BPAP is contraindicated in those with facial traumas not amenable to face mask interfaces and in patient's inability to control their secretions.

BPAP settings start at different levels tailored to various respiratory conditions. Minimal settings are 8 cm H2O for IPAP and 4 cm H2O for EPAP. IPAP is increased by levels of 2 cm H2O to a maximum of 20, whereas EPAP is titrated to a maximum of 10. Providers must be present at the bedside to determine how much titration is indicated to improve the patient's respiratory drive. Caution must be taken as increasing EPAP too much may inadvertently decrease the tidal volume delivered.[27]

COMMON CLINICAL SCENARIOS

Now that noninvasive oxygenation and ventilation modalities have been reviewed, discussion of using them during common disease states can occur. The ATS and the BTS have formulated some guidelines and recommendations for the utilization of NIV in specific disease processes (**Table 2**).

NIV is a modality commonly used in postsurgical extubation. Reintubation rates are generally 20% for all patients but can be 40% following abdominal surgeries due to respiratory muscle dysfunction, which may linger for 7 days.[23] Postoperatively, NIV

Table 2 Types of NIV	
Nasal Cannula	• Delivers oxygen through nasal prongs
Simple Mask	• Oronasal mask interface • Can deliver higher Fi02 with 100–200 mL reservoir
Nonrebreather	• Same interface as a simple mask • Larger reservoir (300–600 mL)
CPAP	• Mask interface • Delivery of continuous pressure
BPAP	• Mask interface • Delivery of IPAP and EPAP

has been shown to increase lung aeration, arterial oxygenation, and decrease atelectasis to counteract the physiologic effects of surgery and anesthesia.

Reintubation is associated with increased mortality. Thus, NIV is a strategy that can be used to prevent or treat postextubation. Options available are HFNC, CPAP, and BPAP, and their use is based on both patient factors and clinical judgment. The ERS and the (ATS) provide guidelines for NIV use in various clinical settings.[8]

Hernandez and colleagues conducted an RCT that demonstrated HFNC not superior to BPAP in patients considered high risk of extubation failure, with reintubation occurring in 60 patients (19.1%) in the NIV group and 66 patients (22.8%) in the high-flow group (risk difference, −3.7%; 95% confidence interval (CI): −9.1% to ∞. Patients who fulfilled at least 1 of their listed criteria were considered high risk, which was not limited to age >/65, heart failure as main indications for intubation, moderate to severe COPD, APACHE II score >/12, BMI >/30, airway patency issues, unable to clear secretions, and prolonged weaning.[28] Another study conducted by Ferrer and colleagues revealed decreased respiratory failure in patients who received NIV immediately after extubation vs those in the control group with Venturi Masks ($P = .029$). Benefits were seen in patients with chronic respiratory disorders and hypercapnia during the spontaneous breathing trial.[29] However, there is no additional advantage in low-risk patients or in patients who developed respiratory failure after extubation.[8]

The trauma population is susceptible to respiratory failure due to the nature of their injuries in conjunction with their comorbidities. Many of these patients present with more than one injury, which contributes to the complexity of their care while placing them at an increased risk for developing hypoxemic respiratory failure. Hypoxemia in these patients is due to ventilation-perfusion mismatch and a right to left shunt from a lung contusion, atelectasis, inability to clear secretions, pneumothorax, or a hemothorax.[30,31]

RCTs have produced insufficient evidence and yielded low-grade recommendations resulting in no established consensus for NIV use in trauma patients.[8,30,32] Nonetheless, an agreement exists for situations in which NIV is not an appropriate option, which includes facial deformities, inability to protect airway or cooperation, upper airway obstruction, respiratory or cardiac arrest, hemodynamic instability, organ failure, severe upper gastrointestinal bleed, and GCS less than 10. The duration of NIV use also remains for further discussion. NIV in trauma patients requires close monitoring as a clinical response is anticipated in 1 to 4 hours. If the patient has a refractory response, the patient should be promptly intubated and ventilated to decrease mortality.[30]

Chronic obstructive pulmonary disease (COPD) is prevalent in our society, and NIV application has been extensively researched. Generally, a patient has compensatory pulmonary mechanisms in chronic COPD. The increased flow resistance impairs full expiration before the next inspiration and produces hyperinflation and use of accessory muscles.[2] However, the patient's compensatory mechanism diminishes during an acute exacerbation. Respirations are compromised as increased respiratory rate leads to low tidal volumes, which increases respiratory acidosis and induces increased energy expenditure and fatigue.[8] NIV provides external PEEP to offset the effects of an acute exacerbation but has been beneficial only in acidotic patients.[8,33] Keenan and colleagues further showed NIV was poorly tolerated in minimally acidotic patients with increased patient discomfort.[34]

Acute respiratory distress syndrome (ARDS) is an inflammatory lung condition that leads to leakage of fluid into the lung spaces causing hypoxemia. The use of NIV for supportive treatment in ARDS is controversial. Ding and colleagues demonstrated that early application with HFNS in patients with moderate ARDS might help avoid intubation.[35] This was also seen in Antonello and colleagues' study that showed NIV reduced the need for endotracheal intubations in ~54% of the time and correlated with a meta-analysis of randomized and observational studies. However, given the heterogeneity of the studies, other outcome measures could not be interpreted.[36,37] Patel and colleagues found NIV delivered via helmet significantly reduced intubation rates than face masks.[38] Frat and colleagues investigated sequential applications of HFNC and NIV and found intubation rates of 36% in patients with a P/F ratio less than 300, including patients with ARDS.[39] It is not uncommon for NIV to be used in 20% to 30% of ARDS patients and most hypoxemic patient.[40,41] The potential benefits of avoiding mechanical ventilation such as complications of sedation, muscle paralysis, pneumonias, delirium, and earlier mobilization have been theorized but the evidence is based on a relatively small sample size. The LungSafe study, which was a prospective, multicentered observational study demonstrated that NIV was used among all ARDS severity categories and that the inspiratory pressures required to improve work of breathing could increase tidal volumes high enough to exacerbate lung injury potentially. It also demonstrated the risk of NIV failure increased with increasing severity of ARDS.[41] The higher inspiratory pressures could also lead to increase mask leaks, gastric distention, and patient tolerance.[42] The ERS/ATS and the BTS mention in their guidelines that the use of NIV has shown to decrease inspiratory effort than no inspiratory assistance but the ERS/ATS guidelines left no recommendation for its use given the small amount of data and the BTS guidelines state that those with the potential failure of NIV should be monitored in the ICU.[42] So while use is common in patients with ARDS, it is recommended that only select patients in carefully monitored units undertake an NIV trial.

Less controversial is the use of NIV in pulmonary edema and, more specifically, cardiogenic pulmonary edema. In cardiogenic pulmonary edema, there is an increase in extravascular lung water, decreased lung volume and lung compliance, and increased airway resistance.[43] Bello and colleagues review of the literature showed that the uses of NIV can decrease the systemic venous return and left ventricular afterload, which would reduce LV filling pressure and limiting pulmonary edema, and that CPAP showed improvement in vital signs of patients and decreased need for endotracheal intubation and hospital mortality than conventional oxygen therapy.[2,44] The BTS guidelines recommend CPAP as it has been shown effective in patient with cardiogenic pulmonary edema and that NIV should be reserved for those for whom CPAP is not successful.[3] The ERS/ATS guidelines recommend either bilevel NIV or CPAP for patients with acute respiratory failure due to cardiogenic pulmonary edema.[8]

The global pandemic of COVID-19 has been deadly, and with some countries and ICUs short of ventilators, the use of NIV has proven helpful, especially with early studies out of China, Italy, and other countries out of Europe showing those who ended up intubated had higher mortality. A study out of Germany suggests that NIV be used as an additional support measure early in the disease course and part of a stepwise algorithm.[45] There are some theoretical concerns about not recommending NIV or HFNC until the patients are cleared of COVID-19 due to transmission risks to health care professionals due to aerosols.[46,49] A study out of China that demonstrated early intervention with HFNC and NIV could lead to lower mortality.[47] The Society of Critical Care Medicine came out with recommendations supporting HFNC and recommended that modality over NIPPV in its 2019 paper, which was not without controversy as some argued HFNC was no safer than NIPPV as most of the work looking at HFNC and NIPPV had been done in SARS and that NIPPV offers a closed system versus HFNC.[48,49]

SUMMARY

It is hoped that this article effectively reviews the most common NIV and oxygenation strategies and modalities used in surgical patients. It is also hoped that the clinical pathologies mentioned in this article serve as a good reference for clinicians who would like guidance on the use of NIV in their patients.

CLINICS CARE POINTS

- NIV is only seen beneficial if used early in the postextubation phase.
- NIV is suggested for use in COPD with those who have acidosis for acute exacerbations of COPD.
- NIV can be used in ARDS but is most successful in patients with mild ARDS. There is an increase in NIV failure rates with increasing severity of ARDS and is associated with worse mortality.

DISCLOSURE

The authors have nothing to disclose.

REFERENCES

1. Jensen MQ, Boatright JE. Respiratory care principles and practice. In: Hass Dean R, MacIntyre Neil R, Galvin William F, et al, editors. Respiratory care principles and practice. Burlington, MA: World Headquarters; 2021. p. 285–302.
2. Bello G, De Pascale G, Antonelli M. Noninvasive ventilation. Clin Chest Med 2016; 37(4):711–21.
3. Non-invasive ventilation in acute respiratory failure. Thorax 2002;57(3):192–211.
4. Mehta S, Hill, NS. Noninvasive ventilation. American journal of respiratory and critical care medicine 2001;163(2): 540-577.
5. Carron M, Freo U, BaHammam AS, et al. Complications of non-invasive ventilation techniques: a comprehensive qualitative review of randomized trials. Br J Anaesth 2013;110(6):896–914.
6. Wepler M, Demiselle J, Radermacher P, et al. Before the ICU: does emergency room hyperoxia affect outcome? Crit Care 2018;22(1):59.
7. Davidson C, Banham S, Elliott M, et al. British thoracic society/intensive care society guideline for the ventilatory management of acute hypercapnic respiratory failure in adults. BMJ open Respir Res 2016;3(1):e000133.
8. Rochwerg B, Brochard L, Elliott MW, et al. Official ERS/ATS clinical practice guidelines: noninvasive ventilation for acute respiratory failure. Eur Respir J Aug 2017;50(2):1602426.
9. Bourke SC, Piraino T, Pisani L, et al. Beyond the guidelines for non-invasive ventilation in acute respiratory failure: implications for practice. Lancet Respir Med 2018;6(12):935–47.
10. Ooi R, Joshi P, Soni N. An evaluation of oxygen delivery using nasal prongs. Anaesthesia 1992;47(7):591–3.
11. Wettstein RB, Shelledy DC, Peters JI. Original contributions delivered oxygen concentrations using low-flow and high-flow nasal cannulas. Respir Care 2005;50(5):604–9.
12. Jensen AG, Johnson A, Sandstedt S. Rebreathing during oxygen treatment with face mask: The effect of oxygen flow rates on ventilation. Acta anaesthesiologica Scand 1991;35(4):289–92.

13. Maggiore SM, Idone FA, Vaschetto R, et al. Nasal high-flow versus Venturi mask oxygen therapy after extubation. Effects on oxygenation, comfort, and clinical outcome. Am J Respir Crit Care Med 2014;190(3):282–8.
14. Soto-Ruiz KM, Peacock WF, Varon J. The men and history behind the Venturi mask. Resuscitation 2011;82(3):244–6.
15. Karras GE. Oxygen therapy in acutely Ill patients. In: Mechanical ventilation e-book: clinical applications and pathophysiology, 149 2007;. p. 418–27.
16. Lodeserto F. High flow nasal cannula (HFNC)-part 1: how it works 2018. https:// rebelem.com Web site. Available at: https://rebelem.com/high-flow-nasal-cannula-hfnc-part-1-how-it-works/. Accessed April 10, 2021.
17. Riera J, Pérez P, Cortés J, et al. Effect of high-flow nasal cannula and body position on end-expiratory lung volume: a cohort study using electrical impedance tomography. Respir Care 2013;58(4):589–96.
18. Sharma S, Danckers M, Sanghavi D, et al. High flow nasal cannula. In: StatPearls. Treasure Island, FL: StatPearls Publishing; 2021. Available at: https://www.ncbi. nlm.nih.gov/books/NBK526071/%20.
19. Möller W, Celik G, Feng S, et al. Nasal high flow clears anatomical dead space in upper airway models licensed under creative commons attribution CC-BY 3.0. J Appl Physiol 2015;118:1525.
20. Mündel T, Sheng F, Tatkov S, et al. Mechanisms of nasal high flow on ventilation during wakefulness and sleep. J Appl Physiol 2013;114(8):1058–65.
21. Frat J, Coudroy R, Thille AW. Non-invasive ventilation or high-flow oxygen therapy: When to choose one over the other? Respirology 2018;24(8):724.
22. Parke RL, McGuinness SP. Pressures delivered by nasal high flow oxygen during all phases of the respiratory cycle. Respir Care 2013;58(10):1621–4.
23. Kacmarek RM. Noninvasive respiratory support for postextubation respiratory failure. Respir Care 2019;64(6):658–78.
24. Aydin K, Ozcengiz D. Noninvasive ventilation in sleep medicine and pulmonary critical care. In: Equinas A, Insalaco G, Duan J, et al, editors. Noninvasive ventilation in sleep medicine and pulmonary critical care. Switzerland: Springer; 2020. p. 285–91.
25. Owens W. The ventilator book. In: The ventilator book. Columbia, South Carolina: First Draught Press; 2018. p. 87–94.
26. Allison MG, Winters ME. Noninvasive ventilation for the emergency physician. Emerg Med Clin North Am 2016;34(1):51–62.
27. Kushida CA, Chediak A, et al. Minimum start- ing CPAP should be 4 cm H 2 O for pediatric and adult patients, and the recommended minimum starting IPAP and EPAP should be 8 cm H 2 O and 4 cm H 2 O, respectively, for pediatric and adult patients on clinical guidelines for the manual titration of positive airway pressure in patients with obstructive sleep apnea positive airway pressure titration task force of the american academy of sleep medicine. J Clin Sleep Med 2008;4(2).
28. Hernández G, Vaquero C, Colinas L, et al. Effect of postextubation high-flow nasal cannula vs noninvasive ventilation on reintubation and postextubation respiratory failure in high-risk patients: a randomized clinical trial. JAMA 2016;316(15):1565–74.
29. Ferrer M, Valencia M, Nicolas JM, et al. Early noninvasive ventilation averts extubation failure in patients at risk: a randomized trial. Am J Respir Crit Care Med 2006;173(2):164–70.
30. Karcz MK, Papadakos PJ. Noninvasive ventilation in trauma. World J Crit Care Med 2015;4(1):47–54.
31. Schreiber A, Yıldırım F, Ferrari G, et al. Non-invasive mechanical ventilation in critically ill trauma patients: a systematic review. Turkish J anaesthesiology reanimation 2018;46(2):88–95.

32. Hua A, Shah KH. Systematic review snapshot does noninvasive ventilation have a role in chest trauma patients? Ann Emerg Med 2014;64(1):82–3.
33. Hess DR. Noninvasive ventilation for acute respiratory failure. Respir Care 2013; 58(6):950–72.
34. Keenan SP, Powers CE, McCormack DG. Noninvasive positive-pressure ventilation in patients with milder chronic obstructive pulmonary disease exacerbations: a randomized controlled trial. Respir Care 2005;50(5):610–6.
35. Ding L, Wang L, Ma W, et al. Efficacy and safety of early prone positioning combined with HFNC or NIV in moderate to severe ARDS: a multi-center prospective cohort study. Crit Care 2020;24(1):28.
36. Antonelli M, Conti G, Esquinas A, et al. A multiple-center survey on the use in clinical practice of noninvasive ventilation as a first-line intervention for acute respiratory distress syndrome. Crit Care Med 2007;35(1):18–25.
37. Agarwal R, Aggarwal AN, Gupta D. Original research role of noninvasive ventilation in acute lung injury/acute respiratory distress syndrome: a proportion meta-analysis. Respir Care 2010;55(12):1653–60.
38. Patel BK, Wolfe KS, Pohlman AS, et al. Effect of noninvasive ventilation delivered by helmet vs face mask on the rate of endotracheal intubation in patients with acute respiratory distress syndrome: a randomized clinical trial. JAMA 2016; 315(22):2435–41.
39. Frat J, Brugiere B, Ragot S, et al. Sequential application of oxygen therapy via high-flow nasal cannula and noninvasive ventilation in acute respiratory failure: an observational pilot study. Respir Care 2015;60(2):170–8.
40. Grieco DL, Menga LS, Eleuteri D, et al. Patient self-inflicted lung injury: Implications for acute hypoxemic respiratory failure and ARDS patients on non-invasive support. Minerva Anestesiol 2019;85(9):1014–23.
41. Bellani G, Laffey JG, Pham T, et al. Noninvasive ventilation of patients with acute respiratory distress syndrome insights from the LUNG SAFE study. Am J Respir Crit Care Med 2017;195(1):67–77.
42. L'Her E, Deye N, Lellouche F, et al. Physiologic effects of noninvasive ventilation during acute lung injury. Am J Respir Crit Care Med 2005;172(9):1112–8.
43. Sharp JT, Griffith GT, Bunnell IL, et al. Ventilatory mechanics on pulmonary edema in man. J Clin Invest 1958;37(1):111–7.
44. Belenguer-Muncharaz A, Mateu-Campos L, González-Luís R, et al. Non-invasive mechanical ventilation versus continuous positive airway pressure relating to cardiogenic pulmonary edema in an intensive care unit. Arch Bronconeumol 2017;53(10):561–7.
45. Windisch W, Weber-Carstens S, Kluge S, et al. Invasive and non-invasive ventilation in patients with COVID-19. Deutsch Ärztebl Int 2020;117(31–32):528–33.
46. Winck JC, Ambrosino N. COVID-19 pandemic and non invasive respiratory management: every goliath needs a david. an evidence based evaluation of problems. Pulmonology 2020;26(4):213–20.
47. Wang K, Zhao W, Li J, et al. The experience of high-flow nasal cannula in hospitalized patients with 2019 novel coronavirus-infected pneumonia in two hospitals of chongqing, china. Ann Intensive Care 2020;10(1):37.
48. Remy KE, Lin JC, Verhoef PA. High flow NC may be no safer than NIPPV. Crit Care 2020;24(1):1–2.
49. Alhazzani W, Møller MH, et al. Surviving Sepsis campaign: guidelines on the management of critically ill adults with coronavirus disease 2019 (COVID-19). Crit Care Med 2020;48(6):e440–69.

Antibiotic Therapy in the Intensive Care Unit

Mehreen Kisat, MD, MS, Ben Zarzaur, MD, MPH*

KEYWORDS

- Sepsis • Infections • Surgical ICU • Antimicrobial resistance
- Antimicrobial stewardship

KEY POINTS

- Appropriate and adequate use of antibiotics remains a challenge in critically ill patients.
- After initiation of empirical therapy, antibiotics should be deescalated to directed, definitive therapy in 48 to 72 hours.
- Source control is an essential component of treatment in surgical patients.
- Emerging technology can help decrease the burden of inappropriate antibiotic use.
- Effective antibiotic stewardship programs can reduce inappropriate antibiotic use and also improve patient safety and clinical outcomes.

EPIDEMIOLOGY

Infections due to antimicrobial-resistant pathogens are responsible for more than 2 million illnesses and 23,000 deaths in the United States every year, a large burden of which occurs in the intensive care unit (ICU).[1] Infection with antimicrobial-resistant organisms are associated with a longer length of stay, ICU admission, and higher mortality when compared with those who do not suffer infections.[2,3] Because of the high risks associated with infections among patients admitted to the ICU combined with the potential development of antimicrobial resistance, ICU providers face challenging decisions regarding appropriate antibiotic use in these complex patients. We know that inadequate initial antimicrobial treatment is associated with worse outcomes,[4,5] and this results in the use of very broad-spectrum agents in critically ill patients even when risk factors for resistance are not present. On the other hand, approximately 30% of the prescriptions for antimicrobial therapy are inappropriate.[6,7] Frequently, antibiotics are started for "treatment" of what turns out to be colonization or contamination, noninfectious physiologic phenomenon (such as systemic

Division of Acute Care and Regional General Surgery, Department of Surgery, University of Wisconsin School of Medicine and Public Health, G5/332A, 600 Highland Avenue, Madison, WI 53792, USA
* Corresponding author.
E-mail address: zarzaur@surgery.wisc.edu

Surg Clin N Am 102 (2022) 159–167
https://doi.org/10.1016/j.suc.2021.09.007
0039-6109/22/© 2021 Elsevier Inc. All rights reserved.

inflammatory response syndrome) or viral infections. Compounding the problem of inappropriate initiation of antimicrobial therapy is the fact that antimicrobial therapy is often used for too long or is too broad for what is needed.

Patients in the surgical ICU (SICU) are typically patients admitted after recent surgery (emergency general surgery or surgery within the preceding 2–4 weeks) or trauma. SICU patients are at the highest risk to have an infection, likely because the infection itself was the cause of admission to the ICU. SICU patients have different sources of infection as compared with general ICU patients. A single-center study demonstrated that most of the patients with severe sepsis in the SICU had an intraabdominal infection. In addition, more than 50% of the cases had infections in multiple locations.[8] Because the sources of infections are different compared with general ICU patients, SICU patients often have a distinct microbiology pattern.

Injured patients represent another patient population that is often found in an SICU. Approximately 1 in 4 trauma patients admitted to the ICU develop an infection during their hospital course.[9] Injury causes systemic inflammatory response, which mimics an infection, and this makes it difficult to differentiate inflammatory response related to injury from infection. Thus, initial treatment of trauma patients manifesting an inflammatory response relies mainly on clinical judgment, until and if more definitive microbiology data becomes available. The purpose of this review is to address the challenge of balancing early diagnosis and treatment of infections in critically ill patients with appropriate antibiotic stewardship. The authors focus on diagnosis, choice of empirical therapy, deescalation strategies, the importance of source control, and antibiotic stewardship best practices.

DIAGNOSIS
Challenges

Typically, SICU patients with infectious complications fall into 2 categories: (1) admitted to the ICU due to an infection or (2) develop an infection during their ICU stay. Both categories have their unique challenges. The diagnostics of infections in SICU patients is challenging, as the tools we tend to rely on are unreliable in many situations. Infections closely mimics systemic inflammatory response syndrome (SIRS) that can normally be expected in critically ill patients. Most patients in the SICU mount an SIRS response to postoperative inflammation, trauma, burns, or other inflammatory process. In addition, signs of impending organ dysfunction in severe sepsis, such as hypotension or oliguria, may be confounded by the presence of other postoperative complications such as bleeding, fluid losses, or underresuscitation.[10]

Role of Traditional Microbiology Testing

Traditional microbiology testing includes Gram stain and culture of various specimen sites, urinalysis and urine microscopy, cellular analysis of bodily fluids (eg, bronchoalveolar lavage, intraabdominal fluid, cerebrospinal fluid), and in vitro susceptibility testing. Gram stains have the potential to aid in decision-making about antibiotic treatment. However, there are inherent concerns regarding the reproducibility of slide preparation and interpretation for Gram stains. Various studies have demonstrated that Gram stain prediction of pathogenic organisms is limited.[11,12] In addition, the negative predictive value of Gram stain is also controversial. A single-center study of trauma patients with ventilator-associated pneumonia (VAP) observed that lack of gram-positive organism visible on Gram stain had a negative predictive value of 83% for gram-positive VAP. However, this was not the case for gram-negative organisms. Gram-negative infections were present in 70% of all VAPs but were not reliably identified by Gram stain.[13] The case is clearer for the usefulness of preliminary studies in the setting of a suspected urinary tract infection. A negative urinalysis can be useful in the decision not to send a urine culture and or/treat for possible urinary tract infection. A negative urinalysis can reliably exclude catheter-associated urinary tract infection in the febrile, trauma ICU patient and also help in redirecting toward other sources of infection.[14]

It takes approximately 48 to 96 hours for identification of a pathogen from a clinical specimen and another 48 to 72 hours for susceptibility results to come back. Thus, patients are started on an empirical antibiotic based on clinical suspicion of an infection and have been on antibiotics for several days by the time full susceptibility is available. In a multicenter study of ICU patients, 50% of empirical antibiotics were continued for at least 72 hours in the absence of adjudicated infection[15]; this represents a large number of inappropriate antimicrobial coverage days that could result in the subsequent development of resistant organisms.

Rapid Microbial Identification and Susceptibility Testing

Emerging technology could help decrease the burden of inappropriate antibiotic use by helping to decrease the time to identification of antibiotic susceptibility as well as improving the speed at which sepsis secondary to bacterial infections can be identified. There are 3 broad categories of assays for pathogen identification and antibiotic susceptibility testing profiling based on their proximity to the specimen source and required assay time.[16] The historical gold standard for blood cultures consists of a 2-step process.[17,18] In the first step, a specimen is cultured with continuous monitoring for growth. In the second step, positive blood culture is evaluated using Gram stain microscopy and subcultures to generate isolates for identification and antibiotic susceptibility testing. 16s sequencing on isolates is used for phylogenetic information. However, the time needed for the first 2 steps and resources on this method make it less ideal for rapid diagnostic applications. The second category involves pathogen identification from culture-positive specimens. Matrix-assisted laser desorption by ionization time-of-flight (MALDI-TOF) mass spectrometry, fluorescence in situ hybridization (FISH), and multiplexed polymerase chain reaction (PCR) fall in this category. MALDI-TOF enables protein-based identification of a bacteria and fungi from cultures samples on the order of minutes. FISH uses fluorescent probes specific to the pathogen of interest to directly stain and monitor its presence via microscopy or luminometer. Multiplexed PCR assays can target multiple organisms simultaneously with limited resistant markers. These methods still require bacterial cultivation as the first step. The third category of assays aims to provide identification and antibiotic susceptibility testing directly from patient specimens without the initial overnight culture step. An example of such an assay is a sample-to-answer multiplex PCR assay, which combines DNA extraction, nested multiplex PCR, and post-PCR melting curve analysis.[19] This assay requires a priori knowledge of the common etiologic agents for the specific infection.

EMPIRICAL THERAPY

Antimicrobial therapy is started while awaiting results of a work-up for a suspected infection. Initial treatment with broad empirical therapy in a patient with high suspicion for infection is appropriate, as use of inadequate antibiotics that do not cover the ultimate identified pathogen accounts for 39% to 51% of excess mortality in ICU patients with various infectious syndromes.[5,20–22] Ideally, empirical therapy should only last 48 to 72 hours. Often, surgeons are faced with a variety of clinical scenarios involving vulnerable patient populations: from the young paraplegic patient due to spine injury after trauma and prolonged ICU stay with ventilator-associated pneumonia to a postoperative abdominal wall reconstruction patient for ventral hernia with necrotizing soft tissue infection of the abdominal wall and an enterocutaneous fistula. Surgeons and intensivist are called on to administer the appropriate antibiotic agents and achieve source control.

The decision for empirical therapy regimen should depend on the following factors[23]:

a. Presumed site of infection and likely pathogen involved
b. Previous antimicrobial exposure and likelihood of pretreatment antimicrobial agent resistance
c. Clinical severity of illness
d. Ability to deliver the agents to the site of infection
e. Risks associated with the antimicrobial therapy
f. Local ecology data and resistance profiles

The unique challenge in initiating the appropriate empirical therapy in the SICU is that many of the patients present with risk factors for multidrug-resistant (MDR) organisms and the usual empirical antibiotic treatment is suboptimal against these organisms. There has been an increased prevalence of surgical infections caused by antibiotic-resistant pathogens, including extended spectrum β-lactamase–producing *Enterobacteriaceae*, *Pseudomonas aeruginosa*, methicillin-resistant *Staphylococcus aureus* (MRSA), and carbapenemase-resistant *Enterobacteriaceae* (CRE) in the past few decades.[24,25] Seguin and colleagues found that in patients who were hospitalized for 5 days or longer and had previous exposure to antibiotics, MDR was present in 38% of the infections compared with 2% when both were absent.[26] We should prioritize identifying patients who are at risk for MDR organisms. When an MDR is suspected, standard empirical therapy based on individual hospital's antibiogram may be inadequate. Rapid identification methods are a potential way to detect MDR organisms. Molecular-based techniques to identify organisms such as MRSA, vancomycin-resistant enterococcus, or CREs as early as 2 hours after a specimen is collected can help in modification of empirical treatment.

DEESCALATION

An antibiotic deescalation strategy combines initially selecting the appropriate antibiotic for empirical therapy with decreasing the time that a patient is exposed to the broad-spectrum therapy. Deescalation is applied in only 40% to 50% of patients, which reflects physician's reluctance to narrow empirical coverage when caring for severely ill patients.[27] There are 3 ways that deescalation can occur.[28] Once the culture and sensitivity data come back, broad-spectrum agents can be changed to a narrower spectrum. However, culture data are often negative in critically ill patients and cannot be used for deescalation. The second way is to use the nonrecovery of certain organisms to narrow the existing regimen. For example, in patients with VAP empirical regimen includes coverage against MRSA and *P aeruginosa*. If the patients are clinically improving, therapy against MRSA and *P aeruginosa* can be stopped if sputum cultures are negative for these organisms.[29] The third possibility for deescalation is to decrease the duration of therapy to the shortest time length necessary to achieve an optimal clinical outcome.[30] An example of shorter duration of treatment is in patients with intraabdominal infection. The STOP-IT (Study to Optimize Peritoneal infection Therapy) trial, which was a randomized clinical trial of patients with complicated intraabdominal infections who had undergone adequate source control, demonstrated that outcomes after fixed-duration antibiotic therapy (approximately 4 days) were similar to those after a longer course of antibiotics (approximately 8 days).[31]

SOURCE CONTROL

In surgical patients, source control is an essential component of the treatment of infections. Source control is defined as removing the cause of the infection and any infected material. It includes drainage of pus and inflammatory material as well as debridement of necrotic tissue. Adequate source control often requires multidisciplinary care and coordination with interventional radiology and infectious disease services. Source control should not be delayed except in circumstances where demarcation of nonviable tissue and infection is preferable, such as pancreatic necrosis, or in situations where source control is difficult to obtain, such as an infected part of a left ventricular assist device. Timing of source control is often debated and should be guided by severity of illness, source of infection, and physiologic status of the patient.[10]

ANTIMICROBIAL STEWARDSHIP APPROACHES

Antimicrobial stewardship (AMS) is defined as "an organizational or healthcare-system-wide approach for fostering and monitoring judicious use of antimicrobials to preserve their effectiveness." The goals of antimicrobial stewardship are to combat the emergence of resistance, improve clinical outcomes, and decrease health care costs. In the ICU, antibiotic stewardship encompasses rapid identification of patients with an infection, appropriate selection of empirical treatment, deescalation once culture results become available, shortening the duration of treatment, and reducing the number of patients treated unnecessarily.[32]

A high volume of inappropriate antibiotic use occurs in the ICUs.[33] Critical care physicians must recognize that antibiotic therapy in the ICU has implications for the unit's microbiome. If antibiotic-resistant organisms are selected by a pattern of antibiotic use, those pathogens can become part of the ICU's ecology and affect other patients. Implementation of effective ASPs reduces inappropriate antibiotic use and improves patient safety and clinical outcomes.[34] The Centers for Disease Control and Prevention (CDC) recommends that all acute care hospitals implement antibiotic stewardship programs. The CDC has defined 7 core elements of this program[35,36]:

1. Leadership commitment: dedicate human, financial, and information technology resources.
2. Accountability: identify a single leader who is responsible for coordinating and reporting of the program. A physician or pharmacist who ideally has training in infectious disease and/or antibiotic stewardship should be considered for this role.
3. Drug expertise: identify a pharmacist leader who is responsible for improving antibiotic use.
4. Action: implement at least one recommended action, such as evaluation of ongoing treatment need after a set period of initial treatment (eg, antibiotic time out after 48 hours).
5. Tracking: monitor antibiotic prescribing and resistance patterns
6. Reporting: regular report on antibiotic use and resistance to doctors, nurses, and relevant staff.
7. Education: education clinicians about resistance and optimal prescribing.

In the ICU, stewardship teams consisting of infectious disease physicians and infectious disease pharmacists can complement the evaluation of patients and provide recommendations on treatment. This multidisciplinary and collaborative team should consist of intensive care physicians, pharmacists, and nurses in addition to infectious disease physicians. The most common reasons for unnecessary antibiotic use are the following: (1) longer than necessary duration of treatment, (2) treatment of noninfectious or nonbacterial syndromes, and (3) overly broad spectrum of activity.[7] A multicenter study that assessed antibiotic appropriateness in 47 ICUs in the United States describes the following intervention strategies to address inappropriate antibiotic use[23]:

1. Require indications on all antibiotic orders and restrict broad spectrum agents.
2. Limit use of intravenous vancomycin when not indicated through educational initiatives, computerized alerts, and prospective audit and feedback protocols.
3. Deescalate broad-spectrum antibiotic regimens after 48 to 72 hours through antibiotic time-outs, antibiotic restrictions, or rapid diagnostics.
4. Implement diagnostic stewardship, including criteria for urine cultures and interpretation of culture results.
5. Improve duration of therapy based on available data through treatment protocols and computerized order sets.
6. Share data at critical care councils of individual hospitals.
7. Ultimately, antimicrobial stewardship enhances antimicrobial therapy. Intelligent and discretionary use of antibiotic regimens can potentially slow antibiotic resistance.

SUMMARY

The SICU remains a challenging environment for the diagnosis and management of surgical infections. The consequences of inappropriate or inadequate treatment of patients with a documented bacterial infection can be life threatening or may result in avoidable complications. At the same time, ICU providers have a responsibility to limit the spread and the emergence of antimicrobial resistant organisms. However, providers often lack to the tools to determine which patients are actually infected with what organisms, susceptible to what antibiotics. Emerging technologies may help future clinicians with this dilemma. Until then, adherence to sound antimicrobial stewardship guidelines will help to reduce the emergence and spread of dangerous drug-resistant organisms.

CLINICS CARE POINTS

- Patients in the SICU often have different sources of infection and distinct microbiology patterns compared with patients in other ICUs.
- In addition to traditional microbiology testing, emerging technologies for rapid microbial detection and susceptibility testing should be used when available.
- Empirical treatment should be started in a patient with a clinical suspicion of an infection.
- Empirical treatment regimen should be individualized based on the patient and ICU/hospital ecology data and resistance profile.
- Identify patients who are at risk for multidrug resistant organisms before starting antibiotic treatment.
- Use culture and sensitivity data for deescalation. If cultures are negative, use absence of certain organisms to narrow antibiotics (eg, absence of MRSA in VAP).

- Decrease the duration of therapy to the shortest time length necessary, for example, 4 days for patients with intraabdominal infections who have achieved source control.
- Source control is essential in surgical patients and requires multidisciplinary care and coordination with other services (infectious disease and interventional radiology).
- Collaboration and compliance with the antibiotic stewardship team is essential to the success of antibiotic stewardship program.

DISCLOSURE

None.

REFERENCES

1. Carlet J, Ben Ali A, Chalfine A. Epidemiology and control of antibiotic resistance in the intensive care unit. Curr Opin Infect Dis 2004;17(4):309–16.
2. Campion M, Scully G. Antibiotic use in the intensive care unit: optimization and de-escalation. J Intensive Care Med 2018;33(12):647–55.
3. Kaye KS, Pogue JM. Infections caused by resistant gram-negative bacteria: epidemiology and management. Pharmacotherapy 2015;35(10):949–62.
4. Hyle EP, Lipworth AD, Zaoutis TE, et al. Impact of inadequate initial antimicrobial therapy on mortality in infections due to extended-spectrum beta-lactamase-producing enterobacteriaceae: variability by site of infection. Arch Intern Med 2005; 165(12):1375–80.
5. Kollef MH, Sherman G, Ward S, et al. Inadequate antimicrobial treatment of infections: a risk factor for hospital mortality among critically ill patients. Chest 1999; 115(2):462–74.
6. Cusini A, Rampini SK, Bansal V, et al. Different patterns of inappropriate antimicrobial use in surgical and medical units at a tertiary care hospital in Switzerland: a prevalence survey. PLoS One 2010;5(11):e14011.
7. Hecker MT, Aron DC, Patel NP, et al. Unnecessary use of antimicrobials in hospitalized patients: current patterns of misuse with an emphasis on the antianaerobic spectrum of activity. Arch Intern Med 2003;163(8):972–8.
8. Cheng B, Xie G, Yao S, et al. Epidemiology of severe sepsis in critically ill surgical patients in ten university hospitals in China. Crit Care Med 2007;35(11):2538–46.
9. Barmparas G, Harada MY, Ko A, et al. The effect of early positive cultures on mortality in ventilated trauma patients. Surg Infect (Larchmt) 2018;19(4):410–6.
10. De Waele J, De Bus L. How to treat infections in a surgical intensive care unit. BMC Infect Dis 2014;14:193.
11. Samuel LP, Balada-Llasat JM, Harrington A, et al. Multicenter assessment of gram stain error rates. J Clin Microbiol 2016;54(6):1442–7.
12. Blot F, Raynard B, Chachaty E, et al. Value of gram stain examination of lower respiratory tract secretions for early diagnosis of nosocomial pneumonia. Am J Respir Crit Care Med 2000;162(5):1731–7.
13. Davis KA, Eckert MJ, Reed RL 2nd, et al. Ventilator-associated pneumonia in injured patients: do you trust your Gram's stain? J Trauma 2005;58(3):462–6 [discussion 466–7].
14. Stovall RT, Haenal JB, Jenkins TC, et al. A negative urinalysis rules out catheter-associated urinary tract infection in trauma patients in the intensive care unit. J Am Coll Surg 2013;217(1):162–6.

15. Thomas Z, Bandali F, Sankaranarayanan J, et al, Critical Care Pharmacotherapy Trials N. A Multicenter evaluation of prolonged empiric antibiotic therapy in adult ICUs in the United States. Crit Care Med 2015;43(12):2527–34.

16. Shin DJ, Andini N, Hsieh K, et al. Emerging Analytical techniques for rapid pathogen identification and susceptibility testing. Annu Rev Anal Chem 2019;12(1):41–67.

17. Jorgensen JH, Ferraro MJ. Antimicrobial susceptibility testing: a review of general principles and contemporary practices. Clin Infect Dis 2009;49(11):1749–55.

18. Lagier JC, Edouard S, Pagnier I, et al. Current and past strategies for bacterial culture in clinical microbiology. Clin Microbiol Rev 2015;28(1):208–36.

19. Leber AL, Everhart K, Daly JA, et al. Multicenter evaluation of BioFire FilmArray respiratory panel 2 for detection of viruses and bacteria in nasopharyngeal swab samples. J Clin Microbiol 2018;56(6):e01945.

20. Leone M, Bourgoin A, Cambon S, et al. Empirical antimicrobial therapy of septic shock patients: adequacy and impact on the outcome. Crit Care Med 2003;31(2):462–7.

21. Luna CM, Vujacich P, Niederman MS, et al. Impact of BAL data on the therapy and outcome of ventilator-associated pneumonia. Chest 1997;111(3):676–85.

22. Ibrahim EH, Sherman G, Ward S, et al. The influence of inadequate antimicrobial treatment of bloodstream infections on patient outcomes in the ICU setting. Chest 2000;118(1):146–55.

23. Trivedi KK, Bartash R, Letourneau AR, et al. Opportunities to improve antibiotic appropriateness in U.S. ICUs: a multicenter evaluation. Crit Care Med 2020;48(7):968–76.

24. Sartelli M, Catena F, di Saverio S, et al. The challenge of antimicrobial resistance in managing intra-abdominal infections. Surg Infect (Larchmt) 2015;16(3):213–20.

25. Sartelli M, Duane TM, Catena F, et al. Antimicrobial stewardship: a call to action for surgeons. Surg Infect (Larchmt) 2016;17(6):625–31.

26. Seguin P, Laviolle B, Chanavaz C, et al. Factors associated with multidrug-resistant bacteria in secondary peritonitis: impact on antibiotic therapy. Clin Microbiol Infect 2006;12(10):980–5.

27. Weiss E, Zahar JR, Lesprit P, et al. Elaboration of a consensual definition of de-escalation allowing a ranking of beta-lactams. Clin Microbiol Infect 2015;21(7):649. https://doi.org/10.1016/j.cmi.2015.03.013, e1–10.

28. Joseph EP, Phillip Dellinger R. Critical care medicine: principles of diagnosis and management in the adult. 5th edition. Philadelphia, PA: Elsevier; 2019.

29. American Thoracic S, Infectious Diseases Society of A. Guidelines for the management of adults with hospital-acquired, ventilator-associated, and healthcare-associated pneumonia. Am J Respir Crit Care Med 2005;171(4):388–416.

30. Hayashi Y, Paterson DL. Strategies for reduction in duration of antibiotic use in hospitalized patients. Clin Infect Dis 2011;52(10):1232–40.

31. Elwood NR, Guidry CA, Duane TM, et al. Short-course antimicrobial therapy does not increase treatment failure rate in patients with intra-abdominal infection involving fungal organisms. Surg Infect (Larchmt) 2018;19(4):376–81.

32. Luyt CE, Brechot N, Trouillet JL, et al. Antibiotic stewardship in the intensive care unit. Crit Care 2014;18(5):480.

33. Singh N, Rogers P, Atwood CW, et al. Short-course empiric antibiotic therapy for patients with pulmonary infiltrates in the intensive care unit. A proposed solution for indiscriminate antibiotic prescription. Am J Respir Crit Care Med 2000;162(2 Pt 1):505–11.

34. Tamma PD, Holmes A, Ashley ED. Antimicrobial stewardship: another focus for patient safety? Curr Opin Infect Dis 2014;27(4):348–55.
35. Pollack LA, Srinivasan A. Core elements of hospital antibiotic stewardship programs from the Centers for Disease Control and Prevention. Clin Infect Dis 2014;59(Suppl 3):S97–100.
36. Fridkin S, Baggs J, Fagan R, et al. Vital signs: improving antibiotic use among hospitalized patients. MMWR Morb Mortal Wkly Rep 2014;63(9):194–200.

Mobilization of Resources and Emergency Response on the National Scale

Jana M. Binkley, MD[a], Kevin M. Kemp, MD[b],*

KEYWORDS

- Mass casualty incident • disaster response • Emergency management
- COVID 19 response

KEY POINTS

- Mass casualty incidents occur when the number or complexity of patients requiring care overwhelms the resources available to provide care
- The most common type of mass casualty incidents in the United States is the mass shooting; however, other mechanisms result in unique injury patterns
- An effective response to a mass casualty incident requires adequate planning, triage, and surge capacity.
- Depending on the scale of the event, a response using national resources may be required

INTRODUCTION

A mass casualty incident (MCI) is an event in which the number of patients exceeds the resources normally available from local resources. The number of patients needed to cause an MCI varies depending on local resources and capabilities. According to a recent survey of the National Emergency Medical Services Information system, just fewer than 10,000 MCI occur annually in the United States.[1] Although this number may seem large, many MCI are not high visibility acts of intentional violence or natural disasters that often come to mind. For example, at a critical access hospital, multiple victims of a motor vehicle crash arriving simultaneously can overwhelm the facility and impair its ability to provide effective care.

Numerous high-profile events have contributed to public awareness of MCI. Images of the September 11 attacks, the Boston Marathon bombing, and numerous active

[a] Department of Surgery, University of Nebraska Medical Center, 983280 Nebraska Medical Center, Omaha, NE 68198, USA; [b] Division of Acute Care Surgery, Department of Surgery, University of Nebraska Medical Center, 983280 Nebraska Medical Center, Omaha, NE 68198-3280, USA
* Corresponding author.
E-mail address: kevin.kemp@unmc.edu

Surg Clin N Am 102 (2022) 169–180
https://doi.org/10.1016/j.suc.2021.09.014
0039-6109/22/© 2021 Elsevier Inc. All rights reserved.

surgical.theclinics.com

shooter events have been seared into our collective memory. Much as advances in trauma care are made in times of conflict, the management of MCI has undergone a subsequent evolution as a result of past events. Best practices are elucidated and experiences shared to improve our response to the next event.

This article reviews the preparation and types of events causing MCI, as well as the injuries to be expected and a framework for mobilizing the resources needed to respond. Should these local resources be insufficient, an overview of the national emergency response will be provided.

PREPARATION BEFORE A MASS CASUALTY INCIDENT

Preparation before the occurrence of an MCI is essential to ensure the best possible outcomes. The planned response for unforeseen disasters is called all hazard preparedness. An all hazards approach focuses on capabilities and capacities that are critical to preparedness for a full spectrum of events. To determine what events are possible to occur, a hazards vulnerability analysis is conducted. This process is specific to a given facility, given their location, circumstances, and surrounding areas. For example, if a hospital is located near a chemical plant, it would be reasonable to consider that an industrial explosion could be a possible event inducing an MCI. Geographic location is also paramount to consider when planning. A hospital on a fault line should consider the aftermath of a massive earthquake, whereas a facility in a hurricane-prone area should plan for operations after a major storm. In these types of events, the hospital itself could be damaged or destroyed by the event, so this contingency needs to be considered as well.

The type of event dictates what resources are necessary to respond. In a mass shooting or explosion, the predominant patient type will be trauma, who will often present to the closest hospital and create a demand on emergency and surgical services. These types of events create a short-term surge in resource demand. However, in a large-scale outbreak of an infectious disease as we have seen in the coronavirus disease 2019 (COVID-19) pandemic, the predominate patient type is medical, patients will present to many hospitals, and the resultant surge can last for months or even years. In the United States, the most common type of MCI event is a mass shooting.[2] Because of this factor, it is imperative that surgeons engage with hospital leadership in the planning and subsequent response to an MCI, should it occur. Owing to the scope of these events, response from law enforcement, emergency medical services, the local government, and surrounding hospitals will need to be considered.

The importance of MCI drills cannot be underestimated. In an article discussing the response to the Boston Marathon bombing, Walls and Zinner[3] outlined the extensive preparation and drills that had taken place at Brigham and Women's Hospital, other area hospitals, and the City of Boston. Influenced by the events of 9/11, a large, city-wide disaster drill simulated the detonation of a dirty bomb and the influx of 72 simulated patients, some of whom required decontamination. In the period between 2006 and 2012, Brigham and Women's Hospital conducted or participated in 73 separate exercises, events, and disaster activations.[3] Physicians and nursing staff from trauma surgery and the emergency department also participated in team training in a simulation center to hone the response of the trauma team. This deliberate practice and drilling likely contributed to a coordinated response and a relatively even distribution of critically injured patients among the area trauma centers; of the patients who arrived alive to the emergency department, none died.[4]

Standardized courses exist to introduce surgeons, physicians, and other members of the health care team to concepts key to response to an MCI. The American College of Surgeons offers the Disaster Management and Emergency Preparedness course, and the Society of Critical Care Medicine offers the Fundamentals of Disaster Management. These courses are similar in concept and seek to introduce participants to the concepts of incident command, triage, different types of MCI events, and expected injuries. Either course would seem to provide some framework and background to surgeons who may find themselves providing care to patients involved in an MCI.

The role of the public in the response to MCI cannot be understated. In response to the Sandy Hook shooting, the Hartford Consensus was formed. The goal of the Hartford Consensus was to provide the public with education and materials that are needed to prevent death from hemorrhage.[5] As a result of this work, in 2015 the national "Stop the Bleed" campaign was rolled out. Bleeding control stations are becoming more visible in public spaces and aim to provide the appropriate equipment to complement a trained provider of basic bleeding control. In response to the blast injuries observed in the aftermath of the Boston Marathon bombing, first responders were forced to apply improvised tourniquets. Six patients arrived at the Massachusetts General Hospital with improvised tourniquets in place, but they were all noted to be venous and therefore ineffective at stopping ongoing hemorrhage. These patients were converted to a Combat Application Tourniquet upon arrival to halt ongoing bleeding.[6] Although none of these patients ending up dying, in a situation where transport times were longer or if care were delayed, this outcome could be anticipated to not be as favorable.

TYPES OF EVENTS CAUSING MASS CASUALTY INCIDENTS

One of the key components to responding to a MCI is classifying the type of MCI present. Local and federal agencies tailor surge plans in preparing for anticipated, progressive, insidious and sudden-onset disasters occurring within the community. Common types of events causing MCI are summarized in this section.

One of the main types of MCI worldwide has been caused by active shooters with the intent of mass killings. Mass shootings have been defined as 3 or more killings in a single event. In the United States, where there has been an intensifying epidemic of violence, the most common MCI is a mass shooter event.[2] The Las Vegas Massacre is the deadliest mass shooting in the history of the United States, with 58 killed and 422 injured. As shown in the aftermath of this particular MCI, mass shootings are subject to a wide array of severity of victims owing to the type of weapon used, the accessibility that the shooter has to the population they are targeting, and the ability of law enforcement to reach the shooter.

Modern warfare has shifted toward civilian arenas and millions worldwide are now at high risk of experiencing an intentional act of harm event.[7] Terrorist attacks are usually described as the intent to harm a large group of the population to achieve a political gain. Different types of terrorist attacks include active shooters, improvised explosive devices, and vehicle attacks. Many of these events lack sophistication and yet have been able to cause large-scale loss of life.

Weapons of mass destruction can certainly cause an MCI on a large scale. These weapons include chemical weapons, biologic agents, and nuclear or radiologic devices. Infectious agents such as anthrax can be leaked purposely to expose people in the masses. Weapons of mass destruction are unique because, once in the environment, they can exist as a combination of solid, liquid, or gas. The method of distribution is an important to consider and ultimately dictates how many people can be affected. Gas or airborne particles such as inhaled anthrax spores result in an immediate response. Skin exposure to liquids or solids may take time to be absorbed directly through the skin or can be transferred to mouth and be ingested. Response to these types of events are often multidisciplinary and require specialized training and equipment.

Natural disasters such as landslides, tornadoes, earthquakes, and tsunamis are a type of MCI where more than 100,000 people are killed around the world and millions more are injured or disabled each year.[8,9] Unfortunately, in most natural disasters, people have either minimal or no time to prepare or seek shelter during these, contributing to the severity of the MCI. Other contributing factors that must be accounted for is the widespread destruction that can affect hospitals and emergency response teams that impairs their ability to respond. This situation was seen in the wake of the catastrophic tsunami in the Indian Ocean in 2004. This disaster highlighted the difficulty in providing medical care without an intact building to do so.

The typical perception of an MCI is associated with a catastrophic event such as a natural disaster, shooting or bombing as described as elsewhere in this article. The COVID-19 pandemic is quite the opposite; it is caused by an unseen virus, yet the effects on the health care infrastructure have been severe. The COVID-19 pandemic has been described as an MCI of the highest nature, straining health care systems across the world owing to continued waves, causing a continued state of surge capacity. It is evident that the management of the COVID-19 pandemic has demonstrated the worldwide challenges of facing a global viral outbreak and, as such, must be described as an unconventional MCI.

Smaller scale MCIs that can affect smaller communities include multiple vehicle or bus collisions and building or bridge collapses. Any of these where 3 or more victims are involved can quickly overwhelm smaller facilities with less surge capacity. Other important MCIs to consider are airplane crashes. Most crashes involve small airplanes and few trauma centers ultimately have experience with triaging victims inured in major commercial airline disasters owing to the historical high mortality rate associated with aviation disasters.

TYPES OF INJURIES

Injuries sustained in an MCI will vary based on the type of event. Because mass shootings are the most common cause of MCI, gunshot wounds can be expected to predominate. Compared with the majority of gunshot wounds often seen in trauma centers across the country, which tend to be inflicted by handguns, patients injured in a mass shooting event have a higher likelihood of being wounded by a firearm discharging a high-velocity projectile. These higher velocity rounds such as those fired by AR-15 and AK-47 type rifles, possess a greater amount of kinetic energy. This greater amount of kinetic energy will create a greater cavitation effect[10] and upon impact with tissue can lead to devastating wounding effects.

An MCI caused by an explosion can result in blast injury to survivors. Blast injury is a caused by 4 separate mechanisms categorized as primary, secondary, tertiary, and quaternary. A primary blast injury results from the dissipation of energy from the blast into tissue. This overpressure can injure hollow structures such as the lungs, hollow viscus, and the tympanic membrane. Secondary blast injury results from the fragmentation effects related to the explosion, which can cause penetrating injuries. Tertiary blast injury occurs when the blast wind propels victims against solid objects, such as a building or the ground. Blunt and penetrating injury can result. Finally, quaternary blast injury are miscellaneous injuries such as a flash burn or crush injury sustained when a building collapses on a patient.

Another injury pattern that can result in an MCI is the dismounted complex blast injury. A dismounted complex blast injury is characterized by high-energy injuries to the extremities, pelvic and perineal soft tissue destruction, penetrating truncal wounds, and fractures to the pelvis and spine. This injury pattern is associated with massive hemorrhage. It is the signature injury pattern resulting from the conflicts in Afghanistan and Iraq. Injuries seen as a result of the improvised explosive devices used in the Boston Marathon attack were similar to those seen in deployed combat settings.[6]

Patients who are pinned or trapped beneath heavy objects such as a building collapse during an earthquake or an explosion can suffer a phenomenon known as crush syndrome. Crush syndrome is characterized by hypovolemic shock, hyperkalemia, and arrhythmias. If not recognized, crush syndrome can result in disseminated intravascular coagulation, acute respiratory distress syndrome, sepsis, multiple organ failure, and death. Three criteria should raise suspicion for crush syndrome, including the involvement of a large muscle mass, prolonged compression (typically 4–6 hours), and signs of vascular occlusion. Before extrication, empiric hydration with saline is essential to prevent the decompensation associated with reperfusion. Mannitol may act as a free radical scavenger and promote diuresis. The use of sodium bicarbonate is somewhat more controversial, but can be considered. Patients suffering from crush syndrome may need hemodialysis. Because an event creating a large number of patients with crush syndrome may exceed the supply of dialysis machines available, peritoneal dialysis can be considered, assuming there are no concomitant abdominal injuries.

The possibility that patients may be contaminated with a hazardous substance or nuclear, biological, or chemical agent should be considered. Coordination with the local fire department hazardous material response team will be beneficial but, depending on the scale of the incident, response to the hospital may be limited to assist. This scenario has many implications, especially for responder safety and to maintain the capability of the facility to continue to function treating patients. The protection of health care workers and the facility is critical. A detailed discussion of the effects of various agents, personal protective equipment, decontamination, and treatment is beyond the scope of this article.

INCIDENT COMMAND

During routine operations, most organizations that would be active in response to an MCI function independent of each other. In a hospital, for example, support from outside organizations is not essential for daily operations. However, if an MCI or other disaster were to occur, a coordinated response from all agencies is essential. The incident command system (ICS) provides the framework for this response. In the ICS, command and control of personnel and equipment are a key tenant, as is the coordination of efforts in response to an event. The ICS exists at the local, state, and national levels, as well as a hospital-based system. At the local level, the ICS is at the core of a coordinated response.

The hospital incident command system (HICS) is the most used arrangement for hospital disaster response. It consists of a command group and 4 sections, which includes operations, planning, logistics, and finance/administration (**Fig. 1**).

The command group of the HICS is responsible for the overall operation and consists of the incident commander, public information officer, safety officer, liaison officer, and medical and technical specialists. The public information office role should not be understated. After conducting a survey of those involved in managing an

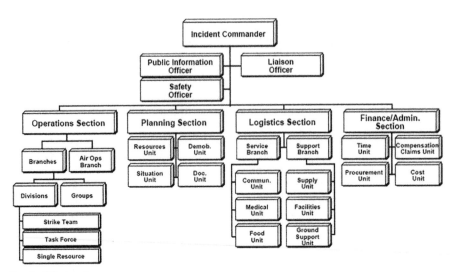

Fig. 1. ICS structure.

MCI at a recent meeting of the American Association for the Surgery of Trauma, one of the most unexpected aspects of the response was demand for information, requests for interviews, and even the arrival of politicians and celebrities while patient care activities were still surging.[11] These issues could be mitigated by scheduled press briefings, providing updates via a website or social media, and setting up a hotline for information requests.

The operations section in the HICS model manages the objectives as given by the incident commander. Within the operations section, there are 5 branches, including staging management, medical care operations, infrastructure operations, security, business continuity operations, and hazardous materials.

The planning section develops an incident action plan by collecting, evaluating, and disseminating various status reports and information. Four units exist within the planning section, which includes resources, situation, documentation, and demobilization.

Necessary resources from both internal and external sources are coordinated by the logistics section. Service and support are the 2 branches under the logistics section.

Finally, finance and administration make up the last section of the HICS. This section develops financial and administrative procedures to support the program before, during, and after the event.

Triage

> Those who are dangerously wounded should receive the first attention, without regard to rank or distinction. They who are injured in a less degree may wait until their brethren in arms, who are badly mutilated, have been operated on and dressed, otherwise the latter would not survive many hours; rarely, until the succeeding day.
> —Baron Dominique Jean Larrey (surgeon-in-chief to Napoleon's Imperial Guard)

The concept of triage is used on a regular basis in surgical practice. Almost daily, surgeons perform triage, whether it is to decide which patient is the sickest and needs to be evaluated first or deciding that an emergent case should supersede a scheduled elective case. Disaster triage is used in an MCI. Its primary goal is to do the greatest amount of good for the greatest number of patients. The goal is not to limit or ration care. In other words, by prioritizing patients, the use of scarce resources can be optimized.

Triage can occur at several points during a given patient's course through the system. Primary triage occurs in the field and is usually performed by emergency medical services personnel using simple criteria. Immediately upon arrival to the hospital, secondary triage occurs by an emergency physician or surgeon, typically. At this stage, the goal is to provide critical initial interventions focused on the airway, breathing, and circulation. Tertiary triage occurs after these interventions and assigns patients to surgery, the intensive care unit (ICU), or radiology. A surgeon, experienced in the care of the injured, will typically perform this role.

Different protocols for triage exist and are applied at different junctions along a patient's path through the system. Historically, most triage protocols in use were intended for primary triage. The Simple Triage and Rapid Treatment system places patients into color-coded group that correspond with a tag that is placed with the patient based on their condition. Three main groups of patients are identified with the Simple Triage and Rapid Treatment triage system. Patients likely to survive whether they receive care or not are classified as green/minimal or yellow/delayed. Those who will benefit from immediate interventions are assigned red/immediate. Finally, those who are likely to die despite maximal therapy are given a black tag. Parameters evaluated to perform Simple Triage and Rapid Treatment triage are respiratory rate, perfusion, and mental status. If a patient has a respiratory rate of more than 30 breaths per minute, capillary refill of more than 2 seconds, or is unable to follow commands, they are assigned to the red/immediate group. The remainder of patients are classified as yellow/delayed. If a patient can walk and move to a designated area, they are assigned a green/minimal tag. Otherwise, a deceased patient is determined by apnea after basic maneuvers to open the airway (**Fig. 2**).

Tertiary triage is somewhat more complex and can also involve patients not injured or affected by an MCI. The goal is to identify patients likely to benefit from treatment as well as those who are too sick to recover despite care. A common protocol in use for tertiary triage is the Ontario protocol, which has contains elements of inclusion criteria, exclusion criteria and minimum qualifications for survival. This protocol uses the Sequential Organ Failure Assessment score.

Triage is an ongoing process and is not static. If a patient's condition changes, their assignment may change. To be effective, there must be a balance between overtriage and undertriage. These terms pertain to the accuracy with which patients are triaged. Undertriage is when the severity of a patient's condition is not recognized, which results in a delay in treatment that can result in death. Overtriage can also increase mortality by depleting resources, fatiguing staff, and impairing patient flow to definitive care.

SURGE CAPACITY

Surge capacity is defined as the ability to respond to an increased number of patients. Capability as it relates to a surge is the ability to address unusual or specialized medical needs of an increased number of patients.

The ability to respond effectively to an MCI requires the ability to provide definitive care. Roccaforte and Cushman[12] wrote that a critical component of disaster planning must be the preservation of definitive care area capability and effectiveness. Definitive care areas were defined as the operating rooms and the ICU.

Expansion of operating room and ICU capacity depends on physical space, staffing levels, and the availability of supplies and equipment. Upon notification of an MCI, any

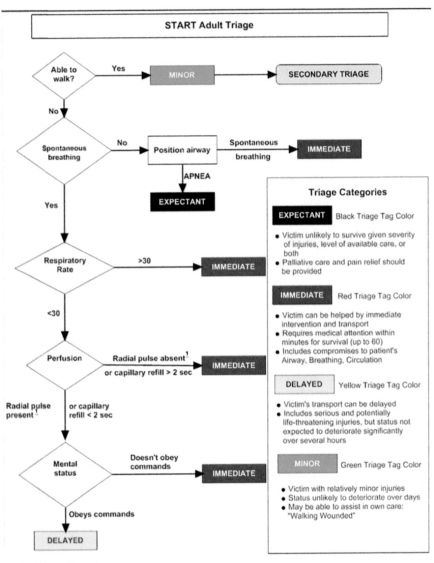

Fig. 2. Triage flow chart.

patients who can be moved from the ICU should be transferred. Elective cases should be canceled. Mobilization of additional staff should commence per the institutional disaster or MCI plan.

During the COVID-19 pandemic, institutions have had to get creative to create surge capacity. Pandemic surge staffing models were put out by Society of Critical Care Medicine, which used non-critical care trained physicians, advanced practice providers, and certified registered nurse anesthetists to care for larger number of critically ill patients than could be managed by a single intensivist. Similar models were used for nursing staff. In teaching hospitals, house staff were taken off elective rotations to form COVID-19 ICU teams. Other institutions created surgeon-led teams to place vascular access and perform other procedures needed in the ICU to offload the medical ICU team.

Depending on the nature of the event, additional critical care spaces can be created from unused operating rooms or the postanesthesia care unit.

Our institution internally developed a protocol using ultraviolet light to decontaminate one-time use personal protective equipment so it could be used multiple times safely. By doing this, the hospital's supply of N95 respirators was able to be extended until some of the stress on the supply chain could be relieved (**Fig. 3**).

SURGICAL CARE DURING A MASS CASUALTY INCIDENT

The surgical care that needs to be provided will depend on the type of event. A recent review of contemporary mass shootings conducted by the Eastern Association for the Surgery of Trauma found that the most common injury among survivors were to the appendicular skeleton. As a result, many patients required interventions that were orthopedic and vascular in nature. Survivors were less likely to have injuries to the head or torso, yet laparotomy was the most commonly performed procedure.[13] Another review evaluating the injury characteristics of the Pulse Nightclub shooting in Orlando found that there were no acute neurosurgical interventions performed in the first 24 hours. The most needed surgical specialists were trauma and orthopedics.[14] This finding is of interest, because many facilities will have back up mechanisms in place for trauma surgery, but may not for orthopedic surgery.

Damage control resuscitation and damage control surgery should be applied liberally in an MCI. Most surgeons who provide trauma care will be familiar with these concepts, but in the context of an MCI, damage control resuscitation is advantageous because it typically results in fewer blood products being transfused, which could limit the strain on the blood bank. Damage control surgery has benefits in the MCI setting because operative times are typically shorter, allowing the limited resource of the operating room to be used to benefit another patient. In additional, because MCI tend to be chaotic, the patient will likely benefit from a second look procedure to help reduce missed injuries or potential complications.

EMERGENCY RESPONSE ON A NATIONAL SCALE

As outlined elsewhere in this article, the initial response to a catastrophic event is primarily local in nature. However, such an event may occur that overwhelms the local response. In this case, additional resources can be made available from the federal government. Multiple federal agencies, including the military, have vast resources at their disposal. These resources will not likely be available immediately owing to the time they would likely take to mobilize.

There are numerous federal agencies involved in a response to a large-scale MCI. Unless the situation is classified as a national security event, a coordinated federal

Common themes identified in responses to military and civilian mass casualty events as described by the panelists
• Assume nontraditional duties
• Make space by any means necessary
• Revisit, review, retriage
• Plan to deal with the media
• Take care of hospital staff

Fig. 3. Common themes identified in response. (*Adapted from* Russo RM, Galante JM, Holcomb. Mass casualty events: what to do as the dust settles? Trauma Surgery & Acute Care Open 2018;3:e000210.)

response does not occur. A state's governor could request a presidential declaration of a disaster, which would allow for response from the federal government. Federal agencies likely to be involved in a national response would be the Department of Homeland Security, the Department of Health and Human Services (DHHS), and the Department of Defense (DoD).

The primary operational arm of the Department of Homeland Security is the Federal Emergency Management Agency. The Federal Emergency Management Agency conducts 15 emergency support functions, several of which would be beneficial in a large-scale MCI, including public health and medical services, urban search and rescue, and emergency management.

The DHHS is another important agency involved in federal disaster and MCI response. Within the DHHS, the Assistant Secretary for Preparedness and Response coordinates disaster response activities. A key asset that is a public–private partnership is the National Disaster Medical System (NDMS). The NDMS is a partnership between the Department of Homeland Security, the Federal Emergency Management Agency, the DHHS, the DoD, the Department of Veteran Affairs, and civilian hospitals and health care professionals. The NDMS serves 2 purposes. It is a backup to military health care operations in case of a war resulting in overwhelming numbers of combat casualties. Second, the NDMS coordinates provision of national health care resources to casualties resulting from disasters in the United States and its territories.

The main operational unit of the NDMS is the Disaster Medical Assistance Team (DMAT). There are approximately 85 DMAT teams throughout the nation. DMAT teams have physicians, nurses, and other allied health care professionals on their rosters and each have approximately 100 members. Teams can deploy on short notice and are designed to be self-sufficient for 72 hours. A DMAT team can operate autonomously, or they can be used to supplement another facility's response. During the COVID-19 pandemic, DMAT teams have been used to augment hospital staffing during times of surging numbers of patients.[15] The NDMS also contains specialty teams such as trauma and critical care teams, disaster mortuary operations teams, and veterinary response teams.

Another important component of national preparedness is the Strategic National Stockpile (SNS). The goal of the SNS is to be rapidly mobilized to provide pharmaceuticals and medical supplies to areas affected by public health emergencies or disasters. Owing to concerns for increased demand, dependence on global supply chains and the just in time inventory practices used by hospitals it is vital to maintain certain amount of essential supplies and equipment.

Contained in the SNS are personal protective equipment, medications, vaccines, mechanical ventilators, and CHEMPACKS. CHEMPACKS are antidotes to nerve agents that are stored throughout the country in such a way that 90% of the population of the United States lives within 1 hour of a CHEMPACK stockpile. Mechanical ventilators deserve special mention as well, especially in the setting of the COVID-19 pandemic. Many ventilators contained within the SNS were not full featured models useful for patients with acute respiratory distress syndrome. Consequently, many hospitals were left to procure additional ventilators that were more suitable for patients with COVID-19 with acute respiratory distress syndrome.

The DoD possesses vast resources and capabilities that can be used to supplement a local response when those resources are overwhelmed. A military response to an MCI is governed by several statutes and laws collectively known as Military Support to Civilian Authorities. The support available from the DoD and military are classified as mass resources or unique resources. Mass resources can be additive to the response provided by other agencies, whereas unique resources can provide

Mass Resources	Unique Resources
Military hospitals (75) and personnel	Deployable public health laboratories
Deployable medical platforms • Air force expeditionary medical support • Navy hospital ships	Specially trained response teams • Army chemical and biological special medical augmentation response team • Navy special psychiatric intervention team • Air force radiation assessment team
Air assets	

Fig. 4. Military resources.

technical assistance and expertise. Although these resources can certainly be impactful, their optimal use requires thoughtful planning and integration into the civilian response. For instance, during the COVID-19 pandemic, the US Navy deployed its 2 hospital ships, the *USNS Comfort* and the *USNS Mercy*, to New York and Los Angeles, respectively. Despite their 1000-bed capacity, the ships were not intended to treat patients suffering from a pandemic illness. Subsequently, both ships treated a small number of patients relative to their vast capabilities during their deployments **(Fig. 4)**.[16]

SUMMARY

An optimal response to large numbers of critically ill or injured patients requires the rapid mobilization of resources. The principles of the ICS, triage, and surge capacity provide a framework to mobilize and apply resources to benefit the most patients. This approach is essential to limit morbidity and mortality in these situations. Large-scale events may require a coordinated response from the federal government if local resources are overwhelmed. Depending on the type of events, the surgeon can expect to play a key role in the response.

REFERENCES

1. Schenk E, Wijetunge G, Mann NC, et al. Epidemiology of mass casualty incidents in the United States. Prehosp Emerg Care 2014;18(3):408–16.

2. Melmer P, Carlin M, Castater CA, et al. Mass casualty shootings and emergency preparedness: a multidisciplinary approach for an unpredictable event. J Multidiscip Healthc 2019;12:1013–21.

3. Walls RM, Zinner MJ. The Boston Marathon response: why did it work so well? JAMA 2013;309(23):2441–2. https://doi.org/10.1001/jama.2013.5965.

4. Biddinger PD, Baggish A, Harrington L, et al. Be prepared-The Boston Marathon and mass-casualty events. N Engl J Med 2013;368:1958–60. https://doi.org/10.1056/NEJMp1305480.

5. Knudson MM, Velmahos G, Cooper ZR. Response to mass casualty events: from the battlefield to the Stop the Bleed campaign. Trauma Surg Acute Care Open 2016;1:e000023. https://doi.org/10.1136/tsaco-2016-000023.

6. King DR, Mesar T. In: Lim RB, editor. "Lessons learned from the Boston Marathon bombing." surgery during natural disasters, combat, terrorist attacks and crisis situations. Springer; 2016. p. 181–9.

7. Bieler D, Franke A, Kollig E, et al. Eur J Trauma Emerg Surg 2020;46(4):683–94.

8. Ritchie H, Roser M. "Natural Disasters". Published online at OurWorldInData.org. 2014. Available at: https://ourworldindata.org/natural-disasters.
9. Choron RL, Butts CA, Bargoud C, et al. Surgeons in surge — the versatility of the acute care surgeon: outcomes of COVID-19 ICU patients in a community hospital where all ICU patients are managed by surgical intensivists. Trauma Surgery & Acute Care Open 2020;5:e000557.
10. Rhee Peter M, Moore Ernest E, et al. Gunshot wounds. J Trauma Acute Care Surg June 2016;80(6):853–67.
11. Russo RM, Galante JM, Holcomb. Mass casualty events: what to do as the dust settles? Trauma Surg Acute Care Open 2018;3:e000210.
12. Roccaforte JD, Cushman JG. Disaster preparedness, triage, and surge capacity for hospital definitive care areas: optimizing outcomes when demands exceed resources. Anesthesiol Clin 2007;25(1):161–177, xi.
13. Sarani Babak, Smith E, et al. MD Characteristics of survivors of civilian public mass shootings: an Eastern Association for the Surgery of Trauma multicenter study. J Trauma Acute Care Surg 2021;90(4):652–8.
14. Smith CP, Cheatham ML, Safcsak KRN, et al. MD Injury characteristics of the Pulse Nightclub shooting: lessons for mass casualty incident preparation. J Trauma Acute Care Surg March 2020;88(3):372–8.
15. County 17. November 30, 2020. *Disaster Medical Assistance Team "a Godsend.* Available at: https://county17.com/2020/11/30/disaster-medical-assistance-team-a-godsend/.
16. Larter DB. The US Navy's hospital ships in the COVID-19 fight badly need replacing. 2020. Available at: https://www.defensenews.com/naval/2020/04/01/the-us-navys-hospital-ships-in-the-covid-19-fight-badly-need-replacing/.

Management of Acute Kidney Injury/Renal Replacement Therapy in the Intensive Care Unit

Salma Shaikhouni, MD, Lenar Yessayan, MD, MS*

KEYWORDS

- Acute kidney injury • CRRT • Hemodialysis • Citrate anticoagulation

KEY POINTS

- Acute kidney injury (AKI) affects up to half of surgical ICU patients. The need for renal replacement therapy is associated with a mortality risk exceeding 50%. This article reviews the current best practices for the management of critically ill patients with AKI, with an emphasis on patients requiring dialysis.

INTRODUCTION

Acute kidney injury (AKI) is a syndrome characterized by an abrupt decline in kidney function. Multiple definitions have been used to define AKI in the past; however, a consensual classification for AKI definition was introduced in the year 2004[1] which defines AKI and its severity based on changes in serum creatinine concentration and degree of oliguria.[2] AKI is a common complication among patients in the intensive care unit (ICU). It is strongly associated with poor patient outcomes including high mortality rates,[3] prolonged hospital stay,[4] increased readmissions,[4] poorer health-related quality of life,[5] and higher likelihood for developing chronic kidney disease and end-stage renal disease.[6–8] This article presents current best practices for the management of critically ill patients with AKI, with an emphasis on patients requiring dialysis.

EPIDEMIOLOGY OF ACUTE KIDNEY INJURY IN SURGICAL INTENSIVE CARE UNITS

AKI afflicts 50% of patients in ICU and is associated with poor short- and long-term outcomes. Nearly 5% of all ICU patients require renal replacement therapy (RRT) with a mortality risk exceeding 50% in these patients.[9] The incidence of AKI in surgical ICUs using the more recent consensus definitions for AKI varies by the reason for intensive care admission and the performed surgical procedure. AKI occurs in

Division of Nephrology, Department of Medicine, University of Michigan, Ann Arbor, MI, USA
* Corresponding author. University of Michigan, 3914 Taubman Center, 1500 East Medical Center Drive 5364, Ann Arbor, MI 48109-5364.
E-mail address: lenar@med.umich.edu

Surg Clin N Am 102 (2022) 181–198
https://doi.org/10.1016/j.suc.2021.09.013
0039-6109/22/© 2021 Elsevier Inc. All rights reserved.

approximately 25% of ICU patients with blunt trauma and 40% of ICU patients with burn injuries.[10,11] Its incidence is approximately 5% following major abdominal surgeries such as gastric, pancreatic, and colorectal surgeries and 50% following major vascular surgeries or orthotopic liver transplantation.[12–14]

PATIENT EVALUATION OVERVIEW

Consensus definitions and staging systems for AKI were introduced and adopted to standardize diagnosis and reporting of AKI. The most recent definition and staging system are the Kidney Disease Improving Global Outcomes (KDIGO) staging system[15] which defines AKI and its severity based on changes in serum creatinine or urine output (**Table 1**). This staging system was adopted from prior definitions of AKI (AKIN[16] and RIFLE[2]). There are several limitations to the KDIGO staging system for AKI. It does not differentiate AKI based on the etiology of AKI. Different causes of AKI may differ in the specific intervention required and in the overall prognosis. To address this limitation, the KDIGO guidelines emphasize the need to promptly identifying the cause. Another limitation is the difficulty in establishing the baseline serum creatinine in patients who do not have a baseline measurement. In such cases, the first documented serum creatinine during hospitalization is often considered the baseline but this may result in delayed recognition of AKI if the onset of AKI preceded the hospitalization. Furthermore, serum creatinine can often be a delayed marker of AKI[17] and urine output may not be accurately recorded. Finally, several factors unrelated to kidney injury may affect serum creatinine, including the loss of muscle mass, large volume shifts, or drug effects.[18]

Blood or urinary biomarkers have the potential to improve the management and outcomes of AKI through stratifying patients for their risk of developing AKI, early detection of kidney injury, and phenotyping the kidney damage to enable a more tailored treatment. However, they have not yet fully made the transition to routine clinical care. Urinary biomarker [inhibitor of metalloproteinase-2 x insulin-like growth factor binding protein 7] is the first biomarker for the risk assessment of AKI to become available for clinical use in the United States. It has shown high sensitivity identifying critically ill patients at risk for developing stage 2 or 3 AKI within the subsequent 12 hours.[19] Two trials have shown a reduction in the incidence of AKI and its severity when preventative strategies (eg, early optimization of fluid status, maintenance of perfusion pressure, discontinuation of nephrotoxic agents) are implemented after cardiac and abdominal surgery in patients identified as high risk with the use of this biomarker.[20,21] The following causes of AKI should always be considered and explored in the surgical ICU setting.

ACUTE TUBULAR NECROSIS

ATN is the most common cause of severe AKI in the critical care setting, and most commonly results from renal ischemia (eg, hypotension or shock, cardiopulmonary

| Table 1 |
| Definition of AKI based on KDIGO guidelines |

AKI Stage	Serum Creatinine	Urine Output
I	increase from baseline OR 1.5–1.9 x baseline	< 0.5 mL/kg/h x 6–12 h
II	2.0–2.9 x baseline	< 0.5 mL/kg/h x 12 h
III	3.0 x baseline OR Requiring renal replacement therapy	< 0.3 mL/kg/h x 24 h OR Anuria x 12 h

bypass), exogenous nephrotoxic insults (eg, iodinated contrast exposure, aminogly-cosides, amphotericin B, vancomycin, or other medications), or endogenous nephro-toxic insults (eg, rhabdomyolysis, hemolysis). ATN is suggested by a history of renal insult and by the presence of granular casts or tubular epithelial cells on the urine sedi-ment. Other supportive tests include urine specific gravity less than 1.015, urine osmo-lality less than 450 mOsm/kg (usually < 350), and fractional excretion of sodium (FENa) is greater than 1% in oliguric patients. FENa may be less than 1% in ATN in the pres-ence of severe hypoperfusion or when ATN is secondary to contrast-induced ne-phropathy and pigment nephropathy (rhabdomyolysis, hemolysis). Treatment is primarily supportive. Hemodynamic abnormalities should be corrected, and poten-tially nephrotoxic agents discontinued. In some patients with severe AKI, dialysis may be required until renal function is restored. Some may remain dialysis dependent for up to 3 months or indefinitely.

ABDOMINAL COMPARTMENT SYNDROME

ACS is characterized by a sustained intraabdominal pressure of greater than 20 mm Hg in the presence of new organ dysfunction. Common culprits include intraabdomi-nal or retroperitoneal hemorrhage, pancreatitis, massive fluid resuscitation, laparos-copy and pneumoperitoneum, and ileus. In critically ill patients, the incidence of ACS may be as high as 12%. Common early signs include tense abdomen, oliguria, elevated airway pressures, and difficulty ventilating. Management is supportive and in-cludes surgical decompression when appropriate. Paracentesis may be needed in pa-tients with tense ascites. Gastrointestinal decompression is required if ACS is due to intestinal distention. Sedation and chemical paralysis (in mechanically ventilated pa-tients) may be required to relax abdominal muscles and to maintain adequate ventilation.

ACUTE URINARY RETENTION

Acute urinary retention may complicate surgical procedures and may lead to oliguria. It may induce vomiting, hyper- or hypotension, urinary tract infection, and arrhythmias. Anesthesia, perioperative medications such as opioids, surgical pain, and destruction of anatomy vital to voiding during pelvic surgeries may all play a role in the develop-ment of postoperative urinary retention. Risk factors include male sex, older age, dia-betes, depression, and prostate hyperplasia. Diagnosis can be made by bladder scan showing more than 400 mL postvoid bladder volume. Management includes early ambulation when feasible and bladder decompression by intermittent or indwelling catheter.

ACUTE INTERSTITIAL NEPHRITIS

AIN generally occurs 10 to 14 days after exposure to a medication (earlier if patient was previously exposed). The most common medications that may cause AIN include beta-lactams, fluoroquinolones, sulfonamides, rifampin, H2 antagonists, proton pump inhibitors, allopurinol, and nonsteroidal anti-inflammatory drugs. Diagnosis is usually made by finding a temporal association between AKI onset and use of known culprit drug, or resolution with discontinuation of a drug. Biopsy may be considered when the diagnosis is not clear or when the withdrawal of a potential culprit drug may affect pa-tient care. Signs and symptoms are nonspecific. The classic triad of fever, rash, and eosinophilia is observed in only 5% of cases. Urinalysis and urine sediment analysis may show proteinuria, glucosuria, white blood cells (WBCs), WBC casts, and red blood cells. Nonsteroidal anti-inflammatory drug (NSAID)-induced AIN may present with nephrotic range proteinuria. Therapy with corticosteroid may be considered in those who have not responded to drug withdrawal. Steroids should be tapered and discontinued if no response is observed after 4 weeks of therapy.[22]

FLUID MANAGEMENT AND ACUTE KIDNEY INJURY

The goal of fluid therapy in the ICU is to optimize intravascular circulating volume and to maintain organ perfusion without causing fluid overload. Excessive fluid administration is associated with poor outcomes including the development of AKI.[23–28] Proposed mechanisms of volume overload causing renal injury include intrarenal compartment syndrome and venous congestion, and oxygen supply/demand mismatch. In patients with established AKI, fluid administration beyond correction of hypovolemia does not improve the possibility of renal recovery.[23] Oliguria should trigger an assessment of volume status but not be regarded as an absolute indication for fluid administration. The need for fluid therapy should be individualized based on the assessment of volume status in patients with signs of ongoing hypoperfusion and guided by hemodynamic indices that inform of fluid responsiveness (eg, respiratory variation of pulse pressure or stroke volume among patients mechanically ventilated or > 15% increase in cardiac output in response to a preload challenge). Patient's underlying diagnosis may also determine the fluid management strategy. For example, a conservative fluid administration strategy is often opted in acute respiratory distress syndrome (ARDS) as this approach has been shown to reduce the duration of mechanical ventilation without increasing the risk of kidney injury.[29] These findings were also applicable to the surgical cohort of patients included in the study.[30] In contrast, fluid restrictive strategy is avoided in the peri-operative settings. Indeed, restrictive fluid management when compared with liberal fluid strategy during and up to 24 hours after major abdominal surgery has been associated with higher risk of AKI and renal replacement requirement.[31]

The composition of crystalloid infusion may potentially impact kidney outcomes. Current evidence favors the use of balanced solutions for fluid resuscitation of patients at risk of AKI who are not hypochloremic, and the use of sodium bicarbonate in patients with moderate to severe AKI. The SALT-ED (Saline against Lactated Ringer's or Plasma-Lyte in the Emergency Department) and the SMART (Isotonic Solutions and Major Adverse Renal Events Trial) cluster randomized clinical trials compared saline to buffered crystalloids and the results support the preferential use of buffered crystalloids over saline.[32,33] Both trials showed a slight yet statistically significant a reduction in major adverse kidney events (a composite outcome of death, need for RRT and persistent kidney dysfunction) within 30 days in those who received buffered crystalloids than saline (SALT-ED, 4.7% vs 5.6%; SMART, 14.3% vs 15.4%). In patients with preexisting moderate to severe AKI and severe metabolic acidosis, the BICAR-ICU (sodium bicarbonate therapy for patients with severe metabolic acidemia in the ICU) clinical trial compared the effect of hypertonic sodium bicarbonate infusion with no infusion.[34] The trial suggested reduction in 28-day mortality and in the onset of one or more organ failures in patients. Interestingly, it also showed a reduction in the percentage of patients requiring RRT during ICU stay and on ICU discharge.

RENAL REPLACEMENT THERAPY
Timing of Dialysis Initiation in Acute Kidney Injury

Early initiation of dialysis based solely on meeting biochemical definitions of AKI has not been shown to provide mortality benefit in three multicenter randomized controlled trials (RCTs).[25,26,35] The STARRT-AKI,[25] the largest and the most recent of the 3 trials enrolled 3019 patients and included a heterogeneous population including surgical patients. Critically ill adults with KDIGO stage 2 or 3 AKI were randomly assigned to either an accelerated RRT initiation (within 12 hours of randomization) or standard RRT initiation strategy based on clinical judgment and guided by a set of recommendations for initiation including (1) potassium level $\geq$ 6 mEq/L, (2) pH $\leq$ 7.20, (3) bicarbonate level $\leq$ 12 mEq/L, (4) Pao_2/fraction of inspired oxygen $\leq$ 200 mm Hg along with clinical perception of volume overload, or (5) persistence of kidney injury 72 hours after randomization. There was no difference in the primary outcome of 90-day mortality between the 2 groups (43.9% in accelerated vs 43.7% in standard; $P = .92$) and across subgroups stratified by sepsis, estimated glomerular filtration rate, type of admission (medical vs surgical), Simplified Acute Physiology Score II, and geographic region. Secondary outcomes that were similar between the 2 groups included the composite outcome of major adverse kidney events at 90 days, serious adverse events, ventilator-free days, and overall hospital length of stay. Interestingly, survivors of the accelerated group experienced greater RRT dependence at 90 days than the standard group (10.4% vs 6.0%; relative risk, 1.74 [95% confidence interval (CI), 1.24–2.43]) and there were more episodes of hypotension and severe hypophosphatemia in the accelerated arm.

In conclusion, the results of the 3 randomized trials do not support preemptive dialysis initiation based on the AKI stage alone. Decision regarding initiation of dialysis should be guided by the broader clinical contexts, the presence or absence of conditions that can be modified by dialysis, and the trends of laboratory abnormalities as advised by the KDIGO AKI guidelines.[15]

PRINCIPLES OF SOLUTE CLEARANCE AND ULTRAFILTRATION

RRT aims to control fluid management and solute clearance in the setting of kidney failure. **Fig. 1** illustrates the basic components of a dialysis circuit. The process of fluid removal is referred to as ultrafiltration. Solute clearance can be achieved by 2 primary means: hemodialysis – which relies on diffusion, or hemofiltration – which relies on convection. Diffusion is the flow of solutes down their concentration gradients across the dialyzer's semipermeable membrane. Diffusion is inversely proportional to its molecular weight in hemodialysis. On the other hand, convection is the process whereby solute is pulled across the dialyzer membrane during hemofiltration by solvent drag. Convection drags solutes regardless of their molecular weight provided the molecular diameter is smaller than the pores of the semipermeable membrane. Any volume removed by hemofiltration is replaced with physiologic fluids to avoid hypovolemia. This fluid is referred to as replacement fluid.

Medium molecular weight solutes such as beta-2 microglobulin, and inflammatory cytokines may be better cleared by hemofiltration as opposed to hemodialysis.[36] However, there is no clinical trial evidence to-date that supports the use of convective clearance (ie, continuous venovenous hemofiltration) over diffusive clearance (ie, continuous venovenous hemodialysis) in critically ill patients with AKI. A systematic review and meta-analysis comparing the 2 modalities in AKI showed no mortality difference, and no effect on RRT dependence or organ dysfunction.[36]

RENAL REPLACEMENT THERAPY MODALITIES

RRT for AKI in critically ill patients may be delivered in 3 different forms: intermittent hemodialysis (IHD), continuous RRT (CRRT), and prolonged intermittent RRT (PIRRT). The choice between the 3 modalities is dictated by the primary goal of therapy,

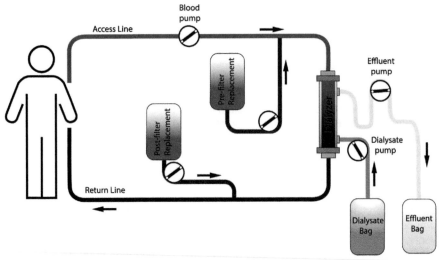

Fig. 1. Schematic illustrating the principal components of a dialysis circuit. Footnote. The patient's venous blood is pumped through the access line toward the dialyzer. In hemodialysis, dialysate flows countercurrent to the blood flow in the dialyzer, allowing for the maximum diffusive gradient between dialysate and solutes in the patient's blood. The dialysate fluid exiting the dialyzer is saturated with diffused solutes from the blood—this is called the effluent fluid. In hemofiltration, solutes are filtered across the dialyzer semipermeable membrane via solvent drag. The volume of fluid that is filtrated must be replaced with an equal amount of physiologic sterile fluid, either before or after the dialyzer.

metabolic disturbances, the degree of volume overload, and the patient's hemodynamics. **Table 2** summarizes the differences between these modalities.

IHD achieves rapid solute clearance and volume removal in a short period of time (typically 3 to 4 h). It is the modality of choice for the treatment of electrolyte derangements and drug poisonings that require rapid correction such as life-threatening hyperkalemia and acidosis, toxic drugs such as lithium, salicylate, and nonvolatile alcohol poisonings. Hemodynamic instability should not preclude the use of iHD with pressor support in metabolic emergencies such as severe hyperkalemia or life-threatening drug poisoning as these are situations that require prompt correction, and most efficiently managed with IHD.

CRRT is generally preferred in patients with hemodynamic instability, elevated intracranial pressures (eg, traumatic brain injury, cerebral edema, or acute liver failure), and severe dysnatremias.[15,37] Slow changes in plasma osmolality afforded by CRRT minimize fluid shifts between body fluid compartments and fluctuations in intracranial pressure. There are several modes of CRRT available, including continuous venovenous hemofiltration (CVVH) which relies on convection alone; continuous venovenous hemodialysis (CVVHD) which relies on diffusion alone; and continuous venovenous hemodiafiltration (CVVHDF) which combines both diffusive and convective modalities. The CRRT modality used at an institution is often dictated by CRRT machine capability and limitations, and protocols developed by the institution.

PIRRT is a hybrid between IHD and CRRT. It encompasses convective and/or diffusive methods of clearance delivery. Examples of PIRRT include sustained low-efficiency dialysis, extended daily dialysis with filtration, and accelerated venovenous hemofiltration or hemodiafiltration. It achieves slow clearance and ultrafiltration over 6 to 12-h periods. It can be helpful in situations whereby a patient may not tolerate hemodialysis but requires frequent interruption of CRRT for procedures.

Table 2
Characteristics of different modalities of renal replacement therapy

Characteristic	Intermittent Hemodialysis	CRRT	PIRRT
Typical blood flow rate (BFR)	400 mL/min	100–300 mL/min	100–300 mL/min
Typical dialysate flow rate	500–800 mL/min	16–40 mL/min	100–300 mL/min
Duration	3–4 h	Continuous	6–12 h
Advantages	• Rapid clearance of electrolytes and toxins: used for severe hyperkalemia and poisonings • Decreases ICU nurse staffing use • Allows time for rehabilitation • Often does not require anticoagulation	• Hemodynamic stability • Effective volume management • Continuous clearance helpful in high catabolic states • Minimizes effects on intracranial pressure	Compared with iHD: • Hemodynamic stability, easier volume management Compared to CRRT: • Decreases ICU nurse staffing use •Allows time for rehabilitation • Allows for more patient treatments per machine per day • May not require anticoagulation
Disadvantages	• Hemodynamic compromise • Volume management more challenging in some cases	• Filter clotting, requires anticoagulation • ICU nursing staff • Limits patient mobility • May not be able to use fistula access in ESRD patients	• Effects on intracranial pressure not well studied

There have been several studies comparing dialysis modalities in terms of mortality and RRT dependence. The studies are limited by selection bias, poor randomization, and high treatment crossover. A Cochrane review[38] and following meta-analysis of randomized controlled trials (RCTs)[39] demonstrated no difference in mortality or RRT dependence between CRRT and IHD. However, the meta-analysis did show that CRRT may be advantageous in minimizing hemodynamic instability and improving volume management. A systematic review of observational trials did show higher rates of dialysis dependence in survivors who were initially started on IHD as opposed to CRRT[40] but this has yet to be confirmed with RCTs. A single-center prospective RCT compared outcomes of PIRRT versus CVVH in ICU patients.[41] There was no mortality difference between PIRRT and CVVH. Patients who received PIRRT had fewer days of mechanical ventilation and fewer days in the ICU and required significantly less nursing care time related to RRT.

ACCESS TO RENAL REPLACEMENT THERAPY

An ideal dialysis access provides effective blood flow rates for RRT with minimal inter-ruptions and recirculation between return and access lines.[42] It should also minimize complications such as thrombosis or infection. The 2012 KDIGO guidelines designate the right internal jugular access as the preferred access choice, followed by femoral catheters and finally left internal jugular catheters.[15] Subclavian access is associated with increased risk of venous stenosis, jeopardizing chronic access options, and is therefore discouraged.[43] Femoral access has traditionally been linked to higher rates of infection, though some more recent studies have shown similar rates of bloodstream infections between jugular and femoral catheters,[44,45] except in patients with an elevated BMI.[46] Studies examining catheter dysfunction or filter life association with the type of access resulted in heterogeneous finding,[47] although there was a trend for left internal jugular access to be most associated with catheter dysfunction and shortened filter life. The length of inserted dialysis catheters should be considered carefully. To provide maximal unimpeded blood flow, a jugular catheter should terminate inside the right atrium as opposed to higher in the superior vena cava.[48]

Uncuffed nontunneled dialysis catheters (NTDC) typically serve as the preferred initial access modality in patients with AKI in the ICU, given the ease and timeliness of their insertion. However, tunneled dialysis catheters (TDC) may be associated with decreased rates of bloodstream infection,[49–51] likely due to the catheter cuff and tunneling under the skin. TDC are also associated with less dialysis interruptions and greater dialysis efficiency than NTDC,[52,53] likely due to the larger bore and catheter tip design, as well as their placement under fluoroscopy ensuring appropriate placement location. A prospective single-center cohort study comparing TDC to NTDC in both IHD and CRRT showed less dialysis interruptions, less mechanical complications, and higher median blood flow rates in the TDC group.[54] If it can be arranged in a timely manner, it is worth considering a TDC-first approach in patients with AKI who may require greater than 1 week of RRT, who have no active bloodstream infection and no significant coagulopathy.

In patients on extracorporeal membrane oxygenation (ECMO) and AKI, CRRT can be delivered either via a separate vascular access or by connecting the CRRT circuit to access points on the ECMO circuits. The CRRT circuit can be combined with the ECMO circuit in various ways. The advantages of each technique have been expertly described by many groups.[55]

DOSE OF RENAL REPLACEMENT THERAPY

Adequacy of dialysis in IHD is typically expressed by the function Kt/V, whereby K is the dialyzer clearance, t is the duration of dialysis, and V is the volume of distribution of urea). In contrast, dose of CRRT is expressed as effluent dose adjusted for body weight (in milliliters per kilogram per hour). Early small studies suggested better survival in patients with AKI with higher doses of dialysis.[56] It was hypothesized that a higher dose of RRT, particularly with convective modes, may help in clearing inflammatory mediators in the setting of sepsis, which may, in turn, translate into a survival benefit.[57]

Since then, 2 landmark studies established the optimal dose for RRT in patients with AKI.[58,59] The VA/NIH acute renal failure trail network (ARFTN) multi-center RCT[58] randomized 1124 patients between an intensive RRT arm (defined as CRRT dose 35 mL/kg/h or IHD 6 times weekly with a delivered Kt/V 1.2–1.4) or conventional therapy arm (CRRT dose 20 mL/kg/h or IHD 3 x weekly with a delivered Kt/V 1.2–1.4). Intensive RRT did not provide an additional benefit in 60-day mortality, duration of RRT or renal recovery. The RENAL trial[59] was another multi-center RCT that randomized 1508 patients between high-intensity RRT (CRRT dose of 40 mL/kg/h) and lower intensity RRT (CRRT dose 25 mL/kg/h). Again, there was no additional survival benefit or RRT dependence between the 2 groups. It is important to note that the delivered dose of

CRRT may not match the prescribed dose of CRRT. In the highly regulated context of these trials, the delivered dose of CRRT was anywhere between 84% and 102% of the prescribed dose. Retrospective studies have shown that, in practice, delivered CRRT can be as low as 68% of the prescribed dose.[60] This is likely due to treatment interruptions for procedures, filter clotting, among other causes.[61] Taking into consideration the time lost due to therapy interruptions, the current therapy guidelines recommend targeting a CRRT dose of 25 to 30 mL/kg/h. Although this guideline applies to most CRRT prescriptions, higher doses may be required in the setting of significant metabolic abnormalities such as hyperkalemia or severe metabolic acidosis which necessitate urgent reversal.

ANTICOAGULATION IN RENAL REPLACEMENT THERAPY

Blood is exposed to thrombogenic surfaces as it travels through the hemodialysis and CRRT circuits. Clotting within the dialyzer or hemofilter may compromise dialysis efficiency and in the event of circuit clotting, approximately 180 to 200 mL of blood may be lost. Therefore, some forms of anticoagulation techniques or periodic saline flushes are typically administered at the time of dialysis to prevent clotting in the blood circuit. For IHD, heparin anticoagulation may be used when not contraindicated. However, many hospitalized patients may be at increased risk for bleeding. Therefore, periodic saline flushes of the dialysis circuit without anticoagulation are considered by many as the preferred method of choice to maintain circuit patency in hospitalized patients. The high blood flow rates and the short duration of hemodialysis treatments (typically 3–4 hours) allow successful completion of the dialysis procedure with saline flushes in most patients.

Maintaining filter patency during CRRT is critical to optimizing delivered CRRT dose. The most commonly used agents for CRRT anticoagulation are regional citrate (RCA) and unfractionated heparin. The main disadvantage of heparin is that it causes systemic anticoagulation in addition to circuit anticoagulation and increases the risk of hemorrhagic complications.[62–64] RCA minimizes the risk of bleeding by restricting the effect of anticoagulation to the dialysis circuit. RCA uss a citrate infusion prefilter to chelate plasma ionized calcium within the dialysis circuit, thus eliminating a critical cofactor in the clotting cascade. The accumulated citrate is then largely cleared with dialysis. A small fraction is returned to the patient, to be metabolized by the liver into bicarbonate. The low plasma ionized calcium is maintained posthemofilter by zero calcium dialysate and/or replacement fluid. Low plasma ionized calcium in the return line is then corrected by calcium infusion either into the CRRT return line or into a central vein via a separate central line (**Fig. 2**).

RCA has been shown by numerous studies to be superior to heparin in terms of circuit life and bleeding complications.[65] However, RCA has not been universally adopted across all institutions administering CRRT.[9] Potential reasons for the slow adoption of RCA may include fear of metabolic complications (eg, hypocalcemia), the need for frequent RCA or calcium infusion adjustments, and the variability in published approaches.[66] Citrate can accumulate in patients with impaired citrate metabolism due to liver dysfunction.[67] In such patients, rising systemic citrate levels chelate calcium which causes low systemic ionized calcium. A total calcium to ionized calcium ratio (both in mmol/L) greater than 2.5 is recognized as an indicator of citrate toxicity.[68] Citrate toxicity is associated with increased mortality.[69] RCA protocols have been designed to completely abrogate the risk of citrate toxicity in patients with absent citrate metabolism, and to maintain systemic iCa levels above 1 mM using a personalized calcium dosing.[66,70] The 2012 Kidney Disease Improving Global

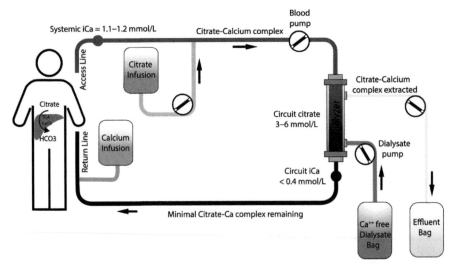

Fig. 2. Schematic illustrating the principals of regional citrate anticoagulation during continuous venovenous hemodialysis. Footnote. The patient's venous blood is pumped through the access line toward the dialyzer. Citrate is infused into the access line of the CRRT circuit. Citrate binds ionized calcium and lowers circuit ionized calcium to less than 0.4 mmol/L and achieves anticoagulation. The citrate-calcium complex is washed out in the dialysate. Anticoagulation in the return line of the CRRT circuit (ie, posthemofilter) is maintained using zero calcium dialysate. Calcium is infused into the CRRT return line to normalize ionized calcium levels just before the blood goes back into the patient.

Outcomes (KDIGO) AKI guideline advocates for citrate as first-line anticoagulation method for CRRT unless citrate is contraindicated.[15]

MEDICATION DOSING ON RENAL REPLACEMENT THERAPY

Retrospective reviews of drug dosing in hospitalized patients with renal dysfunction reveal dosing error rates ranging from 19% to 67%.[71] Such errors can be crucial in the ICU setting, particularly when it comes to antibiotic therapy, as sepsis remains the leading cause of death in the ICU.[72] Kidney failure and RRT introduce unique challenges to medication dosing in the critical care setting. Drug-related factors determining its removal during CRRT include the drug's molecular weight, its volume of distribution (V_d), and degree of protein binding. Drugs with larger molecular weights are removed less than drugs with smaller molecular weights at a given CRRT dose (when diffusive CRRT modalities such as CVVHD are used). The larger the V_d of a drug or the degree of protein binding, the less likely it is cleared by dialysis.

CRRT-related factors determining drug removal include the hemofilter features (eg, membrane, molecular weight cut-off, filter design), CRRT modality (eg, CVVH, CVVHD, or CVVHDF), or the CRRT dose (ie, effluent rate) for a dialyzable drug. A drug must be able to pass through the dialyzer membrane pores to be dialyzable. Drugs that are determined to be dialyzable should be dosed based on the effluent rate, with the guidance of therapeutic drug monitoring when available. Drug dosing should be evaluated on a regular basis in the ICU setting as patient conditions rapidly change. Changes in volume status, dialysis dosing, renal recovery, or transition to IHD should prompt review of the medication regimen and dose adjustment accordingly.

NUTRITION MANAGEMENT IN ACUTE KIDNEY INJURY

AKI generates an overall negative nitrogen balance as it leads to catabolism and muscle breakdown due to insulin resistance, metabolic acidosis, a proinflammatory condition, and the depletion of antioxidants.[73] This hypercatabolic state can be compounded by critical illness. AKI in the ICU puts patients at risk of malnutrition, which has been associated with complications related to wound healing, infections, and increased morbidity and mortality.[74] Nutritional support in patients with AKI should provide adequate macro- and micronutrients to avoid complications during the ICU stay. For patients who are not requiring RRT, standard energy and protein requirements for the general ICU patient applies: 25 to 30 kcal/kg/d with 1.2 to 2 g/kg of protein per day. Electrolyte restrictions depend on the degree of AKI and serum electrolyte profile.[75]

CRRT introduces challenges to nutritional support in the ICU. It is estimated that up to 10 to 15 g of amino acids are lost in 1 day of CRRT therapy. Patients on CRRT, therefore, require at least an additional 0.2 g/kg of protein a day, for a total of 2.5 g/kg/d, to achieve

Table 3
Micronutrients and trace mineral losses and recommended supplementation in CRRT

Micronutrient	Reported Losses in CRRT	Recommended Supplementation in CRRT per Ostermann 2021,[81] Honore 2013[82]
Water-Soluble Vitamins		
Vitamin B_1 (thiamin)	4 mg/d[83]	100–200 mg/d (low risk of toxicity)
Vitamin B_2 (riboflavin)	NR	2 mg/d
Vitamin B_3 (niacin)	NR	20 mg/d
Vitamin B_5	NR	10 mg/d
Vitamin B_6 (pyridoxine)	0.02 mg/d[84]	50–100 mg/d x 3–5 d and recheck levels
Vitamin B_7 (biotin)	NR	200 mg/d
Vitamin B_9 (folic acid)	290 μg/d[79]	1 mg/d
Vitamin B_{12} (cyanocobalamin)	NR	4 μg/d
Vitamin C	59–92 mg/d[79,85]	250 mg - 500 mg/d[a]
Lipid Soluble Vitamins		
Lipid soluble vitamins are typically not dialyzable[c,86]		
Minerals		
Zinc	Lost in RRT but possible positive balance may be due to the contamination of fluids[77,79,83]	5–10 mg/d
Selenium	Loss of 35–91 μg/d[83,85]	50–70 μg/d
Chromium	Loss of 18 μg/d[b,79]	10 μg/d
Copper	Loss of 200–400 μg/d[83,85]	1–2 mg/d

Abbreviation: NR, not reported.
[a] Avoid oversupplementation with vitamin C due to risk of oxalosis
[b] Despite losses with RRT, chromium is renally excreted, and some studies show higher levels in patients on CRRT.
[c] Reported cases of vitamin A toxicity and hypercalcemia in those receiving multivitamin with parenteral nutrition. Cautious with supplementation in the setting of kidney failure.

the appropriate nitrogen balance.[75] CRRT does provide additional caloric support through dextrose, lactate, or citrate that may be present in dialysate and replacement fluid therapies or acid-citrate-dextrose infusions. A prospective study of 10 ICU patients on CVVH estimated that an average of 512 kcal/d was delivered to the patients through the acid-citrate-dextrose formula A solution used in RCA.[76] The exact nutritional support delivered to the patient depends on the dialysate fluid composition and the CRRT prescription.

CRRT likely also leads to ongoing micronutrient vitamin losses. This is especially true for water-soluble vitamins which are more readily dialyzable, depending on their size. A retrospective study of patients on CRRT who had a micronutrient level measured during their hospital stay showed that several patients had evidence of below normal levels of thiamine and pyridoxine, as well as low levels of ascorbic acid, folate, zinc, and copper.[77] This was a retrospective study, so there was no opportunity to confirm that these micronutrients were lost in the effluent fluid. A prospective study by Ostermann and colleagues[78] investigated amino acid and micronutrient losses in patients in the ICU with severe AKI with or without CRRT. Patients on CRRT did have lower levels of citrulline, glutamic acid, and carnitine. Several amino acids were low among patients with AKI, both with or without CRRT. This was also noted in a prior small prospective study.[79] These findings do suggest that acute illness and AKI may lead to micronutrient deficiency independent of losses from CRRT. ESPEN guidelines[80] do recommend supplementation of water-soluble vitamins (particularly thiamine), selenium, and attention to serum calcium and magnesium levels in patients undergoing CRRT, though evidence for the clinical significance of this practice is lacking. **Table 3** provides reported losses of various micronutrients and their recommended daily supplementation during CRRT.

Enteral feeding electrolyte composition in the setting of CRRT depends on the serum electrolyte profile. Most patients can maintain appropriate serum potassium and phosphorus with no restrictions whereas on CRRT unless they have underlying cell or tissue breakdown. Patients will require phosphorus supplementation if the dialysate fluid does not contain any phosphorus. When transitioning from CRRT to hemodialysis, care must be taken to ensure that their diet is changed to a renal-restricted diet.

SUMMARY

AKI is a common complication among patients in the ICU. It is strongly associated with poor patient outcomes. Future study efforts should focus on measures to prevent AKI and develop tools for its early diagnosis. This would allow more prompt intervention to prevent worsening renal injury and improve outcomes. Observational studies and clinical trial data have provided some evidence-based guidance to best practices of care of patients with or at risk of AKI. However, many questions remain unanswered. We provide a summary of these studies as well as clinical practice recommendations that are guided by the conclusions of these studies.

CLINICS CARE POINTS

- Fluid therapy in the ICU should aim to optimize intravascular volume status and maintain organ perfusion, all while limiting volume overload which is associated with adverse outcomes.
- Current evidence favors the use of balanced solutions for fluid resuscitation of patients at risk of AKI who are not hypochloremic, and the use of sodium bicarbonate in patients with moderate to severe AKI.

- Priority should be made for a right internal jugular access site when placing a dialysis catheter. Subclavian access should always be avoided.
- Hemodialysis is the dialysis modality of choice for patients with severe hyperkalemia or acidosis, regardless of hemodynamic stability. Pressors can be used to support the patient while correcting metabolic abnormalities.
- CRRT is the dialysis modality of choice for those who are hemodynamically unstable or those at risk of cerebral edema or herniation.
- The current therapy guidelines recommend targeting a CRRT dose of 25 to 30 mL/kg/h
- Regional citrate anticoagulation is the preferred method of anticoagulation with CRRT.
- Dialyzable drugs should be dosed based on effluent rate, with the guidance of therapeutic drug monitoring. Changes in renal function or dialysis modality should prompt the review of medication dosing and schedule.
- Standard energy and protein requirements apply to patients with AKI who are not requiring RRT. We recommend against protein restriction in these patients.
- The daily nutritional requirements for patients on CRRT should account for their high energy demands, as well as amino acid and micronutrient lost in CRRT effluent. A protein requirement of 2.5 g/kg/d is anticipated. Supplementation with water-soluble vitamins is also necessary.
- When transitioning patients from CRRT to IHD, ensure that their diet is changed to a potassium, phosphorus restricted diet. Their medication regimen should be reviewed and appropriately dosed for hemodialysis.

DISCLOSURE

The authors have nothing to disclose.

REFERENCES

1. Kellum JA, Levin N, Bouman C, et al. Developing a consensus classification system for acute renal failure. Curr Opin Crit Care 2002;8(6):509–14.
2. Bellomo R, Ronco C, Kellum JA, et al. Acute Dialysis Quality Initiative w. Acute renal failure - definition, outcome measures, animal models, fluid therapy and information technology needs: the Second International Consensus Conference of the Acute Dialysis Quality Initiative (ADQI) Group. Crit Care 2004;8(4):R204–12.
3. Nisula S, Vaara ST, Kaukonen KM, et al. Six-month survival and quality of life of intensive care patients with acute kidney injury. Crit Care 2013;17(5):R250.
4. Bedford M, Stevens PE, Wheeler TWK, et al. What is the real impact of acute kidney injury? BMC Nephrol 2014;15:95.
5. Wang AY, Bellomo R, Cass A, et al. Health-related quality of life in survivors of acute kidney injury: The Prolonged Outcomes Study of the Randomized Evaluation of Normal versus Augmented Level Replacement Therapy study outcomes. Nephrology (Carlton). 2015;20(7):492–8.
6. Rimes-Stigare C, Frumento P, Bottai M, et al. Long-term mortality and risk factors for development of end-stage renal disease in critically ill patients with and without chronic kidney disease. Crit Care 2015;19:383.
7. Thakar CV, Christianson A, Himmelfarb J, et al. Acute kidney injury episodes and chronic kidney disease risk in diabetes mellitus. Clin J Am Soc Nephrol 2011; 6(11):2567–72.
8. Ishani A, Xue JL, Himmelfarb J, et al. Acute kidney injury increases risk of ESRD among elderly. J Am Soc Nephrol 2009;20(1):223–8.

9. Uchino S, Bellomo R, Morimatsu H, et al. Continuous renal replacement therapy: a worldwide practice survey. The beginning and ending supportive therapy for the kidney (B.E.S.T. kidney) investigators. Intensive Care Med 2007;33(9): 1563–70.

10. Bihorac A, Delano MJ, Schold JD, et al. Incidence, clinical predictors, genomics, and outcome of acute kidney injury among trauma patients. Ann Surg 2010; 252(1):158–65.

11. Folkestad T, Brurberg KG, Nordhuus KM, et al. Acute kidney injury in burn patients admitted to the intensive care unit: a systematic review and meta-analysis. Crit Care 2020;24(1):2.

12. Mizota T, Yamamoto Y, Hamada M, et al. Intraoperative oliguria predicts acute kidney injury after major abdominal surgery. Br J Anaesth 2017;119(6):1127–34.

13. Ostermann M, Cennamo A, Meersch M, et al. A narrative review of the impact of surgery and anaesthesia on acute kidney injury. Anaesthesia 2020;75(Suppl 1): e121–33.

14. Kundakci A, Pirat A, Komurcu O, et al. Rifle Criteria for Acute Kidney Dysfunction Following Liver Transplantation: Incidence and Risk Factors. Transplant Proc 2010;42(10):4171–4.

15. Kidney Disease: Improving Global Outcomes (KDIGO) CKD Work Group. . KDIGO Clinical Practice Guideline for Acute Kidney Injury. Kidney Int Supplements 2012;2:1–138.

16. Mehta RL, Kellum JA, Shah SV, et al. Acute Kidney Injury Network: report of an initiative to improve outcomes in acute kidney injury. Crit Care 2007;11(2):R31.

17. Waikar SS, Bonventre JV. Creatinine kinetics and the definition of acute kidney injury. J Am Soc Nephrol 2009;20(3):672–9.

18. Thomas ME, Blaine C, Dawnay A, et al. The definition of acute kidney injury and its use in practice. Kidney Int 2015;87(1):62–73.

19. Vijayan A, Faubel S, Askenazi DJ, et al. Clinical Use of the Urine Biomarker [TIMP-2] x [IGFBP7] for Acute Kidney Injury Risk Assessment. Am J kidney Dis 2016; 68(1):19–28.

20. Meersch M, Schmidt C, Hoffmeier A, et al. Prevention of cardiac surgery-associated AKI by implementing the KDIGO guidelines in high risk patients identified by biomarkers: the PrevAKI randomized controlled trial. Intensive Care Med 2017;43(11):1551–61.

21. Gocze I, Schlitt HJ, Bergler T. Biomarker-guided Intervention to Prevent AKI or KDIGO Care Bundle to Prevent AKI in High-risk Patients Undergoing Major Surgery? Ann Surg 2018;268(6):e68–9.

22. Raghavan R, Eknoyan G. Acute interstitial nephritis - a reappraisal and update. Clin Nephrol 2014;82(3):149–62.

23. Garzotto F, Ostermann M, Martín-Langerwerf D, et al. The Dose response multi-centre investigation on fluid assessment (DoReMIFA) in critically ill patients. Crit Care 2016;20(1):196.

24. Wang N, Jiang L, Zhu B, et al. Beijing acute kidney injury trial W. Fluid balance and mortality in critically ill patients with acute kidney injury: a multicenter prospective epidemiological study. Crit Care 2015;19:371.

25. Investigators S-A. Canadian critical care trials G, Australian, et al. timing of initiation of renal-replacement therapy in acute kidney injury. N Engl J Med 2020; 383(3):240–51.

26. Gaudry S, Hajage D, Schortgen F, et al. Initiation strategies for renal-replacement therapy in the intensive care unit. N Engl J Med 2016;375(2):122–33.

27. Zarbock A, Kellum JA, Schmidt C, et al. Effect of early vs delayed initiation of renal replacement therapy on mortality in critically Ill patients with acute kidney injury: The ELAIN randomized clinical trial. JAMA 2016;315(20):2190–9.

28. Bouchard J, Soroko SB, Chertow GM, et al. Fluid accumulation, survival and recovery of kidney function in critically ill patients with acute kidney injury. Kidney Int 2009;76(4):422–7.

29. National Heart L, Blood Institute Acute Respiratory Distress Syndrome Clinical Trials N, Wiedemann HP, et al. Comparison of two fluid-management strategies in acute lung injury. N Engl J Med 2006;354(24):2564–75.

30. Stewart RM, Park PK, Hunt JP, et al. Less is more: improved outcomes in surgical patients with conservative fluid administration and central venous catheter monitoring. J Am Coll Surgeons 2009;208(5):725–35.

31. Myles PS, Bellomo R, Corcoran T, et al. Restrictive versus liberal fluid therapy for major abdominal surgery. N Engl J Med 2018;378(24):2263–74.

32. Self WH, Semler MW, Wanderer JP, et al. Balanced crystalloids versus saline in noncritically Ill adults. New Engl J Med 2018;378(9):819–28.

33. Semler MW, Self WH, Wanderer JP, et al. Balanced crystalloids versus saline in critically Ill adults. New Engl J Med 2018;378(9):829–39.

34. Jaber S, Paugam C, Futier E, et al. Sodium bicarbonate therapy for patients with severe metabolic acidaemia in the intensive care unit (BICAR-ICU): a multicentre, open-label, randomised controlled, phase 3 trial. Lancet 2018;392(10141):31–40.

35. Barbar SD, Clere-Jehl R, Bourredjem A, et al. Timing of renal-replacement therapy in patients with acute kidney injury and sepsis. N Engl J Med 2018; 379(15):1431–42.

36. Friedrich JO, Wald R, Bagshaw SM, et al. Hemofiltration compared to hemodialysis for acute kidney injury: systematic review and meta-analysis. Crit Care 2012; 16(4):R146.

37. Yessayan LT, Szamosfalvi B, Rosner MH. Management of dysnatremias with continuous renal replacement therapy. Semin Dial 2021.

38. Rabindranath K, Adams J, Macleod AM, et al. Intermittent versus continuous renal replacement therapy for acute renal failure in adults. Cochrane Database Syst Rev 2007;(3):CD003773.

39. Bagshaw SM, Berthiaume LR, Delaney A, et al. Continuous versus intermittent renal replacement therapy for critically ill patients with acute kidney injury: a meta-analysis. Crit Care Med 2008;36(2):610–7.

40. Schneider AG, Bellomo R, Bagshaw SM, et al. Choice of renal replacement therapy modality and dialysis dependence after acute kidney injury: a systematic review and meta-analysis. Intensive Care Med 2013;39(6):987–97.

41. Schwenger V, Weigand MA, Hoffmann O, et al. Sustained low efficiency dialysis using a single-pass batch system in acute kidney injury - a randomized interventional trial: the REnal Replacement Therapy Study in Intensive Care Unit PatiEnts. Crit Care 2012;16(4):R140.

42. Huriaux L, Costille P, Quintard H, et al. Haemodialysis catheters in the intensive care unit. Anaesth Crit Care Pain Med 2017;36(5):313–9.

43. Schillinger F, Schillinger D, Montagnac R, et al. Post catheterisation vein stenosis in haemodialysis: comparative angiographic study of 50 subclavian and 50 internal jugular accesses. Nephrol Dial Transpl 1991;6(10):722–4.

44. Marik PE, Flemmer M, Harrison W. The risk of catheter-related bloodstream infection with femoral venous catheters as compared to subclavian and internal jugular venous catheters: a systematic review of the literature and meta-analysis. Crit Care Med 2012;40(8):2479–85.

45. Ge X, Cavallazzi R, Li C, et al. Central venous access sites for the prevention of venous thrombosis, stenosis and infection. Cochrane Database Syst Rev 2012;(3):CD004084.

46. Parienti JJ, Thirion M, Megarbane B, et al. Femoral vs jugular venous catheterization and risk of nosocomial events in adults requiring acute renal replacement therapy: a randomized controlled trial. JAMA 2008;299(20):2413–22.

47. Brain M, Winson E, Roodenburg O, et al. Non anti-coagulant factors associated with filter life in continuous renal replacement therapy (CRRT): a systematic review and meta-analysis. BMC Nephrol 2017;18(1):69.

48. Morgan D, Ho K, Murray C, et al. A randomized trial of catheters of different lengths to achieve right atrium versus superior vena cava placement for continuous renal replacement therapy. Am J Kidney Dis 2012;60(2):272–9.

49. Timsit JF, Sebille V, Farkas JC, et al. Effect of subcutaneous tunneling on internal jugular catheter-related sepsis in critically ill patients: a prospective randomized multicenter study. JAMA 1996;276(17):1416–20.

50. Randolph AG, Cook DJ, Gonzales CA, et al. Tunneling short-term central venous catheters to prevent catheter-related infection: a meta-analysis of randomized, controlled trials. Crit Care Med 1998;26(8):1452–7.

51. Maki DG, Kluger DM, Crnich CJ. The risk of bloodstream infection in adults with different intravascular devices: a systematic review of 200 published prospective studies. Mayo Clin Proc 2006;81(9):1159–71.

52. Klouche K, Amigues L, Deleuze S, et al. Complications, effects on dialysis dose, and survival of tunneled femoral dialysis catheters in acute renal failure. Am J Kidney Dis 2007;49(1):99–108.

53. Crosswell A, Brain MJ, Roodenburg O. Vascular access site influences circuit life in continuous renal replacement therapy. Crit Care Resusc 2014;16(2):127–30.

54. Mendu ML, May MF, Kaze AD, et al. Non-tunneled versus tunneled dialysis catheters for acute kidney injury requiring renal replacement therapy: a prospective cohort study. BMC Nephrol 2017;18(1):351.

55. Van Dyk M. The use of CRRT in ECMO patients. The Egypt J Crit Care Med 2018; 6(3):95–100.

56. Ronco C, Bellomo R, Homel P, et al. Effects of different doses in continuous venovenous haemofiltration on outcomes of acute renal failure: a prospective randomised trial. Lancet 2000;356(9223):26–30.

57. Ronco C, Bellomo R. Acute renal failure and multiple organ dysfunction in the ICU: from renal replacement therapy (RRT) to multiple organ support therapy (MOST). Int J Artif Organs 2002;25(8):733–47.

58. Network VNARFT, Palevsky PM, Zhang JH, et al. Intensity of renal support in critically ill patients with acute kidney injury. N Engl J Med 2008;359(1):7–20.

59. Investigators RRTS, Bellomo R, Cass A, et al. Intensity of continuous renal-replacement therapy in critically ill patients. N Engl J Med 2009;361(17):1627–38.

60. Venkataraman R, Kellum JA, Palevsky P. Dosing patterns for continuous renal replacement therapy at a large academic medical center in the United States. J Crit Care 2002;17(4):246–50.

61. Claure-Del Granado R, Macedo E, Chertow GM, et al. Effluent volume in continuous renal replacement therapy overestimates the delivered dose of dialysis. Clin J Am Soc Nephrol 2011;6(3):467–75.

62. Kutsogiannis DJ, Gibney RT, Stollery D, et al. Regional citrate versus systemic heparin anticoagulation for continuous renal replacement in critically ill patients. Kidney Int 2005;67(6):2361–7.

63. Monchi M, Berghmans D, Ledoux D, et al. Citrate vs. heparin for anticoagulation in continuous venovenous hemofiltration: a prospective randomized study. Intensive Care Med 2004;30(2):260–5.

64. Betjes MG, van Oosterom D, van Agteren M, et al. Regional citrate versus heparin anticoagulation during venovenous hemofiltration in patients at low risk for bleeding: similar hemofilter survival but significantly less bleeding. J Nephrol 2007;20(5):602–8.

65. Bai M, Zhou M, He L, et al. Citrate versus heparin anticoagulation for continuous renal replacement therapy: an updated meta-analysis of RCTs. Intensive Care Med 2015;41(12):2098–110.

66. Yessayan L, Sohaney R, Puri V, et al. Regional citrate anticoagulation "non-shock" protocol with pre-calculated flow settings for patients with at least 6 L/hour liver citrate clearance. BMC Nephrol 2021;22(1):244.

67. Kramer L, Bauer E, Joukhadar C, et al. Citrate pharmacokinetics and metabolism in cirrhotic and noncirrhotic critically ill patients. Crit Care Med 2003;31(10): 2450–5.

68. Schneider AG, Journois D, Rimmele T. Complications of regional citrate anticoagulation: accumulation or overload? Crit Care 2017;21(1):281.

69. Link A, Klingele M, Speer T, et al. Total-to-ionized calcium ratio predicts mortality in continuous renal replacement therapy with citrate anticoagulation in critically ill patients. Crit Care 2012;16(3):R97.

70. Szamosfalvi B, Puri V, Sohaney R, et al. Regional citrate anticoagulation protocol for patients with presumed absent citrate metabolism. Kidney360 2021;2(2): 192–204.

71. Long CL, Raebel MA, Price DW, et al. Compliance with dosing guidelines in patients with chronic kidney disease. Ann Pharmacother 2004;38(5):853–8.

72. Braber A, van Zanten AR. Unravelling post-ICU mortality: predictors and causes of death. Eur J Anaesthesiol 2010;27(5):486–90.

73. Druml W. The renal failure patient. World Rev Nutr Diet 2013;105:126–35.

74. Dempsey DT, Mullen JL, Buzby GP. The link between nutritional status and clinical outcome: can nutritional intervention modify it? Am J Clin Nutr 1988;47(2 Suppl):352–6.

75. McClave SA, Taylor BE, Martindale RG, et al. Guidelines for the provision and assessment of nutrition support therapy in the adult critically Ill patient. J Parenter Enteral Nutr 2016;40(2):159–211.

76. New AM, Nystrom EM, Frazee E, et al. Continuous renal replacement therapy: a potential source of calories in the critically ill. The Am J Clin Nutr 2017;105(6): 1559–63.

77. Kamel AY, Dave NJ, Zhao VM, et al. Micronutrient alterations during continuous renal replacement therapy in critically Ill Adults: a retrospective study. Nutr Clin Pract 2018;33(3):439–46.

78. Ostermann M, Summers J, Lei K, et al. Micronutrients in critically ill patients with severe acute kidney injury – a prospective study. Scientific Rep 2020;10(1):1505.

79. Story DA, Ronco C, Bellomo R. Trace element and vitamin concentrations and losses in critically ill patients treated with continuous venovenous hemofiltration. Crit Care Med 1999;27(1).

80. Cano N, Fiaccadori E, Tesinsky P, et al. ESPEN guidelines on enteral nutrition: adult renal failure. Clin Nutr 2006;25(2):295–310.

81. Ostermann M, Lumlertgul N, Mehta R. Nutritional assessment and support during continuous renal replacement therapy. Semin Dial 2021.

82. Honore PM, De Waele E, Jacobs R, et al. Nutritional and metabolic alterations during continuous renal replacement therapy. Blood Purif 2013;35(4):279–84.

83. Berger MM, Shenkin A, Revelly JP, et al. Copper, selenium, zinc, and thiamine balances during continuous venovenous hemodiafiltration in critically ill patients. Am J Clin Nutr 2004;80(2):410–6.

84. Fortin MC, Amyot SL, Geadah D, et al. Serum concentrations and clearances of folic acid and pyridoxal-5-phosphate during venovenous continuous renal replacement therapy. Intensive Care Med 1999;25(6):594–8.

85. Lumlertgul N, Bear DE, Ostermann M. Clearance of micronutrients during continuous renal replacement therapy. Crit Care 2020;24(1):616.

86. Gleghorn EE, Eisenberg LD, Hack S, et al. Observations of vitamin A toxicity in three patients with renal failure receiving parenteral alimentation. Am J Clin Nutr 1986;44(1):107–12.

Printed and bound by CPI Group (UK) Ltd, Croydon, CR0 4YY

03/10/2024

01040400-0002